IN BLACK GRANITE

GRANITE

A novel

William Stuart Gould, M.D.

WMG
WMG Ltd. Publishers
288 Lexington Avenue
Suite 6-F
New York, New York
10016
wmg.ltd.publishing@gmail.com

For information about WMG Ltd.'s Speakers Bureau or discounts for bulk purchases, please email: wmg.ltd.publishing@gmail.com

ISBN: 978-0-9912237-2-5 (ebook)
ISBN: 9780997980400 (paperback)
ISBN: 0997980400

ALSO BY BILL GOULD

At Yonah Mountain
Captain Iron Mustache
C.O.L.A.
A Heart Wind from the Desert
Raphael's Blanket
Lincoln Friday

To Aiden and Ezra:
My Gems
No father was ever so lucky

PROLOGUE

Along the Little Salmon River
Outside Cedar Springs
Rocky Mountains
Mid-1990s

A Kokanee sprang from the rapids to light upon an eons-worn slab of black granite. Scarlet oozed from the stump where her dorsal fin had been rasped away by the upstream fight home. She arched and twisted desperately, struggling to continue her battle.

J.W. Weathersby watched the drama from his black silk hammock, a tattered remnant unearthed in Viet Nam, from within a Viet Cong tunnel, some thirty years before. As often as he'd laundered his wartime memento in perfumed soaps, a musty odor still clung to the shiny material, the scent of that star-crossed land impossible to wash away. He imagined the ragtag Viet Minh raiding the base camps of French Airborne Legionnaires in the early Fifties, the barefoot, communist soldiers commandeering munitions to fight the white invaders. They would also make off with parachutes to cut into strips and fashion the hammocks that would serve their jungle army against the French, and a generation later, against the Americans. He wondered if the enemy soldiers who had slept on that very strip of silk were still alive, and if they were, could they close their eyes and fall to sleep without remembering the war.

J.W. lay on his porch, swinging gently in the hammock, glancing sideways at the river, trying to decide if his story should be told, or if he should follow Seltzer's advice and let it die, allow the crimson scars to fade, and finally move on.

PART I

CHAPTER ONE

Philadelphia, Pennsylvania
Early 1970s

Roosevelt Medical College, the fourth of five interviews he had managed to talk his way into, differed only in its dean of admissions, a man more rotund than the other administrators before whom J.W. Weathersby had stood, hat in hand, over the past year. Pointing with the plump Cuban cigar he'd pulled from the breast pocket of his white medical coat, the dean motioned indifferently toward a straight-backed wooden chair. As his assistant, a pale, dirty blond, bent forward to place an ashtray by the old man's hand, an inch of silk blouse pulled from her skirt. The slightest hint of her milky skin captured J.W.'s attention. The dean noticed that J.W. noticed, and as the man's jowls tightened, he nodded impatiently for the assistant to take her seat in the corner. Notebook in hand, she sat stiffly, legs uncrossed, thighs squeezed tightly together.

The yellow-gray swell of cigar smoke did not obscure the dean's disinterest in J.W.'s saga of combat in Viet Nam, the two

Purple Hearts, the stint as a P.O.W., and then the years of graduate study at the Sorbonne in Paris.

"I really want this, sir," J.W. groveled, but the dean cut him off with a swipe of the cigar.

"You say you want to be a doctor, but you haven't done anything to convince us you can handle it. Look at your undergraduate grades at Sterling College. Do you know what people do to get into medical school? How perfect your record has to be? One blemish and forget about it." He inhaled deeply from the cigar and nipped before J.W. could catch his breath, "No, you don't, do you? You need to go back to graduate school. Earn a PhD in biology or something." He waved the cigar in front of his face. "Prove your mettle. Maybe some school somewhere, I don't know, Mexico, Grenada, will forgive the grades." He puffed deeply again as he reclined with a satisfied smile, eventually grunting as he righted himself in preparation for rising.

"But, sir, I'll be forty by the time I get around to medical school. Fifty when I hang out my shingle."

The dean lifted himself creakily and considered J.W.'s protest. "And seventy when you're done paying off the school loans. Fifty's not dead. Just that much closer to being turned into a cadaver for our anatomy lab. And I hope you'll remember us when the time comes."

As the dean turned toward the door, his assistant snapped into seated attention, her thighs squeezed even more snugly. A faint chuckle belched from the dean's generous midsection, his final judgment on J.W.'s appeal. That brought a tightening of the assistant's hand on her never-opened notebook and her formal inquiry. "Have you any questions?" But without waiting for an answer, she whisked J.W. into the hallway. "Thank you for your interest in Roosevelt."

J.W. found his way off the campus, drifting through the grimy streets of Philadelphia, embedded in a crater so murky, he was barely aware of the legions of passing figures. At a corner, several pedestrians jostled him, and he slipped from the curb, twisting an ankle. He thought about hollering at the fools, perhaps even pushing back, but he knew by their cold, urban faces it would be of no purpose. Instead, he wondered if they were subject to the ironclad laws of human destiny, the ones at which he had wagged his tongue for so long. He shook his head, surprised that he had actually begun to accept the immutable principles that were asserting themselves in his life. Despite his dreams and the years of work, it was becoming clear, as he had always suspected and feared, that he was headed nowhere. His head dropped even lower as he chastised himself to accept the truth: he did not possess the brains, the strength, or the karma to honor his final promise in Viet Nam. The image of that last night with Vu Van Khai swelled in his heart. He could feel the mortar rounds pounding and hear his vow to return as a doctor, to wipe the slate clean.

His gut clutched in humiliation thinking back to the naysayers he had sassed—uncles, friends, neighbors, and even his parents—unenlightened souls who had fluttered their eyes solemnly, quoting the three-hundred-to-one-odds a man well over thirty faced applying to medical school. And he remembered declaring to the frail of spirit that he would never be dissuaded by mere numbers. He had tasted of life, he had been a combat soldier, and he would carve his own path.

He had shouted that refrain so many times, he had actually begun to believe he was capable of the impossible. But slowly, with each of the deans of admission, his shout had become more and more muffled, until even he could no longer hear it. Now, he found himself walking alone in the city, lost, tired, and frightened that his future would be mired in dark obscurity.

At the Walnut Street Bridge, he dropped onto a forgotten, splintered bench along the trash-strewn banks of the Schuylkill River. As eddies splashed, J.W. was lulled into a shallow sleep, dreaming of the law of cause and effect, wondering where he had faltered, why his life had struck so impenetrable an obstruction. The laughing pilot of a passing gasoline barge blasted his horn to startle the dozing man in the fancy suit, but J.W. ignored the rusted tub and stared, instead, across the bridge over the green water of the Schuylkill toward the campus of the University of Pennsylvania's medical school. He consoled himself that if even one of the deans had been minimally positive about a future in medicine, J.W. would have heard that as a covenant and trotted off half-cocked, eager to waste thousands of dollars and thousands of hours on pre-med courses, prepared to ride back triumphantly in two years and demand his promised place in medical school.

But not one of the deans had proffered even the slightest encouragement. And though their rejections had been subtle before Roosevelt, J.W. asked himself which of those deans had really been kinder.

He set off across the bridge and spied a school of sunnys loitering in the muck of midstream, thirty tiny fish dispersing in panic as one by one of their number disappeared into the jaws of a striped bass. But the bully passed with the current, and the sunnys drew together again, to give the river another chance, J.W. supposed, though he could not think of a reason why.

He wandered, broken-spirited, through the streets of West Philly, skirting the red-brick walls of Penn's medical school, finding himself eventually in the University Book Store, facing the volumes of medical texts through which the next generation of the chosen would travel its gilded road. He remembered the dreaded hard science volumes that had been dull brown and green fifteen years before when he had left them unopened. But now, even the nuclear physics text was shiny bright, its cover etched in bas relief with atoms smashing together so viciously, mu-mesons, neutrinos, and pastel sub-atomic fragments flew at the speed of light from violated nuclei. J.W. picked the book off the shelf to read about particles so new, they had not been dreamed of during his undergraduate years. On a shelf below were the modern biology, chemistry, and physics tomes he had abandoned at Sterling College for the football playbook and the fraternity songbook.

A prematurely balding man next to J.W. rubbed his chin thoughtfully, nodded comfortably, and pulled a chemistry text from the shelf. Before opening it, he took an innocent sidestep toward J.W., whispering, "I see you're consulting a nuclear physics book. Are you a scientist?"

"Nope."

"A doctor?"

"Nope."

"You know anything about science?" he asked, inching closer.

"Nope."

"Then why the hell are you reading a nuclear physics book?"

"I used to know something about science."

"Used to?"

"I got a degree in engineering, but it's from a long time ago."

"Look," the man declared abruptly, "Let me be frank. I got this problem. I'm trying to sell some machines." He nodded at a handsome leather briefcase by his feet. "But, I don't know a thing about 'em. Take a quick look at one, would ya? Give me a rough idea how it works. I'll slip you twenty bucks for your time, and I'll leave you alone."

J.W. considered lashing out at the man, but he reflected upon the day's outcome and on his rule that every action begat another of parallel ilk. He turned away and drifted to the ancient literature section, pulling *Beowulf* from a shelf, engrossing himself in what was far more unintelligible than even the laws of quantum mechanics.

Thirty seconds later, however, the man with the briefcase was staring at him through the stacks, sucking in a deep breath for round two, so J.W. shuffled out of the store and into the corner A&P. The man caught up with him at the cheese section.

"Hey, I'm sorry. I'm not trying to sell you anything. Honestly, I just need some help."

"What can I do for you, pal?"

"Look, I need some advice from a professional. I waited in the science section for two hours before anyone mature showed up."

"Mature?" J.W. turned and faced him. "What the hell does that mean?"

He ignored J.W.'s bristling. "I just got a job selling machines that measure toxic particular matter, that's, ah, dust, in the workplace. I told 'em I'm an engineer. I'm not. Come on, I'll buy you lunch. Just take a look at one of these things. I'm sure you're very busy, but thirty minutes isn't going to kill you, is it?"

He led J.W. into a local pub where medical students in short white coats sat under curling posters of rustic watering holes in Paris and Madrid. J.W. drifted toward a seat near them, but the man tugged at his sleeve and chose a sticky table in a darkened corner. In a fluid set of practiced movements, the man rolled a cigarette with a pinch of grainy tobacco spread carefully into a sheet of Zig Zag paper. It looked like the joints J.W.'s troops had passed around in Viet Nam.

The man sucked in a generous billow of the acrid smoke and shook his head in disbelief. "They hired me because I told 'em I graduated from N.Y.U. in mechanical engineering. Can you believe that shit? So, I'll buy a transcript, mail it to 'em in the morning, and in the meantime, I'm on the payroll."

With the arrival of the cheese steaks and beer, the man's eyes brightened. He consumed the fare with gusto, relit his cigarette as if it were dessert, leaned back, and became pensive.

J.W. watched wide-eyed as his new friend tilted forward and laughed to himself in a gritty, Flatbush inflection, tugged on his smoke twice more, and fell back, eyes closed, head bobbing limply.

J.W. considered a mad dash to the door, a hard pivot to the left, and back to the bookstore to hide in the stacks. Steeling himself for the escape, he ruminated aloud about fat deans, weirdoes in bookstores, and the time and spirit he'd already squandered on his foolish dream. A wave of helpless anger swept over him, and he started to rise, muttering, "What the hell am I doing here? I quit."

Though the man's eyes remained shuttered, he spoke suddenly in a gravelly, breathless voice. "Have a seat. Quit what?"

"You're alive! Great. Medical school."

"You're in medical school?"

"No, I am *not* in medical school. I can't get in."

"Why not?" the man objected as he receded into his stupor.

As J.W. dropped back into his chair, he reflected upon his atrocious grades as an undergraduate at Sterling College, a stain admission committees had uniformly counseled so indelible, it could not be expunged, even by his stellar performance at the Sorbonne. The man was motionless as J.W. pattered on about deans and secretaries in front of whom he had prostrated himself, and he remained inert when the waitress flipped the bill in front of J.W., her live customer. So, this was the modus operandi, J.W. nodded to himself. He quietly shifted his seat backward, waiting for the waitress to turn away.

But as J.W. lifted out of the chair, the man's jaw sagged, and he grumbled inarticulately, "You quit because some fat guy who smokes cigars inside a hospital told you to? Pretty gutsy. And why'd you tell him about your grades at Sterling College? You tell all the deans? You tell all of them about Viet Nam, too?"

"Yeah. I didn't know you were listening."

"Brilliant. You don't tell people about that stuff. He's probably screwing the blond," the man laughed with revulsion. "Figure he's gonna tell you? Hell, no. And another thing, people don't wanna hear about Viet Nam anymore. That shit's passé. Get over it. You gotta come up with a new gig." His eyes opened. "Look, these deans got a good thing going, and so do you. You look the part. That's why I asked you to gimme a hand. Thinning a little on top maybe, but look at you, still in great shape. You an athlete?" Without pausing, he went on, "The jerk's probably worried to leave the office, afraid you're gonna toss him into the Schuylkill. He's probably saying to himself, 'Crazy fuckin' Viet Nam vet.' Maybe you should lighten up, act like a doctor. When was the last time a real doctor told you he was lucky he didn't fail thermo?"

"You think I've blown it?"

"Well, you ain't going to Roosevelt, but you said you got one more interview, right? Marimore, right?"

"I didn't think you heard that."

"Marimore's a good school. It's in the bowels of Philly, right? Who lives there? Think about it."

"I don't know. Lotta poverty."

"Exactly. Is that who you want to serve? Think about it!"

"I grew up in a tough neighborhood in New York. Yeah, that's what I want to do."

"Yeah, well, tell the guy tomorrow you need a place in his school. Tell 'im that's why you chose Marimore—nowhere else'll do. And, for Christ's sake, don't spill your guts about the mistakes of the past. Get off the past. Stop tripping over it. Think about it."

The man took another rich draught, held it for thirty seconds, and J.W. watched his eyes swim as he let the vapors escape in tiny puffs. The man ordered two more beers, but his head fell forward, and he ceased all movement. J.W.'s host had died.

Without opening his eyes or moving his head, though, the man groped for his briefcase and pulled the tooled leather onto the table. He drew from the neat innards a camera-sized device, a small black box covered with toggle switches, knobs, and a meter. He thrust it across the table. "Just take a quick look at it, would ya? Open it up if you need. No problem."

"You got any tools?" J.W. asked sarcastically.

"Nope."

"I'm shocked." J.W. picked a butter knife off the table and loosened the four screws, but one had been stripped in production and fell to the floor. The last was so tight, the head torqued off, launching hair-thin coils past J.W.'s face. "You should 'a told me the thing was spring-loaded." But the man was again comatose.

Clumps of untidy resistors and capacitors now hung from the case. "What you have here is a twelve-hundred-dollar transistor radio. Where was this thing designed? Lemme guess—the happy engineers of Pango Pango."

There was no answer, and J.W. tugged at the spaghetti-like tangle of components until another spring flew from the device and bounced off his companion's forehead. The man barely twitched but droned, "How does it work? Just gimme the essentials."

"What's it supposed to do again?"

"Like I said, it measures pollution in the workplace. There's that new thing, the EPA. Environment or something."

"I know about the EPA. Thank you."

"Well, it has standards, ya know. That's marked on the dial with this red line." The tip of his index finger wagged through the air, seeking to home in on the meter.

J.W. flicked the master switch and directed the man to blow some of his powerful smoke at the intake port. The needle budged a bit and began a slow crawl, as if mired in molasses, nudging to a stop at three-and-a-half, well within the green arc. But it vibrated once and drooped back to zero. "Is this thing supposed to measure the gaseous component of smoke or particulate matter?"

"What? I don't know. That's why we're here."

"In other words," J.W. commented under his breath, "the average worker could be stoned to Mars, and that's okay with your EPA."

The man blew one more volley of exhaust toward the intake port. This time the needle barely brushed three. He sat poker-faced for a moment but brightened and asked, "Okay, there are no problems in life, just solutions. So, what do we have to do to get this thing working?"

"It's got potential. They just need to make it more sensitive, you know, spread the scale out, change the resistors. You got a multimeter with you?"

The man patted his pockets. "Fresh out. You're sure that's all it'll take?"

"I think so."

"Good. Why don't you write it down? I'll have a talk with the company in the morning. I'll get 'em to raise my commission for the information. So, which circuit does that?"

The man shoved a pad and pen in front of J.W., who scribbled some sentences and spelled several of the words phonetically for his student. As he pushed the paper back across the table, J.W. watched the man's eyes open momentarily then reclose dreamily.

J.W. grunted dispiritedly, "I don't even know your name, and we're already involved in industrial espionage."

The man snapped to life and shot his hand across the cluttered table. "Bernie. And, not to worry. I've never seen you before in my life. And yours?"

J.W. hesitated and considered the tab sitting halfway across the table, where Bernie had surreptitiously pushed it. "What the hell. Weathersby, J.W. Weathersby."

Bernie stared at J.W.'s face. "Weathersby? Kind of a big nose for a Weathersby. Gimme your number. I'll call 'em in the morning and get back to you. Maybe we can get you in on this thing," he added matter-of-factly.

Bernie did not make a move toward the tab as he leaned back, stretched, and rubbed his belly contentedly. When he lifted his hands from his stomach, he patted his hip pocket, searching disappointedly for the billfold he knew he hadn't brought. He stood to leave.

J.W.'s face tightened, but he picked up the check and reached for his wallet. Bernie's hand, though, jutted forward to grab the bill. Without looking at it, he dropped a twenty and a five peeled from a bulging wad he'd slipped from his front pocket. The money was held together by a single, purple rubber band, one that had started life holding together stalks of broccoli at the A&P.

He took J.W. by the arm and steered him to the door without waiting for change.

Outside, J.W. extended his hand, but Bernie put his arm around J.W.'s shoulder. "And I'm gonna call ya."

J.W. grunted, "Uh huh."

"No, I mean for sure. Really." Bernie grinned as he turned and walked toward the taxi stand.

J.W. watched as his new friend bent forward to speak to the cabbie. Though Bernie was in jeans, they were pressed with a sharp crease, and when he turned to wave, it was the first time J.W. noticed the heavy gold necklace and the mat of thick, black hair foaming over the "V" of his cashmere sweater. The last thing J.W. saw as the cab drove off was the sparkle from the nubbin of gold in Bernie's left earlobe.

Over dinner, Krista reacted with a sarcastic twist of her lips when J.W. reassured her that neither Bernie nor medicine was likely to become part of their lives.

"Yeah, right."

"I'm serious. I gave it my best shot. I'll do something else for Viet Nam."

"No, I don't mean becoming a doctor, I mean your friend. We're not done with him. What did Barnum say? Or was it Bailey? Sounds like he's got more on his mind than dust machines. A little light in the loafers, 'ay what? That turn you on?"

J.W. stared back silently. His wife's Nordic features had lost their sharpness. The high-boned cheeks had grown puffy, the blond hair dull at the roots. He had not noticed the change before, probably because he had not looked, really looked, at Krista for a long time.

It wasn't until eight that the phone rang. Krista half-covered the receiver and whispered loudly, "It's Dust Man. You remember, the one with the earring."

J.W. moved a chair beside the phone, fortifying himself for a long conversation on the merits of shielding workers from industrial poisons, and surely a plea to borrow his sheepskin, but Bernie just offered softly, "Hey, have fun tomorrow at Marimore. You won't forget what I told you, will ya?" J.W. could feel Bernie smiling into the phone. "Good luck. You, of all people, deserve it." While waiting for the other shoe to fall, the line clicked off.

J.W. spent much of that night awake, angry ahead of time at the bastard with whom he'd meet at Marimore. "I'll chew his ass if he gives me any crap. I'm not taking it anymore. I got nothin' to lose. Feels good to be free. And that's *if* I even bother to show up."

CHAPTER TWO

He knocked gently on the door of Marimore Medical College's administrative offices. He was an hour early. The inside was nearly as austere as the waiting room in the Philippines, where he'd gone through the same drill a year before at his first interview—the University of the Pacific Rim, eight thousand miles from home.

⊨⊧

He tried to forget how he'd placed himself on a hard bench in the torpor of Manila, on a set of wooden planks outside the dean's office—for two days, from 6 AM to 6 PM, eyes down, never letting his gentle, deferential smile fade. Seeking but a three-minute audience, J.W. was afraid to leave the musty, open-air waiting room to go to lunch, or even to the bathroom. J.W. wanted the man to see the crew cut, rosy-cheeked American who had waited so patiently outside his office. The dean would be moved; how could he not? The man was a doctor, noble, all-knowing, and saintly. He would be so impressed with the applicant's tenacity, J.W. would be invited to lunch. They would share rice, *adobo, calamanci,* and *patis* in a tropical garden, and shake their heads at the plight of the wretched. In the end, after a warm shake of hands, a place in the medical school would be carved for him. He would work hard, learn the diseases of the tropics, and return to Viet Nam to fulfill the promise.

And precisely at noon both days, the dean did indeed emerge from his office, but he passed J.W. in a rush without acknowledging him then quickly bounced down five flights of mildewed stairs. J.W. watched as he slipped into a shiny, new Mercedes, drove to the end of the university driveway, and gallantly opened the door for a magnificent, waiting Filipina. When the dean dragged himself back, alone, two hours later, J.W.'s face brightened. But the man shuffled past, J.W. still invisible.

At the end of the second day, hearing the zipper of the dean's briefcase close, J.W. swallowed a large gulp of the foul, humid air, rose slowly, skirted the receptionist, knocked, sucked in another deep breath, and opened the door slightly. "Excuse me, sir. May I have a minute of your time?"

The dean rose, mouth agape. His petite secretary squeezed between J.W. and the door. Though the woman apologized with her eyes, the dean nodded silently for J.W. to enter. The man was an aesthetic figure, standing imperially, though defensively, behind the protection of a large mahogany desk. J.W. quickly perused the air-conditioned, teak-paneled office, his eyes settling on a print of the dean shaking hands with President Marcos. He was in the same banana-fiber barong he'd worn in picture. The man waited as J.W. studied the photo before nodding toward a bench in the corner. J.W. sat at attention as the dean rearranged knickknacks on his desk.

In a single, distilled sentence, J.W. told him how badly he wanted to attend medical school in the Philippines, and that he was committed to tropical medicine after his time in Viet Nam. The dean's eyes rose from the desk and stared at J.W. for a moment before drifting upward in thought. Eventually, he nodded to himself and shuffled through his desk, handing J.W. a smudged business card with ratty corners. "Premier Auto" was lettered in red along the top. "Mr. Maldonado" and an address in Los Angeles were in smaller print below.

"Go see this man. He will help you. He takes care of all of our American friends. That is how we do it," he assured as he escorted J.W. from his office.

Twenty-four hours had passed on the bench, and thirty seconds inside the great man's office. It would have been as futile to persist, to ask the dean for more, as if he had appealed to the slats of worn wood that had supported him for two days. The moment was an epiphany, for it was the first time in his life J.W. understood how little his heart meant to the world outside it. Nonetheless, he bought a ticket for California

In Los Angeles a week later, J.W. went to Premier Auto to find the dean's Mr. Maldonado. As J.W. walked into the parking area of the used car lot, he was halted by vociferous shouting, and he took a step back onto the street. A salesman tore from the showroom, sprinting up to an immense, indigent, furry blond man who had parked himself behind the wheel of Mr. Maldonado's personal XKE. A customer in a Corvette had also just turned into the lot and honked impatiently for J.W. to move out of his way. Though Weathersby stepped aside, the car moved ahead only a few feet before it had to stop again, this time for a tattered pack and bedroll flopped in the middle of the driveway. J.W. looked at the derelict in the Jaguar and recognized the unit patch on the greasy, army field jacket. J.W. walked up to the XKE. "You with the First Cav in the Nam?"

"Fuckin' A. You?" he asked seriously, broodingly, but suddenly laughed and offered J.W. a drink from a bottle in paper bag.

J.W. blurted, "You know the 33rd Mech?" then took a breath to tell him about the time he had been loaned to the Cav to fly out wounded GIs, but another salesman rushed over and took J.W. by the arm, tugging him into the showroom. When J.W. asked for Mr. Maldonado and showed him the card, the employee pursed his lips and nodded stiffly for J.W. to follow into a shabby office. Maldonado looked up. J.W. introduced himself.

"Quite frankly, Mr. Weathersby, there are very few places left in our Philippine medical schools for foreigners. Those days of nearly free medical education for Americans in Manila are gone. It would require a very substantial donation to the building fund to be considered. I'm sure you understand."

"Yes, of course." J.W., still standing, added, "I've saved a lot of my army pay. I don't care what it costs. I'm going to do it."

Maldonado's pupils narrowed to pinpoints as they began a mad dance, darting about like bats. Admission to medical school hovered in front of J.W.'s eyes. All he had to utter was, "Yes, sir!" and the prize was his. He would graduate from the foreign school then fight for a slot in an American residency program, like a million foreign graduates before him. And when residency was over, he would be absorbed into the mainstream of American medicine, his medical school of no consequence. All he had to do was agree, but he was able to produce only a squeak and a dry gurgle. Maldonado stared and held his breath.

Be cool. Think objectively, J.W. demanded silently of himself. What do you want most in the world? "Whatever it takes, sir."

"Oh, this is very good," Maldonado exhaled and took a gulp of his coffee. "Do you live in L.A.?"

"No, sir. Philadelphia."

Mr. Maldonado became very serious. "You have traveled far. You must want to be a doctor very badly. Now, you must contact

Mr. Ramirez in Cherry Hill, New Jersey, for the actual transaction. Mr. Ramirez is a very trusted member of the Board of Directors of the University. He will help you." J.W.'s face deflated, but Maldonado shook his head. "It is the way it is done, the *transaction*."

"Transaction, sir?"

"It is only seventeen thousand U.S.," he blurted. "And that is a bargain, my friend. Just last month, a student from Michigan, his father, he donated twenty thousand *and* a car, a Mercedes, for the dean's office. To take around important visitors. We have many, you know."

"Does that include room and board, sir?"

"Oh, no. The *transaction* is only a donation to the University. Room and board and tuition are the student's responsibility."

Mr. Ramirez's business card was blank, aside from his name and telephone number. Every time J.W. sat down to contact him, the calluses on his butt from the bench in Manila chafed. He never made the call.

⚊⊹ ⊹⚊

And now, a year later, J.W. sat outside another dean's office, on another wooden bench, this time at Marimore Medical College, the name of the institution perhaps more ornate, but the planks as hard. He had studied Bernie's dictum, especially the part about avoiding the subject of Viet Nam, and wondered why he was bothering, for nothing else beside his war experiences distinguished him from the masses. Without that, what *did* he have to offer? Zero. So, why was he about to waste the time of a famous doctor who could be in the hospital saving lives? He was selfishly chasing an absurd dream and doing harm along the way.

It was better, he allowed, when the vision had all but vaporized. He relished the relief he had enjoyed after Manila and the meeting with Mr. Maldonado, when he simply accepted that he would not attain the unattainable.

That quiet acceptance had lasted nearly a year, until the night his daughter was born. J.W. was thirty-one. The doctor who delivered his little girl was twenty-seven. "I've never seen anyone smile so much," the redheaded obstetrician shook her head after the delivery. "You know something I don't?"

J.W. babbled on about his love for the drama of medicine, the old lives going, the new arriving, his daughter's pristine lungs unfolding for the first time. It was the thought of the delicate, pink tissue, and the first beams of light shining into the yet unsullied crystal blue eyes.

"Ever think about becoming a doctor?" she mumbled as she sutured Krista's wounds. J.W. sighed and shook his head. She looked up at him and asked seriously, "Why don't you just go to medical school and get it over with?"

J.W. started to tell her about the dean, the bench, and Maldonado and Ramirez, but he was embarrassed, so he shrugged and muttered defensively, "By the time I'd be done with medical school and residency, I'd be damn near forty."

She screwed up her face, tied a last surgical knot, jumped up, and pulled off her gloves. She started to dart off to the next delivery but called back, "What are you going to be doing in ten years that's so important?"

And she was gone. Though J.W. did not see her again, nor even learn the name of the woman who had delivered his jewel, the flame he believed had been long extinguished began to glow faintly. As hard as he tried to ignore the dull orange ember, it emitted a peculiar heat all that day, the first day of his daughter's life, every time he watched her suckle. The need to study medicine, or at least try again, had rekindled itself.

J.W. was shaken out his reverie by the gentle hand of the dean's secretary, who escorted him toward an office smaller than at Roosevelt. As they walked, J.W. accepted that, though he was going through the motions, the flame had darkened for the last time, smothered by the reality of advancing adulthood, and Krista's constant reminders about the needs of a little girl whose future demanded work and money, not dreams. He knew very well she was right.

A tiny man in a pin-striped suit greeted him with a handshake so powerful, J.W. grimaced. "I am James McNamara. It is a pleasure to meet you, Captain Weathersby." The dean pulled his chair to the side of the desk and sat across from J.W., who was struck with the intensity of the man's eyes, and with his dour expression. Nonetheless, J.W. began to relax and casually unbuttoned his suit jacket. Dr. McNamara's eyes happened to drop to J.W.'s waist but quickly darted back to his guest's face. J.W. stiffened; his fly must be open, and he had probably forgotten underwear. Reticent to look, but overcome with the need to know, J.W. forced his own eyes into his lap. He wasn't wearing a belt.

How can a man expect to be considered for so lofty a station in life as student of medicine if he can't remember to dress himself? J.W. squirmed and shifted, trying to close his jacket, to hide a transgression that had already been broadcast to the free world. His last chance was over before it had begun.

But Dr. McNamara had likely blocked out fifteen minutes for the interview, and as a man of integrity, despite the foregone outcome, J.W. would get that time. The dean played his role politely, asking why J.W. was interested in medicine so far down the path of life. Though J.W. tried to formulate an answer, all he could do was wonder why the dean didn't just get it over with and ask J.W. how he planned to keep his pants up skating from exam room to exam room treating patients.

Accepting that all was lost, J.W. ignored Bernie's maxim and told the dean about Viet Nam. The man stared at him silently, listening intently, but in lieu of the customary promenade to the door at that juncture, he leaned toward J.W. and fired question after question. "Why did you choose to spend your combat tour living in a remote Vietnamese village? What possessed you to drive wounded civilians from that hamlet, at night, along deadly roads, to hospitals hours away? What did the peasants teach you? Do you remember any of those lessons? Do you use them?" J.W. wanted to move on, but the dean pursued Viet Nam, intrigued with the image of a captain in a combat unit learning and doing, not shooting.

J.W., having never understood how much he had absorbed in the little hamlet west of Saigon, hesitated before answering. It had all seemed so simple at the time. Dean McNamara, however, would not let his fish off the hook, and they spent two hours together, trading evenly. The dean had been drawn to a side of the war in South East Asia few had seen, and J.W. had forced himself to think, to dig and search for answers and images that never could have been revealed on a formal application.

As Dean McNamara walked J.W. to the door, J.W. was struck by how a man of such small stature could loom that large. "It's really quite simple," he advised, "if you want to go to medical school, really want to go, you will. Take the MCAT and let me know how you do."

"MCATs, sir? That's going to be hard to do without having taken the courses it's based on."

"I know The Medical College Admission Test is hard. I don't care if you've aced all your pre-med chemistry, physics, biology, and organic chemistry. And there's math and general knowledge, too. Mr. Weathersby, it is a weeding out exam. It's designed to see just who really wants to go to medical school—who's willing to master everything there is to know about those subjects at the college level. It's going to be especially challenging if you haven't taken the courses. Actually, impossible. I've never heard of anyone doing it. So, you're going to need to find a way to get it done. Most of our applicants score in the high six-hundreds, but that's not cast in stone. As I said, let me know how you do. Oh, and thank you for having had the courtesy to dress appropriately. Most of the young people headed for medical school these days would have shown up in jeans and running shoes."

⚊⊹ ⊹⚊

J.W. raced to the bookstore, hoping to find Bernie browsing, but he saw only kids in their early twenties hurriedly pulling medical texts from the shelves, cursing the prices and bitching about the coming semester's unending hospital rotations. J.W. chose the newest, crispest chemistry, physics, and biology textbooks; a sheaf of notebooks; a good fountain pen; and a handful of MCAT review books. He carried the load home on his bicycle, several hundred dollars of future work and vision tucked neatly into a shopping bag.

Krista greeted him with wide-open eyes. "Plastic bag man, what 'cha got?"

She watched as he extracted his treasures then placed the back of her hand on his forehead to check for a fever. "Never saw you treat the printed word quite like that before; maybe a new football, or a steak, but not a book," she laughed nervously.

"Listen," he suggested, as he opened each tome for the first time, as if the crack of the virgin covers heralded a new world. "I'm excited! Aren't you?"

"You're serious about this? I thought you were done with the medical school thing," she answered barely audibly as she turned toward the kitchen.

"I don't know. The guy I met today at Marimore, the dean, he said I could do it if I wanted. Just gonna take a lot of work."

"And a lot of money. But, whatever you want, if you think we can manage."

She disappeared before he pulled the last of the books from the bag.

J.W. sat in the sparsely furnished living room inscribing names, Krista's, Khai's, and his, on the title leaf of each book. Krista stuck her head out, watched him for a moment, raised her eyes in disbelief, and asked, "You want Stroganoff for dinner, Dr. Schweitzer?"

"Yeah!"

"Then run out and get a stick of butter."

J.W.'s '58 Dynaflow Buick, a hand-me-down relic of his father's less energy-conscious days, slowed to a stop at the corner, the headlights silhouetting a man in a wheelchair waiting near the curb. A scruffy blanket protected the invalid's legs, and despite the winter cold, only a tee-shirt covered his chest. With the light of J.W.'s car, the chair began a creep toward the street, but the man lost control and vaulted off the curb. His body spilled out of the chair onto the frozen road.

As J.W. jumped from the Buick, the man turned several revolutions and rolled to a stop under the front wheels. He looked up and clamored about J.W. having knocked off his legs. J.W.'s eyes searched the intersection and under the car for the man's lower half. He found nothing. The victim was, though, slurring so unintelligibly, J.W. cursed, "Shit, the guy's got brain damage."

As J.W. scanned again for a pair of legs, another car pulled up to the stop sign from the opposite direction. Its lights played on the overturned wheelchair and the quivering body, which had wedged itself even more tightly under the Buick. The driver screamed out of his window, "Hey, what the hell's going on?" but as J.W. tried to explain, the other driver yelled, "Bullshit. I'm callin' the cops."

J.W. returned to his victim, who had ceased even a flicker of movement. J.W. assumed the lifeless heap had suffered a heart attack, or perhaps a stroke, and died. J.W. gulped, realizing he was suddenly a candidate for admission to prison on felony manslaughter, not for admission to medical school. "Back away. Run!" he cried to himself, but another car pulled up to the stop sign and the driver asked if he needed help.

"Nah, just some old drunk," he laughed. "I got it under control."

J.W. knelt and touched the skin of the cadaver's face. Despite the freezing air, it was still warm, and the man's hand shot up to brush J.W.'s fingers from his face. A reverberating snore burped from his throat, along with the stench of both stale and freshly chugged alcohol. J.W. jumped away, though as the foul breath dissipated in the freezing wind, J.W. stepped back toward the derelict. An explosive passage of intestinal gas sent J.W. several yards into retreat.

"Where the hell you goin', honkey? You gonna make good for takin' my mutha fuckin' laygs. You dig?"

"Hey, my man, why don't you get back in your chair and go home before you freeze to death?"

"Now how the fuck you want me to do dat?"

"I'll put you in your chair and get you home. Where do you live?"

"I donno. Lemme move in witch you."

"Look, man, like I said, I'm gonna put you back in your chair and point you home."

"You can't do that. I ain't got no home. And you da one who done knocked me off my chair, took my mutha fuckin' laygs"

"Look, pal, I didn't do anything to you. You're goin' home. End of story." J.W. righted the wheelchair and lifted the mendicant by the armpits, struggling with the one-hundred-and-fifty pounds. "Stop wiggling around," J.W. hollered as he yanked up hard and popped the man back in the chair. As the full weight of the torso dropped onto the seat, there was a loud snap as one of the axles cracked, and the wheelchair collapsed. The man rolled back into the street.

"Hey man, you tryin' to kill me or somethin'? Told ja, movin' in witch you!"

More lights approached from the bottom of the hill. As he seized his new friend by the armpits again, J.W. cursed, "Shit, I am going to live to regret this. Hey, man, stop your wiggling." J.W. maneuvered him into the Buick and laced the shoulder strap around the man's chest, but let the lap belt hang because his victim didn't have a lap. The body rocked precariously as J.W. shoved the seat forward to make room for the wheelchair, motions that precipitated a spasm of seasickness and the retching of a purple fluid that was most certainly blood, despite the odor of putrefied wine. Abandoning further manipulation of his passenger, J.W. gave up and squeezed the wheelchair behind the driver's seat. He drove scrunched against the steering wheel, so far forward, he was barely able to shift the car into drive or use his arm to steady the man, who toppled at every corner until J.W. lashed him into the seat with a jumper cable.

Weathersby followed the garbled directions to the center of one of Philadelphia's myriad decrepit enclaves. The duo cruised the darkened streets of burned-out tenements in North Philly. J.W. ignored the crumbling bars at which the nearly stuporous man begged J.W to. pull over. He rallied, though, as they crawled past a dilapidated, single-family house whose entrance sat atop a steep flight of crumbling, cement steps.

"Dat's da place, dat's da place!" he howled and rolled out of the jumper cable harness tilting onto J.W.'s lap.

J.W. negotiated the stairs gingerly, picking through the detritus, trudging fifty feet up to the doorway. Most of the boards had rotted through on the porch, several directly in front of the entrance, and he had to lean forward with one hand on the peeling door to steady himself as he knocked. A large, angry man snatched it open, and J.W. fell forward.

"What? What the hell you doin' on my gotdamn door, fool?"

"Well, sir, I have a man in my car who says he lives here."

"Yeah, so?"

"Well, what do you want me to do with him, sir?"

"He got legs?"

"No, sir, he does not."

"Don't want dat sumbitch here no more. Got it, honky?"

J.W. gazed past his unwilling host into the grimy living room, bare save for a shredded couch and a stained, once-green rug upon which were sprawled several young men and a woman. They weren't particularly active; in fact, they weren't moving at all, apparently, victims of a pandemic that came with living in that house. With his medical hopes newly revitalized, J.W. viewed the needles and syringes lying around objectively and presumed they had all succumbed to diabetic comas.

"Look, sir, I don't want no trouble. I picked him up on the street. He fell out of his wheelchair. He's drunk as shit."

He turned and asked his guests, "You 'all want dat muh fuckah Preston anymoh?"

The council did not move.

"Well, sheeet," he spat. "Breeng da muh fuckah up here."

J.W. thanked him and returned to the street. His passenger had opened the car door and fallen, head first, into the gutter. J.W. picked him up and tried to put him back in the car so he could take the wheelchair up first, but the man was flailing so angrily, J.W. could not get him past the doorjamb. Instead, J.W. steeled himself, flung the near-corpse over his shoulder, and began the trek to the house, a Sherpa, or The Saga of Gunga Din in reverse. At the porch, J.W. put him down on the frozen wood and went back for the wheelchair, but when J.W. dragged himself back up, Preston was gone.

Krista was sitting by the window in the rocking chair, nursing Khai. J.W. waited for the, "Where the hell have you been?" but she just kept on swaying back and forth, mentioning offhand-edly that the police had canvased the neighborhood asking questions about a hit-and-run accident. She was surprised, but only because, in the end, J.W. had forgotten the butter. She went back to feeding Khai.

"Your friend Bernie called," she commented disinterestedly with her pinkie extended.

By the time J.W. finished the conversation, it was late, so he made firm plans to arise before the sun, open the books, and start his new life.

CHAPTER THREE

For a kid cultivated on the streets of the Bronx, Viet Nam had been a world far beyond rifles and rockets. Guns, J.W. had seen at home, but the tropical forests and endless kilometers of emerald rice paddies were images only from books and movies. Then, one day early in his combat tour, he found himself out in rural Kien Tuong Province, at the northern reaches of the Mekong Delta. The scent of water buffalo wallowing in mud pens often came to J.W. after the war, their odor redolent of the elephants his pop took him to see at the circus in Madison Square Garden.

On slow days in the war, J.W. landed his helicopter in the paddies near a hamlet and forced his crew to help the villagers shuck rice or pitch hay. "Builds character," he assured them as they sweat in their flack vests, chicken plates the fliers called them, until the stiflingly humid bogs took their toll, and J.W. allowed his men to strip to the waist. For the second half of his tour, he convinced his commanding officer, Colonel Sanford T. Bierlein, the most decorated officer of World II, to allow him to live in one of those tiny hamlets, My Co, alone, to build a school, a market, and a dispensary for the peasants. He was told to go out and win their hearts and minds.

My Co was the first place J.W. ever saw a dead body, a Viet Cong soldier, a local teenager, who had been shot in the chest during an enemy raid. The next morning, the boy's rigid body lay in the dust of the hamlet road, just as he had died, alone. One of the old ladies shuffled by under the load of a carrying pole but dared not stop, glancing only sideways at the stony, pain-contorted face. She shook her head and murmured that she remembered the day he was born, fifteen years before, under the blistering sun of My Co.

J.W. waited all day, but no one buried the child, or even acknowledged the corpse, until late in the afternoon, when an old man rode in on an ancient bicycle. He wept over the bloated body. As J.W. helped the old man load the body on the bicycle, the peasant mumbled it was his grandson.

J.W. stared at the boy's eyes, frozen open and clogged with dust. J.W. thought he saw a flicker of the kid's finger but had to accept the child was gone, something squandered in the world that could not be put back right. The boy had been an elusive, dangerous enemy the night before, but as the body was wheeled away, J.W. sensed the loss, realizing he wasn't much beyond fifteen himself.

Lieutenant Weathersby had also forged a union with the hamlet chief of My Co, and several of villagers as well, a bond that would alter J.W.'s life. On the final day of his tour, J.W. thanked the villagers for what they had given him from their world, the vista of a gentle society, a realm he never dreamed could endure in the eye of such a storm. He delivered a speech in broken Vietnamese to the gathered elders.

"Ladies and Gentlemen, you taught me much about a world I did not know. You treated me with kindness and respect, though you could have thought of me as the enemy. I promise I will come back, I hope as a doctor, and repay the debt I owe you. I will never forget you."

The old men were silent. Perhaps they hadn't understood his Vietnamese, to say nothing of his sentiments.

CHAPTER FOUR

Late in December, on a frigid Philadelphia afternoon, J W.
stopped at a street vendor's cart for his customary Tuesday afternoon hot pretzel. The mustard sprayed from the ice-clogged
squeeze bottle onto his jeans, prompting Mr. Papadimitriou,
the proprietor, to tear a sheet from his Philadelphia Enquirer to
sop up the yellow ooze. The word "Vietnam" in a small headline
caught his eye. Children's War Relief was looking for a staffer to
work in a tiny hospital deep in the Mekong Delta.

To save the dime, J.W. ran home. The pre-med texts lay unopened, gathering dust under his rickety desk. Next to the books
were stacks of Xeroxed copies of the returned application forms
J.W. had submitted to volunteer agencies still working in Viet
Nam. Stapled to each was the rejection letter every one of them
had drawn like a powerful magnet.

"Kris, guess what! I found an organization looking for someone to go to Viet Nam!"

"Great. So how did the job hunting go?"

"Same-o same-o, left a few applications. You have any luck?" Without allowing her to answer, J.W. dialed the phone, letting it ring a dozen times.

"This is Elizabeth Marie Hollingsworth-Proctor."

J.W. covered the receiver and laughed to Krista, "It's a law firm," then spoke into the phone. "I'm sorry. I thought I was calling Children's War Relief."

"This is CWR," an impatient voice countered. "How may we help you?"

"Could you tell me about the position in Viet Nam?"

"My friend, it is five on Christmas Eve. Please call next week."

"But, Mrs. Proctor..."

"We find that title offensive."

"Miss, Ms.?"

"We find titles offensive."

"Betty?"

"Elizabeth Marie Hollingsworth-Proctor."

"Ma'am. Sorry. Look, I'm an ex-GI, and I made this promise to come back to Viet Nam and do something positive this time. I've applied to a hundred-and-six volunteer organizations. Everyone's shutting down programs in Viet Nam."

She listened and offered boorishly, "That's very noble of you. Are you aware this is an *anti-war* organization? We don't hire former GIs. We provide war relief, not absolution to guilty soldiers."

"But I speak Vietnamese," J.W. protested. "I know about medicine, too."

"I'm very sure you do. Try your church. And, Merry Christmas."

J.W. granted CWR a two-day reprieve then called again, and again, and again. By mid-January, they had agreed on a monthly salary of ten dollars for Krista, ten for him, and five for Khai, though CWR would provide housing, business-related travel expenses, and food. There would be no problem with visas, they were assured, for CWR was highly honored across the world. In early February, Krista, Khai, Marc Banter, the operations director for CWR, and J.W. drove from Philadelphia to the Vietnamese Embassy in Washington to present their credentials to Mr. Nguyen, the distinguished, silver-haired, liaison officer.

He seemed pleased to see them. "We are so extremely encouraging, you come Viet Nam. Yes, we need you training. This wonderful," he beamed as he signed and stamped their applications before placing them in an official-looking envelope. He placed the packet in front of the receptionist and patted it paternally. The woman took the papers to another desk. That employee lifted the phone, spoke in hushed tones, and yet another of the embassy's staff appeared from behind a door to carry the documents away.

Mr. Nguyen played gently with Khai and remarked, "That could be Vietnamese name. Very interesting."

J.W. explained it was the given name of a man with whom he had spent much of his time in Viet Nam, the village chief of My Co. He had promised to name his firstborn after the man the night the two had barely survived a vicious mortar attack. And he had kept his word.

Mr. Nguyen walked the petitioners to the door and spoke softly. "Thank you, Captain, for what you do in Viet Nam then, and what you do now. Thank you."

Marc advised the Weathersbys to vacate their tiny apartment and be ready to leave for Viet Nam at a moment's notice. CWR would provide a room at the Center City Paris Inn for the few days it would take to process the papers.

By late February, their visas had not arrived. "There have been many changes in our country. You must be patient," Mr. Nguyen's voice smiled. "We are so happy you are come to our country to help," he laughed nervously after each of J.W.'s biweekly calls.

⇥⊹⊱

Room 360 at the Paris Inn was economy lodging. The subtly faded wallpaper was light green with originally off-white, now cigarette-smoke stained, yellow flowers. The sheets on the two single beds were changed on Thursday, the day Krista and J.W. found the beds pushed out to their separate positions. The bright side was that Khai finally had a room of her own, a teepee of blankets and hanger wire pilfered from the maid's cart. Five dollars a week left on Khai's crib sealed the housekeeper's lips.

At first, eating out was a treat. The brand "Philadelphia" on the cream cheese was there, not because the populace of the City of Brotherly Love had invented or loved fat-laden fare, but because Philly was famous for good food. After two months of eating out, however, the Weathersbys had been politely discouraged from returning to every eating establishment within three miles of Center City, the rejections a function of Khai's vocal displeasure at being strapped in restaurant highchairs three times a day. Krista and J.W. began to crave home cooking and a meal away from a waitress, an angry maître d', and their screaming child.

Life at the Paris became one squabble after another until Krista came up with a two-point plan. The first component was to send J.W. out on forays to buy restaurant meals; the second involved reheating the selections on the room radiator, from which J.W. had temporarily disabled the fan. The grill sizzled heartily late each afternoon as it heated cans of soup and tinned beef stew. It also charred toast, setting off the smoke alarm, until J.W. found the breaker box in the hallway and disabled the entire floor of fire-detecting devices, but only for the half-hour each

35

night the Weathersbys boiled, roasted, poached, fricasseed, and griddled the evening meal. The major drawback was that the intense heat burned the paint off the top and sides of the radiator.

Cold comestibles, on the other hand, were stored in a plastic bag outside the window. Aesthetically, the rudimentary refrigerator did not have a negative environmental impact, as their window faced a four-foot alley and the ancient brick wall of the Kreutzer Piano Factory. On Thursday mornings, before the maid arrived, J.W. touched up the burned patches on the radiator with white paint, into which he had dumped tablespoons of soot scraped from the wall outside the window. That rendered the grill a hue matching the rest of the radiator, though the paint smelled like paint and remained wet and sticky for the day, forcing them to leave the window open, exposing the food bag. The maid hinted that their behavior was not in keeping with the standards of the Paris Inn, though her concerns were mitigated when the weekly tip rose to seven-fifty.

⟫⟪

By early April, two months after the Weathersbys had moved into the Paris, they spent their evenings watching the news on the tiny hotel TV. Each night was one more page in the diary of the worsening calamity in Viet Nam, a recapitulation of the cultural and political humiliation of an ancient society. With victory after victory, the communist soldiers consolidated their hold on the nation. Doors were being drawn shut tighter each day. J.W. began to wonder why they were languishing in Philadelphia, fretting away their lives. These were supposed to be the great years, watching their little girl grow, not time clouded with his need to return to Viet Nam, the demon that could harm the one beautiful creation of his life.

"If you ever hurt his baby, I'll destroy you," Krista cried bitterly one night as the television news from Viet Nam worsened.

"Hey, Goddamnit, you wanted to go, too," J.W. snapped back.

"Take my child into a war? Why are you making us go?"

"You never said you didn't want to go. You never said a goddamn word!" J.W. screamed until his throat hurt, until he tasted the bitterness of his own tears. Khai had begun to fuss as well. Her high-pitched whine rose louder and louder, until it was an uncontrollable, screeching cry. Krista rocked her by the grimy window, but the baby's face became scarlet, and her brow glistened with sweat. She drifted slowly into listlessness, her eyes soon becoming crusted with crystals of yellow pus. A CWR pediatrician arrived at midnight. He hemmed and hawed before blurting, "We should hospitalize this child. Just for observation, mind you. Just one night, that's all."

Krista's face reddened. "You're not taking my baby away to some sick house," she sobbed.

As Khai was being discharged from the pediatric ward in the morning, they met with her doctor. "What's going on with you two? You want to know why Khai's sick? Simple. You guys are hurting. You haven't disguised that very well. Khai knows. Kid's aren't stupid."

CHAPTER FIVE

As hard as J.W. tried to carry the load, to discipline his thoughts, he woke each morning at three or four, relieved for a few seconds, convinced it had all been just a bad dream. But as he focused on the gritty curtains of Room 360, his chest clutched, for it was true—he was about to hurl everything he cared about into a pilgrimage to atone for a wrong he had not done. No, it was worse: the poison that infected his heart was as toxic as if he had been sentenced to prison for a crime he had not perpetrated. But to the penitentiary he would go, and the wait to report there would be a turmoil of unbroken dread.

And, he was also putting Krista through it as well.

The newscasts from Viet Nam just worsened. After a week of nightmares, J.W. made a private decision that if the visas did not arrive the next day, he would put an end to the madness. As he feared, and hoped, the mailman came and went leaving nothing but ads. J.W. paced the room, driven by instinct and emotion, no longer by reason. His hand reached out to call CWR, to tell them

he and Krista could not honor their contract; he would find
something else to do for Viet Nam. But as his fingers grasped the
cold plastic of the receiver, J.W. was startled from his trance by
a shrill ring. The voice, though vaguely familiar, surprised him
with its unexpected jauntiness.

"Hey, Doc, guess who!"

Bernie was calling from New York. He had moved on from
Philadelphia and the environmental phase of life to men's apparel,
opening a mod shop on the lower East Side. "Hey, J.W., I love my life.
Can you dig crawling over sleeping drunks to unlock the barred
doors of my shop every morning? The crazies. Are you kiddin' me?
It's a parade. The rich and the poor, the sane and the psychotic. I
can't tell who's who without a program. I got great people working
for me. I treat them well; they treat me well. God, I love it!"

For a moment, J.W. thought Bernie was setting the stage to
dun him into a loan, perhaps an active partnership, but Bernie's
patter slowed and softened. "Which medical school have you decided to grace with your presence?"

J.W. laughed sarcastically, "Ya know, Bernie, I haven't opened
the books. There's just not enough inspiration in the air, or
something."

J.W. related the saga of the CWR fiasco, but Bernie stopped
him. "Look, we're heading down to Philly tomorrow. Just for the
day. Mind if we stop by? We'll talk over the options. There's always options, J.W., *always options.*"

"We?" J.W. asked lightheartedly, fearful of Krista's reception
should Bernie's friend arrive with a beard in need of a trim.

"Didn't I tell you? I moved in with a social worker. Clients
all over the City, borough to borough, doing follow-up investiga-
tions on sexually transmitted diseases. Exciting work! Hey, see ya
tomorrow."

Though J.W. had assumed Krista was asleep, she looked up
and grunted. "Dust Man cometh—VD lover follows."

Bobbie Jo was full of street savvy from her days in New York chasing down leads on strains of VD that hadn't yet made it into J.W.'s unopened medical books. But she still had the innocent smile that remained from her childhood years in North Dakota. And she was tall and stately, but had not lost her farm-girl shoulders. To J.W. it looked as though she wasn't wearing a bra under her cowboy shirt, but he saw Krista watching, and he dropped his eyes to her snakeskin, Frye cowgirl boots. As they walked through the door of Room 360, her eyes were half-a-foot above Bernie's bald spot. Krista invited Bobbie Jo into Khai's corner, where they played with the baby. Bobbie Jo's legs were so long, when she lay on her back on the floor holding Khai, her boots were near the center of the room.

Bernie was mostly silent as he and J.W. walked to buy dinner at one of the better delis from which the Weathersbys had been banished weeks before. J.W. trusted the owner wouldn't recognize him, but as they crossed the threshold, the proprietor leapt through the kitchen's swinging doors to glare at J.W.'s back. J.W. remembered the owner's growled admonition, "You don't belong in here. My clientele don't haul their children in knapsacks. As a matter of fact, my customers don't haul their issue around at all. The kids stay at home with the maid, where they belong."

Bernie wiggled his index finger to call the proprietor aside. He spoke softly, gesticulating and smiling until the man went to the kitchen and fetched two burnt sienna roast chickens, their juices streaming so copiously, the brown wrapping paper grew translucent as they walked the frigid Philadelphia streets back to the Paris.

The foursome sat around the Weathersby's dining room table, the squat dresser. Krista covered the chipped plastic-wood veneer with newspaper while Bobbie Jo served beer, wine, and the sides Bernie and J.W. had gathered. Bernie inhaled most of the first chicken, stopping only to play with Khai, but when he plunged into the second bird, Bobbie Jo tapped him on the hand with the tines of her fork and took his plate, dumped the heap of slick-cleaned bones into a paper bag, and put the plate in the bathroom sink, where she and Krista did the dishes.

They drank and talked until early morning, when Bernie yawned deeply and glanced at his watch. Bobbie Jo smiled, "Bernard, let's let our friends get some sleep. They have a kid."

But the infusion of oxygen from Bernie's yawn triggered a second wind and he asked, "Where were you five years ago at this very moment? Viet Nam, right? Do you remember the story you told me about the little propaganda leaflets the Viet Cong dropped all over that hamlet you lived in?"

"Yeah, I was somewhere in Viet Nam. In My Co, I guess. And?"

"And, I'm talking about the leaflet quoting Benjamin Franklin. 'Success is ten percent inspiration and ninety percent perspiration.' Even the peasants know that," he laughed. "You gonna wait for 'inspiration' to get your ass in gear and open the books? Or, you just gonna get it done?

"And this abject fear over going back. You two need to cool your jets. You're not going to be out in the boonies, crawling through mine fields. The cities are okay. You told me that yourself. Sure, it's a calculated risk, but not a single civilian Western child has been harmed during the whole war. Shit, I wish we were going. It's safer than Bruckner Boulevard."

"How do you know that?"

"I made some calls after we talked yesterday, okay?" he smiled. "Be patient. Open the books and get your butt on a stick."

Bernie yawned loudly, and Bobbie Jo poked him in the ribs. "Did I say something wrong?" he stammered, pointing to himself with both index fingers. "Okay. Guess it's time to pack it in for the night, what'a ya say?"

Krista stood before Bernie could change his mind. She insisted, "Please, you guys sleep in the beds. We'll camp out next to Khai."

Bernie chuckled. "No chance. J.W., tell me, where you gonna be sleeping in a week? Think about it." Bobbie Jo took Bernie's hand and led him to the bathroom, where he curled up in the tub, and she on blankets lining the tile floor, her feet sticking a foot out of the door. At eight the next morning, they emerged smiling, rested, and showered.

As J.W. walked through the door from dropping Bernie and Bobbie Jo off at the 30ᵗʰ Street train station, Krista handed him an envelope postmarked, "The United Nations, Embassy of the Republic of Viet Nam, New York City." Three tissue-thin visas were enclosed, ornate documents embossed with the exotic script of a culture that had buffered the Chinese and Indic worlds for millennia. J.W. held the delicate papers to the light, staring in wonder at the elaborate watermarked crests. He pondered if these visas were any different than those the Vietnamese emperors had been fooled into issuing over the millennia. How many times had foreign dignitaries entered Cochin China legally, only to go on and violate that trust by using its people as slaves to strip the land of its natural wealth? Perhaps J.W. was just another of the interlopers, with nothing to offer the Vietnamese in return for the exorcism he so badly needed.

"We still need to think about this," J.W. said, hoping Krista would explode again and refuse to go, but she was silent as they drank beer and watched the worsening news flowing out of Southeast Asia.

PART II

CHAPTER SIX

They awoke during the descent, squashed together as the airliner made a tight turn onto final approach. Hong Kong was to be the penultimate leg of their journey to Viet Nam. Krista opened her eyes just as her window filled with a feline silhouette carved from the jagged granite mountains separating free Hong Kong from Communist China. She gripped J.W. with one hand and held Khai tightly with her other. An ancient Chinese lady with skin as craggy as the peaks pointed to the figure and whispered to her Eurasian grandson, "Lion Rock Mountain. We are finally home."

Their 747 passed over the stubby tin and reed squatter's huts on the Kowloon side of the mountain and, just seconds later, dipped between the tall, austere, cinder block tenements, miles of gray concrete swathed in a hundred thousand scraps of clothing never drying in the unspeakable humidity. Two hundred yards before touchdown at Kai Tak Airport, they beheld the teeming masses at the Kowloon City market. Not a soul bothered to look up at the screaming jet just feet above their lives.

They stayed their first night at the Chinese YMCA, which sat in a grimy alley in the bowels of the city. Their room that made them yearn for Suite 360. There were no blankets to steal to make a room for Khai, and no corner large enough to set up her tiny portable crib. As they dropped their baggage in the room, a little man in a stained gray suit with a Mandarin collar knocked on the door. He pushed it open without waiting for an invitation. "You go desk," he commanded as he disappeared even faster than he had emerged from the mildewed hallway.

Marc Banter had telexed from Philadelphia.

"SAIGON COLLAPSE STOP GO NO FURTHER STOP
STAY HK STOP RENT FLAT STOP WAIT FOR
WORD STOP"

They rushed from the Y to the lobby of a nearby Western hotel. On the TV were satellite clips of North Vietnamese tanks lurching along the streets of cities J.W. had walked with impunity just a few years before. The next scenes were images of panicked farmers, hordes of them, clawing their way onto rusting barges headed down-country to the false security of Saigon. Kowtowing peasants begged the self-appointed, rifle-toting ships' stewards to bring their water buffalo, pigs, and dogs aboard, all that was left of their life savings and their lives.

Finally, Hong Kong Television broadcast film of great, olive drab American helicopters evacuating the cities, flying out to sea, and landing on U.S. aircraft carriers to belch inconceivable numbers of peasants onto the rolling decks. A moment later, the choppers were pushed overboard so waiting helicopters running low on fuel could land. Some of the aircraft just ditched in the rolling seas near ships of any flag. The human cargo harbored such profound fear, they were willing to chance the ocean to await rescue, rather than return to the imminent victory of the Vietnamese Communists.

⋙ ⋘

Krista had never been to Asia, nor had she ever dreamed her life would be dictated by twelve telexed words. And she had never imagined street odors so pungent, nor human swarms of such density. Her face and shoulders sagged over the smells, the heat, and the crowding, but she breathed not a word. Late in the afternoon, she asked if J.W. would be hurt if she and Khai retired early. As Krista closed her eyes, she whispered, "Are we going to stay?"

"I don't know. What do you think?"

"As long as it's not in this room."

"You sleep. I'll find us a place to live."

The man at the desk, the messenger in the gray suit, wrinkled his face in confusion when J.W. asked if he knew of any apartments for rent. "Apartments, a-p-a-r-t-MENTS?" J.W. queried again several decibels louder than necessary. The man smiled and nodded. He brought from under the sticky counter a glass ashtray with cellophane-wrapped, red-and-white-striped candies.

"MENTS," he announced proudly, but more to an older man sitting in a corner of the beastly hot lobby reading a wilted newspaper.

J.W. shook his head and left the building. He wasn't twenty feet into the muggy afternoon before he was stopped by the sights and smells in the ancient alley. While Krista had found them repugnant, to J.W., they culled recollections of My Co, the tiny Vietnamese village in which he'd spent much of the war. Though that year had tattooed him deeply, it had also engendered a painful rebirth, one that wiped away much of the sadness that had woven itself through his young life. He had come away from that star-crossed land believing his life had been given purpose, and even promise, for he had learned of the gift he'd been granted to soothe the demoralized and the fearful.

It was the first moment in all those years he understood the lesson he'd absorbed in Viet Nam. He only wished he had known it when Dr. McNamara, the dean at Marimore, asked what he'd learned there.

For a moment, J.W. was paralyzed by the revelation, to the point he had forgotten where he was standing. It was just a gentle tap on his shoulder, but he shuddered and turned, ready to fight. The Caucasian man who had been reading the paper in the corner of the YMCA lobby jumped back two feet.

The man drawled, "I'm so sorry, sir. Excuse me."

J.W. calmed and smiled. "No, *I'm* sorry. Just got here. Really tired."

"You know, I overheard you asking the clerk if there were any apartments for rent."

"Yeah, I did. Don't think he understood."

"Well, if you're looking for a place to rent, I can...I'm sorry. I'm Harlan Flowers. Mission Church has a number of flats to let. If you're interested."

"Thank you, Mr. Flowers, but we're not really church folks, sir. We're here temporarily, just waiting to go back to Viet Nam."

He chuckled sadly. "And I'm still waiting to go back to China. For twenty years, I've been here waiting. Come on up and take a look at the flats. That's what we call apartments here in the Colony. We can work out a month-by-month if you need it."

They rode his Harley through the shadowy, dank streets of Kowloon, along alleys with mobs of rats diving in an out of piles of garbage, and men squatting, gambling noisily at cockroach fights. Flowers turned onto Waterloo Road, a wide boulevard lined with lofty tropical hardwoods and the magnificent homes of Hong Kong's fabulously wealthy. A block later, he rolled the motorcycle into Mission Hospital's parking lot. The mountains by which they had flown a few hours before rose out of the far end of the hospital's lush gardens. Harlan Flowers gazed into the mauve sky casting its final, dusky flickers on the Nine Dragons, the mountain chain after which Kowloon was named.

"I'm going to miss Lion Rock someday." He was quiet for a bit then added, "I need to check on a patient. Just take a moment. Ever been in an Asian hospital? Before J.W. could answer, Flowers went on, "You're welcome to come in."

"You're a physician?"

"Does that surprise you?"

"No. I mean, I can't believe it! I'm trying to get into medical school. That's one of the reasons I came here. To study for the MCATs."

"MCATs?"

"Well, sir, you see, I'm going to become a doctor. I've got all the books, and a place at Marimore Med School. Just a matter of busting my ass now."

Flowers winced. "What's MCATs?"

"That's the Medical College Admission Test. It's a bear. Everyone's got to take it. Didn't you? Lucky if you didn't."

"Nah, it was easier in my day. When I got home from the War—I was in the Pacific—I decided I wanted to be a doctor. So, all I had to do was finish high school. Then I went to college for a few years, and I had to tell my mother I wasn't going to keep the farm. Now, that part wasn't so easy. Come on, I'll show you the hospital I built."

They toured the brick and concrete building, stopping to rest in the surgeons' lounge. Over toast and tea, Dr. Flowers told J.W. of his boyhood home in rural Alabama, near Marian Military

Institute, and of his two decades as a surgeon in Hong Kong. He had first come to Asia a quarter-of-a-century before, director of his church's plan to fund a hospital in Mainland China. But those were the days of Mao's Communist Revolution, and soon after the hospital was opened, he and his family were expelled. They were lucky to have gotten out with their lives. Nonetheless, Harlan Flowers was still petitioning for a visa to go back.

He was quiet for a minute. "I guess you treat a patient here, you treat one there, it's all the same. Don't matter where you do it, just as long as you do it." He was quiet again, eyes on the ceiling, but quickly blurted, "I know just the place for y'all." His jowled face brightened. "Let's go."

They left the hospital and rode the residential streets of Kowloon Tong, past the walled enclaves of military officers, doctors, barristers, businessmen, and government officials. On the top of each rampart sealing off the multi-million dollar homes, shards of broken glass were set in beds of concrete. Some of the barriers were laced with barbed wire. Dr. Flowers nodded to the walls and shook his head. "We got a real robbery problem here. Drugs. Just like at home." They finally rolled up to an impenetrable wrought iron gate, which a doorman opened obsequiously, allowing the motorcycle into a vestibule of handsome flats.

"What 'a y'all think?"

"Looks expensive. We're living on a shoestring, you know."

"Shoot, two-thousand a month? On Paris Road? That's the most reasonably priced accommodation in the Colony. Better snatch it up! I ain't foolin'."

"Paris Road? Seems like every place we've lived in the last five years has had the name Paris in the address."

"Told ya. It's in the stars. But Paris?"

"Yeah, The Sorbonne, the nickname of the University of Paris."

"When were you there? What'd you take?"

"It was right after Viet Nam. I went to study Vietnamese and Chinese literature. I was going to go to Paris for a year, but it turned into four and a Ph.D. After I got my degree, it was the Paris Inn, in Philly, waiting to go back to Viet Nam."

"Sounds like a checkered past," he laughed.

"My British friends at the Sorbonne called it 'spotty.'"

At nine that night, J.W. called Marc at CWR in Philadelphia. "Contact Mr. Chou Van Hong in Saigon by telex. Good man. Find out what he wants for the refugees still in Viet Nam. Buy it and ship it. There's no money limit."

"Marc, you got a rich uncle die or something? Last week we were making twenty-five dollars a month."

"You still are. The American public's gone crazy. All the pictures of Vietnamese farmers living on the roads, livestock gone, houses gone, nothing but the clothes on their backs. We've collected a million bucks. Spend it. All of it. Plan on staying in Hong Kong for two years. And, for Christ's sake, take the apartment from Dr. Flowers. Everybody knows Harlan. Best guy in Hong Kong's giving you the best deal in Hong Kong. Say hello to Stella for me."

By noon the next day, Khai's crib was set in a spacious, airy room off the dining area. J.W. opened the door of what appeared to be a closet at the other end of the apartment. It was an eight-foot-by-eight-foot storage area with a window in which teetered a rusting air-conditioner. He staked out the space as his office, taping a handwritten sign on the door:

DR. WEATHERSBY – DO NOT DISTURB

He arranged the pre-med books in a neat row on the moldy wicker desk and cracked the cover of the biology text. He allowed himself a minute of dreaming about how he would sit in his office, study for hours, day after day, take the MCATs right there in

Hong Kong, return to America with top tier scores, and receive offers of admission from six medical schools. Who could resist so committed a student? And, J.W. had an in with the dean of a great university. He had said it; J.W. had heard him. "Let me know."

J.W. stuck his head out of the office. Krista and Khai held each other on the couch, gazing out through the barred living room window into the lush greenery of Paris Road. They were more peaceful than he had ever seen them, and J.W. settled back to Chapter One of the biology book, to enter the world of the single-celled organisms. He filled the fountain pen from the bottle of Pelican ink they had carried halfway around the world, opened the spiral notebook, and placed the nib on line one. As his life began anew, the air tensed with excitement and, also, with a gentle vibration that filtered through the clanking air-conditioner. In seconds, though, the hum built to a rumble, and abruptly to a shattering thunder so furious, the ink bottle vibrated off the table and splattered onto the mildewed linoleum floor.

J.W. tore from the office. Krista stood at the front door, her arms wrapped desperately about Khai to calm her screaming. He grabbed them and ran into the courtyard, sure the open space was safer than the house that was about to collapse. The roar came closer, and the sky darkened. He screamed to Krista, "Typhoon—get on the ground. Cover the baby!"

She did, and he dove on top of them spread-eagled, desperately sheltering as much of his family as he could. With the ground shaking, J.W. turned his head toward the sky. Expecting a swirling cloud of Asian debris, he was even more shocked to witness the fuselage of a Boeing 747 passing feet above their heads, close enough, it seemed, to touch.

J.W. had not witnessed an airplane crash since Viet Nam, and he shook with the picture of a white-glowing aircraft melting on the ground just half-a-mile away. He could smell the plane engulfed in oily flames. Worse, J.W. heard the pleading of victims still belted into their mangled seats. He could feel the coming disaster in the stifling heat of the Kowloon afternoon. It was as if his last crash had been only yesterday. J.W. began to hyperventilate.

Krista and J.W. squeezed Khai between them to shield her from the explosion, and they waited like that, anticipating their punishment for having ventured so far from the script. But all that came seconds later, exactly thirteen, was the proper squeal of landing aircraft tires. The fireball and the shrieks did not come, and they rose to their feet to stand in the yard until the scenario repeated itself, this time a 707 sweeping over. This plane's beaten jet motors speared Kowloon Tong with a high-pitched whine that made the 747's engine noise a melody of ocean surf. Two minutes later, the sky blackened yet again, and the roar of down-spooling turbines on a Tri-Star shook the house.

A DC-10 was next, its wing tip vortices blasting into the Weathersby's flat via the barred living room windows. It swept documents and clothes off the table and through the grille of the far window. The next vortex bounced around before exiting, a mere breeze, its energy dissipated under the doors that Krista had slammed shut. It left behind only thick, kerosene-laced, tropical air.

Seventy flights had passed over their house by sunset, when the wind shifted to the north, and landing planes approached the emerald of the South China Sea over Hong Kong Harbor instead of Paris Road. J.W. sat in the quiet at his desk and reopened the biology book to page one. He was ready to begin, again, but the phone rang—Dr. Flowers asked if they had settled in, if they needed anything. "J.W., I got a little problem. My partner just left the Colony on emergency leave. I need someone to assist me in surgery tomorrow morning. You have the time? Have you out of there by eight."

"I'll sweep your office. I'll do the windows. I'll do anything, if I can just hang around and watch. You mean real surgery?"

"J.W., I know that. That's why I asked. Hey, I'm sorry, but it's not that exciting, just a routine kidney operation."

While J.W. knew the kidneys made pee, and that a kidney punch hurt like hell, exactly where they were in the greater scheme of things, where the renal organs sat in the body, was still a grand mystery. His new biology book had a section on nephrology, so J.W. skipped ahead and spent the rest of the night with his head buried in that chapter.

In the morning light, Mission Hospital seemed smaller. Inside, however, even at 6 A.M., it teemed with those who had run for their lives from the madness of the Communist Revolution in South China's Canton Province. The hospital that Dr. Flowers had built some twenty-years before treated the Cantonese, all Cantonese, rich and poor, anyone who presented for care.

That morning's patient was an elderly woman, a Yau Ma Tei boat person, who had lived and slept every one of her eighty years on a sampan in the typhoon shelter of Hong Kong Harbor. In the surgical waiting room, Dr. Flowers talked with her family in Chinese and asked how long it had been since she had set foot on land.

"Twenty years," the son answered matter-of-factly.

Dr. Flowers believed Mrs. Shou had a blocked ureter. He told the family he was going to aspirate from her kidney a few drops of urine, a specimen to send to the lab for an analysis that would tell him where and what the trouble was. "I really need that urine," he advised the family several times.

"Why do you need her water?" one of the elder men asked, looking askance at Dr. Flowers. "We Chinese throw away a person's water. Right into the harbor. We just don't save that stuff.

Do you foreigners also save the brown stuff? We've seen you blow your nose and save snot on rags that you put back into your pockets. We Chinese just blow it out into the street where it can't do any harm. We Chinese just don't save all that stuff you foreign devils do."

Dr. Flowers answered poker-faced. "I'm sorry we have to do an operation just to get her water, but that's what my medical books say must be done. He opened the thousand-page, English language medical text he had carted along and pointed to a paragraph of very large print at the beginning of the book.

THIS VOLUME MAY NOT BE REPRODUCED WITHOUT THE EXPRESS PERMISSION OF THE PUBLISHER.

He fanned through the innumerable pages, finally coming back to the words at the beginning. He tapped them three times as the family stared. The spokesman nodded submissively, bowed slightly, and left J.W. and Dr. Flowers to their work.

J.W. mumbled, "What if they can read English?"

"They can't read English, or Chinese, or anything for that matter, these fishermen. But the funny thing is, when you invoke the concept of the written word, you automatically get respect. The bigger the book, the more powerful its words. Can you imagine? I told them, 'It says so right here,' and now they're going to let us take off all her clothes and cut her open."

Dr. Flowers shook his head, as if after all the years, he still didn't understand why he had been granted that terrible power of life and death. Perhaps that was because he knew the healer rarely changed the course of disease, helping most of the time just to manage it. And yet he held the inconceivable power to whisper the words, "Just lay down here lady and let me slice you up with a knife, and when we're done and you hurt worse than

you ever did before in your life, you dang well better thank me—
and give me money."

Flowers' reverie broke, and he nodded J.W. toward a point
down the hallway. J.W. followed into a sterile, green room where
a slip of a human being lay on the stainless steel operating table.
The neat bun of Mrs. Shou's silver hair was partially covered with
a sterile cap as she stared at the ceiling in perfect, unflinching
silence, waiting for the mask-covered foreigners to do with her
what they would.

This was the first time J.W. had seen Dr. Flowers uneasy, and
he spoke quietly toward J.W., but not to him, "This lady's so delicate, she may not make it through the anesthesia." He took her
hand gently, closed his eyes, and whispered a prayer seeking
guidance in his mission to help her, and for all in the operating
room to be exceptional that day.

The anesthesiologist, a diminutive Nepalese woman whose
fingers and wrists were crusted with Asian gold and peanut-sized
diamonds, nodded for Dr. Flowers and his wide-eyed assistant
to leave the room and scrub. They retired to the porcelain sink
in the hallway, rubbing iodine-soaked, pig-bristle brushes over
their hands and arms, and under their nails, over and over until their halogen-stained skin shriveled. After three minutes of
scrubbing, J.W. asked Dr. Flowers how long the ritual was to last,
and Flowers laughed, "Every other place on Earth, it's a three-
minute scrub, but our illustrious chief of surgery, Milton Wong
has decreed, because our water isn't as pure as in the States, we
do five minutes."

"Wait a minute," J.W. challenged, "Three minutes, five minutes, seven hours—dirty water's dirty water. What's the difference? What does water get, clean with age?"

"You're from New York, aren't you?" Without letting J.W. answer, he continued, "Don't ask me, ask Dr. Wong. And don't you

dare. I just built the place and pay all the bills, including his salary."

Dr. Flowers led J.W. back into the operating room, sterile paws in front of them, pushing backwards through the swinging door. The nurses wrapped the two in flowing, thick cotton, green surgical gowns that smelled of bleach and a peculiar soap from somewhere in J.W.'s distant Asian memory. Dr. Flowers nodded at the operating table, nonchalantly handing J.W. a hissing plastic tube coupled to a pump under the table. J.W.'s teeth clenched so hard, his head ached; they closed even harder as the surgeon put his scalpel to Mrs. Shou's flank and made the initial incision.

The blood was scarlet under the operating theater lights, far more stark than any battlefield red, though here it spurted in tiny fountains from neatly separated capillaries, not in gushes from brutally violated arteries. Dr. Flowers calmly picked off each minuscule bleeder, one by one, with tiny hemostat clamps. He called in Mandarin for Mrs. Wong, the scrub nurse, to hand him instruments. She tendered tools from her perch atop three stacked wooden boxes barely high enough to lift her even with the surgeon.

Dr. Flowers tied surgical knots to stop the bleeders and had J.W. snip the ends of the suture material with scissors. He'd mutter how long he wanted the stubs to be, but after each of J.W.'s attempts, he'd cluck impatiently, "Too long," or, "Too short."

After forty-five minutes, J.W. asked, "Dr. Flowers, would like them too long or too short?" The surgeon's eyes smiled.

There was so little to Mrs. Shou's substance, they arrived at her kidneys after a short journey through layers of mysterious, paper-thin tissue. Isolating the ureter, Dr. Flowers placed a tiny hypodermic needle into the bloated tube and withdrew a teaspoon of the precious urine. His shoulders began to loosen, but the anesthesiologist mumbled in a nearly unintelligible tongue, "Doctor, her blood pressure. You must hurry-hurry fast."

Dr. Flowers, without looking up from the surgical field, smiled again with his eyes, then gingerly placed the syringe on Mrs. Wong's instrument table. The tension in the OR thickened as he instructed the staff, first in Mandarin, "*Bu yao chu mo;*" and then Cantonese, "*But yiu jok mo;*" and finally to J.W., "DO NOT TOUCH IT!"

The stress bore deeper as the anesthesiologist shifted in her seat, nervously pulling multicolored vials of chemicals from her bag, injecting each with a more frantic push into Mrs. Shou's IV. After each, she urged, "You must work faster, Doctor!"

Aside from Harlan Flower's suturing and the involuntary, muscular twitch of J.W.'s hand on the scissors, nothing in the room stirred. Suddenly, though, the anesthesiologist blurted, "You must go fast-fast now! Fast-fast, Doctor. Fast-fast!"

J.W. considered dropping his suction device and bolting from the room—he had never wanted to be a surgeon in the first place. Psychiatry or pathology would be ideal specialties. Dr. Flowers, however, did not lift his eyes from his work. "Ever heard of Barry Manilow? Saw him on TV last night. Guy's great," he beamed, and went on operating on his dying patient, humming *I Write the Songs*. He must have also seen the quivering of J.W.'s hand, for he whispered calmly in his deep southern drawl, "Just hold what you got, Hoss. Y'all's doin' fine."

But Dr. Flowers' eyes had become tense slits. He sutured layers quickly, now working in silence. When the last stitch was placed, and Mrs. Shou's skin drawn together precisely, he took a deep breath and stood up straight for the first time in over an hour.

Now the anesthesiologist's flitting slowed, and the OR staff came together around the operating table, closing on the patient as if petals of a Venus Fly Trap. They prepared to shift Mrs. Shou onto a gurney, and when the anesthesiologist settled back into her seat, Mrs. Shou's cot was wheeled out to the recovery room. Before the doors could swing shut, a platoon of little old Chinese ladies from housekeeping swept into the OR, mopping and scrubbing furiously for the next soul on Dr. Flowers' docket.

A young, incredibly thin, six-foot-tall Asian man, Mr. Wong, approached Dr. Flowers obsequiously. The doctor pulled off his surgical gloves, his mask and gown, and gently picked the glass syringe of urine off the scrub table. He handed it painstakingly to Mr. Wong. "We need to get this to micro lab right away. Please hurry, but *be careful*." He repeated the instructions in Cantonese and Mandarin.

J.W. asked, "Hey, Dr. Flowers, I can say it in Vietnamese if you want." The surgeon's lips tensed. He barely shook his head.

With the five-hundred-dollar-per-teaspoon pee on its journey through the halls of Mission Hospital, and having beaten the clock with Mrs. Shou, Dr. Flowers sighed deeply, let his shoulders relax, and invited his new assistant for tea and wheat toast in the doctors' lounge before starting on rounds. As in all buildings in Hong Kong, the rooms in Mission Hospital were of pygmy dimension. Dr. Flowers, a muscular, stocky man, maneuvered with little ease past the ends of the bed in room 308, where another slip of an ancient Chinese woman recuperated from yesterday's surgery. As breakfast was wheeled in behind them, taking up most of the room, J.W. and the doctor shuffled onto the verandah. Flowers drew in a deep breath of the ocean air blowing off the South China Sea. "That breeze's 'bout as therapeutic as any of the procedures or medicines we dispense around here, J.W."

He turned back to acknowledge the charge nurse, who had appeared at the door of Room 308 whispering his name. They were separated by only the breakfast tray. She mumbled a message to the doctor in English, subtly lowering her face as she spoke. "You know Mr. Wong? He very skinny. That Mr. Wong."

"Yes, I know Mr. Wong," he answered impatiently.

"He send urine test tube by pneumo to lab. I tell you now," she continued, taking a step backward out the door, her head dropping thirty more degrees, "She not put test tube in messenger tube. She to send tube by self."

"She? You mean he?"

"Yes, yes, he not put test tube in messenger tube. She to send tube by self."

"Well, where is the urine now?"

"It at bottom pneumo."

"Well, let's go retrieve it, shall we?"

"It very broken."

She opened the towel in her hand to display the remains of still-wet glass. There was a brief hiatus in the conversation. Dr. Flowers proceeded through a silent metamorphosis of hues, ending with a shade of carmine J.W. before observed only in his commanding officers.

"WHERE IS MR. WONG?"

"Mr. Wong, he go home."

Harlan Flowers turned back toward the verandah and took a step through the doors, sucked in a grand calming breath, eyed the spectators, those in the room and the half-dozen peeking around the doorway, smiled tightly, snatched the tray of breakfast, lifted it as if to fling it at them—every head in the room dropped, a church congregation in sudden prayer, including the near-lifeless patient—and with a fluid, though violent swing, twisted about and hurled the meal over the railing. The porcelain dishes must have accelerated at several multiples of the speed of ordinary gravity, for they crashed, four stories below, into the parking lot, with such a blast, nurses poured from the emergency doors to see which of the propane tanks had exploded this time. Dr. Flowers looked over the veranda, grasped the railing, and bellowed, "BLOODY HELL!"

J.W. rushed out to help. He followed Harlan's eyes to the pavement. The breakfast tray had landed on Dr. Flowers' motorcycle, smashing the headlamp. Despite the deepening crimson of his complexion, he took two slow paces back into the room. He took an ancient stethoscope out of his back pocket, warmed it in his palm, and listened to his patient's heart. His face relaxed. "I feel better now."

They looked in on Mrs. Shou in the recovery room, and the family asked him what her water had shown. Dr. Flowers took his patient's hand and patted it reassuringly. She smiled up at them then closed her eyes and slept.

J.W. walked beside Dr. Flowers to the lounge for another cup of tea. "J.W., I shouldn't be keeping you here this long. You've got work to do for Children's War Relief. That's more important than standing around watching me make a fool out of myself. Get goin'. I'll call ya."

"No, sir, I don't want to leave. I've got all day to get my work done. I'll work late tonight and make up the time. I don't care."

A spate of minor operations followed: a hemorrhoid excision; a circumcision on a middle-aged British businessman who'd read in a magazine that the clipped life was far more pleasurable; and another infected hemorrhoid. At noon, Flowers and J.W. dressed in their street clothes and walked to the parking lot.

The doctor asked, "What y'all gonna do with all that money they's a given ya?"

"Buy what the new government in Viet Nam wants for the refugees."

"How you gonna get it to 'em? You know anything about spending a million dollars?"

"Krista does."

Flowers laughed and put a hand on J.W.'s shoulder. "Shoot, y'all know any shipping companies in Hong Kong? You know the regulations? Think you're gonna be home in no time, sittin' in medical school, don't cha? I think you're gonna learn a lotta surgery before you're done in the Colony." He nodded and turned to his bike, grinding his teeth as he flicked congealed bacon and eggs off the windscreen. He kicked the fragments of glass into a corner. "Gimme your hand." He wrote the number of a shipping company on J.W.'s palm, then invited J.W. back for surgery the next morning, calling as he turned onto Waterloo Road, "Nothin' excitin', just a gall bladder."

As J.W. jogged the mile back to Paris Road, the first of the day's airliners banked hard to avoid Lion Rock Mountain. At the house, Khai lay in the courtyard on her back in the playpen, cooing at the endless procession of planes. Inside, Krista had buckets of soapy water spread over the living room, scrubbing the veneer of years of spent jet fuel from the walls and ceiling fans. A twenty-five-pound barrel of Chinese detergent sat in the middle of the floor, scenting the room with the same aroma as the surgery gowns.

———

The Weathersbys boarded the 7-A for the harbor. The double-decker bus crawled the teeming streets of Kowloon, a two-mile voyage that took nearly an hour. Then they sailed across Victoria Harbour on the Star Ferry. They chose second-class, steerage, for three cents, to save CWR the two additional pennies to ride in style on the upper deck. Khai, in the carrier on J.W.'s back, grabbed chicken coops and tethered, squealing pigs as the Weathersbys were shoved fore and aft on the lower deck. But in five minutes, the journey was over, and the ferry bumped its way into the berth on Hong Kong Island.

Half-a-dozen short, wiry men donning but threadbare, baggy, dark blue shorts, without underwear, materialized from the bowels of the ferry. Another team of grizzled men stood from their hunkers on the pier and tossed hand-rolled cigarettes aside impassively. The two squads of stevedores numbly drifted to their duty station with such practiced apathy, J.W. tensed, fearing the massive ferry would crash into the terminal. He jumped behind Krista to insulate Khai from the coming crash. But the ship's bell clanged, and so began the perfect docking ballet the sailors danced forty times a day. Some tossed worn hawsers that weighed twice what they did; others caught those ropes, using the momentum of the cables to spin themselves around and loop the ends fluidly over the pier's stanchions. The movements were so elegant, it was hard to tell if a single calorie had been consumed securing the ferry to the dock. When it was done, the men picked their cigarettes off the concrete and squatted to stare into Hong Kong Harbour.

First in the queue to disembark was squealing livestock. Grimy men, not terribly taller than Khai, toted carrying poles, trussed to which were upside down wiggling pigs, calves, goats, and lambs. Next came a dozen diminutive men pushing mounds of plumbing supplies, rugs, bricks, crates stuffed with ducks and chickens, and boxes and boxes of tinned goods, all loaded on beaten bicycles. Finally came Krista, Khai, and J.W., who were shoved into line and carried with the tide through the mildewed passageways of the terminal. Surfacing in the street, they threw up hands for shade against the blistering, Southeast Asian sun. Krista took a diaper from Khai's bag and wiped sweat from the baby's face.

Krista stopped as soon as the last bicycle man had shoved his way past her. She caught her breath and waved a finger in J.W.'s face. "Next time, we go first class. It's a nickel, Dr. Schweitzer. I'm not doing that again."

"Yes, Dear."

They placed Khai in her fold-up stroller and walked the two blocks to shipping company Dr. Flowers had recommended. The office was high in Connaught Centre, the mighty, cylindrical creation that sat above the port of Hong Kong. Its round, cobalt-blue tinted, convex windows peered five hundred feet above the shore into a hazy distance. From the waiting room, they could just make out the blurry mass of Lion Rock Mountain and the specks of jet liners that dipped between the buildings of Kowloon City seconds before touching down at Kai Tak. Beyond that, almost obscured by the clouds of store-front-factory contamination, were the forbidden mountains of Guang Dong Province in southern China—the real China.

DeStahl Shipping welcomed their latest customers with the finest Earl Grey tea and the declaration, "We will be happy to deliver Children's War Relief's material to Viet Nam, or anywhere else on Earth you and Mrs. Weathersby so desire. It is a pleasure to be part of so important a humanitarian effort. Special consideration will be given, considering the nature of your financing. It's the least we can do."

J.W. smiled inwardly in quiet triumph at the life skills he had polished, at his sophistication, to arrive halfway around the world and within forty-eight hours have accomplished so much. CWR would be amazed at their luck in having found the Weathersbys. He continued to glow until Mr. Simeon quoted his price in Deutche marks, and J.W. calculated the conversion to dollars. J.W. added and multiplied, subtracted and divided for several minutes, grinning plastically each time he punched the equal sign. He whispered to Krista, "Hey, check numbers," then asked Mr. Simeon to write the amount down so there could be no misunderstanding based on the latter's proper British accent.

"Are you sure these figures are correct, sir?"

Simeon recalculated and penned numbers on a sheet of fine linen letterhead. "Oh, yes, there is a slight error." He turned the paper toward J.W. The amount was now eight dollars higher.

"Oh, my God," J.W. blurted. "You rounded up! No, we won't pay that. It's a pirate's ransom. We could buy the ship for that much." He collected Khai's toys and loaded her in the backpack, grabbed Krista's hand, and dragged his family back across Victoria Harbour, First Class, into the alleys and doorways of Mong Kok and Lei Cheng Uk, gathering the names of longshoremen available at short notice to load ships. Later, he towed Krista and Khai through half-a-dozen government offices, laying out piles of cash for the red stamp allowing transshipment of goods through the colony. The bureaucrats were unmoved by J.W.'s noble purpose, for his exports were, they grimaced, bound for the communist bullies in Viet Nam.

The next morning after surgery with Dr. Flowers, J.W. cabled a CWR contact in Taiwan and ordered a load of acrylic sweaters for the children of Central Viet Nam, in the mountains, where it got colder during the winter than in Buffalo, New York, or so the American soldiers who had fought there swore.

J.W. assumed he would have to organize offloading the sweaters from the Taiwanese boat once they arrived in the Colony, store them in a warehouse, then load them onto a ship for Viet Nam. Nurse Wong at the hospital had a cousin, Mr. Wong, whose brother-in-law, Mr. Wong, was a waiter, but also dabbled in the illegal import and export of Communist Chinese goods. In the back of a sweating kitchen, J.W. haggled with Wong over shipping rates to Viet Nam, but after a few minutes, the man scowled, waved the back of his hand, and left the kitchen with an order of fried noodles. J.W. called him back and slipped five-hundred American dollars into his fist. Wong wrote the name of a Communist Chinese freighter due in Hong Kong shortly after the sweaters were scheduled to arrive. J.W. was to pay the captain the balance after the cargo was loaded. No set amount was ever spoken, but there were repeated handshakes and pats on the shoulders. It was the way business was done in China, J.W. supposed. He did not realize until he stepped off the bus on Paris Street that there hadn't been exchanged a receipt or single signature.

Several weeks later, when he received a cable from CWR in Philadelphia that the sweaters had arrived, he rushed into the back alleys and gathered his platoon of stevedores, standing them at near attention in the warehouse parking lot. As he briefed the men that a ship in the harbor held his goods, and that they were to stack the bales neatly inside, several of the crew muttered that they had already crammed the warehouse with bales of sweaters from Taiwan, and hadn't been paid very well. A laborer grabbed J.W. by the wrist and took him inside. Five tons of garments sat swathed in a veneer of green bat guano. Stenciled to the burlap was "CHILDREN'S WAR RELIEF." On the bill of lading, Sol found a note that CWR had already paid for the goods to be offloaded and stored.

He muttered to the dockhands' leader, Mr. Wong, "Nice of them to tell me."

The man spoke in Mandarin, "Yes, very nice. Your CWR pays very good."

Mr. Wong's platoon of laborers, however, grumbled that Waiter Wong was a greedy turtles egg, and they demanded recompense for having been shortchanged on the original off-loading job, and then some more for having been snatched from their families and cockfights to shape up for nothing that day. J.W. smirked and rolled his eyes, but Mr. Wong took him by the arm back into the warehouse. He smiled, "Foreign devil, you see these rats flying around all over the place?" J.W. nodded. "They're Hong Kong rats. Very smart, not like the communist rats up north. But they are very hungry. My men, they may just tell the rats it's okay to eat your precious sweaters, burlap sacks and all. Maybe tomorrow, not even a thread of your stuff'll be left."

J.W. handed each man four dollars.

⇥⇤

Waiter Wong drove up to J.W.'s house at 5 A.M. the next morning on a bicycle. The Communist Chinese freighter with whom he had an illicit business arrangement had rasped into Hong Kong Harbor. J.W. collected Mr. Wong, the coolie chieftain, who collected the bearers, one of whom had a cousin, Mr. Wong, whose brother-in-law, Mr. Wong, owned a sampan in Hong Kong Harbour. Within two hours, the sweaters were loaded aboard the lighter, and J.W. found himself squatted amongst the coolies, trying not to let his shoulders touch the slimy acrylic. The sampan lighter captain dropped anchor, a Chevrolet transmission, at Buoy No. 67. J.W. looked up. Moored there, listing, was an enormous, rusting ship marked with the ghosts of Chinese characters. Though the heat was unbearable, the ship's crew wore long-sleeved, blue Mao jackets and blue Mao hats, each sewn with a little red star. They stood over the main deck rail and hooted as J.W. climbed the rotting Jacob's ladder and, hanging from the top rung, requested permission to come aboard. He was escorted through the narrow, musty corridors below decks to the captain, whose black eyes sparkled and exuded an air of leadership reminiscent of the better officers under whom J.W. had served in Viet Nam. The captain's accent was aristocratic Pekinese as he offered fragrant jasmine tea. The two men chatted in Mandarin, the crew flitting in and out of the miniscule compartment, awestruck by the foreign devil's Chinese.

As the stuffy cabin filled, J.W. inquired of the first mate, "Sir, who's topside loading the acrylic bound for your communist brothers in Viet Nam?"

The first mate squinted questioningly and deferred to the captain, who sucked a deep breath through his teeth, shook his head, and lamented, "Sir, I would like to take your cargo to our comrades in the lesser dragon of Viet Nam, but this boat must go to Senegal, to our struggling brothers in Africa."

"Africa? You're not going to Viet Nam? So where are you taking the sweaters?"

J.W. plucked from his hip pocket a shredded copy of the *South China Morning Post* and pointed to the listing under Buoy No. 67. The captain plucked half spectacles from his Mao jacket, consulted J.W.'s English-language edition, then retrieved from his own hip pocket a soiled copy of the *Hong Kong Daily*, Chinese language edition. The captain pointed apologetically, "*Bu hao yi si, bu hao yi si, tung bao,* I am so sorry, comrade. You see, sir, the ship you are looking for, the People's Hope, is anchored at Buoy No. 76. You are aboard the People's Salvation, a much superior vessel, if I do say so myself. I'm afraid your newspaper is wrong. Come topside. We'll get things fixed. No problem."

On deck, however, the second mate, who had taken charge of the situation based simply on the instructions J.W. had issued in Chinese when he first struggled aboard, announced proudly to his captain that all the sweaters had been loaded. The captain lit a foul-smelling cigarette and snapped orders for the lowering of the launch. He took J.W. and both the first and second mates on a choppy excursion beneath the behemoth ships of the world to the People's Hope, another rusting tub with barely distinct Chinese characters stenciled on the bow.

The captain greeted them warmly, inviting them below decks for jasmine tea. Here, too, the crew gathered in the commander's quarters, dressed to a man in blue Mao jackets and blue Mao hats with little red stars, each drawing deeply on rancid cigarettes. The two captains, the four first and second mates, and several of the lesser crew, motored back to the People's Salvation, where a summit was convened on deck. Both skippers, the owner of the sampan lighter, the coolie leader, and J.W. Weathersby entered a dialogue that began politely. Eventually, the sampan captain who had brought the acrylic to the first ship smiled that he would be happy to accept the cargo back aboard, and even deliver it to Buoy 76, but the transfer was naturally going to require a recalculation of the contract. He growled, hemmed and hawed for five minutes, borrowing the captain's abacus, and finally wrote the supplemental charge in the margin of his own copy of the South China Morning Post.

J.W. grunted, "Bullshit. No way, pal."

"Look, foreign devil, I was hired to load one ship, and only one ship. My people are very tired. They've done enough work for three days, and anyway, I don't like communist governments, like that new one in Viet Nam, or, to be honest, the one I escaped from in China." He snarled at the two Mainland Chinese captains and waved the back of his hand dismissively as he turned his face away.

The two captains' mouths curled down. "You are a capitalist roader, a running dog of the imperialists. Off the ship of the great People's Republic of the PURE China before we arrest you and execute you for treason."

The coolie leader, assuming the socialist mariners had no power to execute him in Hong Kong Harbour, jumped out of his hunker and screamed at his men, "Leave this rotting ship and go squat on the lighter. You are not to touch another piece of this tainted, communist-bound trash."

J.W. slithered behind one of the lifeboats and counted his money then reappeared and offered the coolie chieftain triple the fee to resume his labor, but the captain of the second Chinese ship called J.W. a capitalist dog for offering money over principle, and for bribing an enemy of the revolution. All work ceased. It was after five. The sun was growing large and orange, the lower edge of its rim just touching the mountains of Lan Tau Island to the west.

The two captains bantered back and forth—a compromise was struck, but only because of J.W.'s passable Mandarin. The captain of the 76 would sail the sweaters to Viet Nam if they were loaded aboard his vessel, but the coolies were banned from setting foot on the Chinese vessels. J.W. agreed and enjoined the sampan captain to sail back to shore and drop the sweaters and the gang of capitalist roaders off on dry land. He would find another sampan, gather a politically mature delegation, and return to get the sweaters aboard the 76 before 3 A.M., when the ship was to set sail.

The coolie leader had also only recently escaped from the communist regime in China and warned that he, too, was tired of this American fire drill, and that if J.W. didn't get on with it, they would sail off, and J.W. would swim back to shore dragging the sweaters behind him.

Surrounded by over one hundred unyielding faces, J.W. dropped into the hull and opened the massive steel door to hatch Number 3. A nest of cat-sized rats watched curiously, completely oblivious to the bar of steel J.W. flung at them. The crew, however, pondering the banging and jangling in the bowels of their ship, slid down thick hemp ropes to observe.

An antediluvian, deep green Cadillac limousine had just been lowered into the hold, blocking access to the sweaters. The captain ordered the vehicle slung to the ship's derrick and lifted out, but it was raised in fits and starts, dropping down half-a-foot each time the mechanism came to the missing gear tooth in the decomposing block and tackle. With no place to store the car while the sweaters were off-loaded, the captain gave further orders for it to be left dangling over the hull. Nuts, bolts, and small parts fell sporadically from the undercarriage, clanking next to J.W. as he dragged bale after bale of acrylic fiber out of the hold. The crew tried to lend a hand, but the captain kept appearing over the edge of the hold, shooting enemy-of-the-revolution stares.

J.W. grabbed each bale with a steel loading hook, ripping the burlap and extruding bright pastel tufts of sweater material. One of the crew members grabbed the hook from J.W. and ranted in Cantonese, pointing angrily to the Chinese characters stenciled on the side of the bales, the few not obliterated by the bat guano. J.W. apologized in Mandarin that he did not speak the man's dialect, so the sailor shrugged and climbed the rope out of the ship's belly. When the bales were loaded aboard the lighter, J.W. sat back on the deck to rest in the dark. The sun had disappeared behind Lan Tau.

On the 76, putrid, oil-slicked water pooled in the hold. Expired rats floated back and forth in the muck as the ship rolled gently. The last bales were lowered, and J.W. struggled with the cargo hook to pull them into storage. Several of the crew yelled at him and pointed angrily at the barbed metal rod until one of the crew told him in English that the Chinese characters on the bales read, "Use No Hooks."

It was past midnight when the lighter arrived back at the docks of Kowloon and tied up at the end of a long line of sampans, their occupants asleep on straw mats lining the moldy decks. J.W. tiptoed his way across a dozen boats, Chinese faces staring up at the apparition, their worst nightmare come true. J.W. was angry at these people and cursed under his breath at the ignorance of those who found anyone unlike themselves abhorrent.

On shore, though J.W. searched for a bus or taxi, he reminded himself that the freighter captains, the lighter captain, and the coolie captain had sucked from him his last Hong Kong dollar. He stuck his thumb out to hitch. A Westerner stopped, but when he rolled the window down and looked more closely at J.W., the man paled and drove off, squealing his tires. J.W. began the five-mile walk to Paris Road. He passed a downtown shop, catching a frightening glimpse of a sepia freak staring at him through the store window. The features were somehow familiar, and he took a second look—his face and clothing were stained deeply with bunker oil and filth.

J.W. turned onto Paris Road at three A.M., minus the front door key that was now on its way in a ship's hold to ports unknown. Nor did he have a key to the iron gates, so he settled exhaustedly on a pile of tropical leaves in the alley behind the house and slept until dawn.

＊＋＋＊

Krista woke him for dinner that night. Khai was in her highchair, as quiet as J.W. had ever heard her, the hamburger bits already half-gone, and without a single threat about not getting dessert. Krista commented on how hungry Khai had become the last few days. "Must be a growth spurt—common in kids this age," J.W. added, but a 747 passed over, and Krista shut her eyes tightly and covered her ears. She missed the comment. Khai stole a look at her blinded mother and dropped shreds of hamburger and carrot bits onto the floor. She giggled.

J.W. looked under the table, expecting mounds of meat and mashed carrots; in fact, the carrots were there, but he caught just a glimpse of the last trace of meat being devoured by a dusty brown rat with patches of missing hair. J.W. gasped but shut his mouth abruptly, electing to kick at the creature, sending it off before Krista opened her eyes.

The next day, J.W. woke early and asked to have a cup of coffee with Krista before Khai climbed out of her crib. "Sweetheart, would you go into Hong Kong and discuss a deal with that dick, Simeon, at DeStahl? He's got us by the balls, and he knows it."

J.W. watched through a crack in the window as she boarded the 7-A bus. He sprinted to the phone and called the Hong Kong Department of Exterminators. A Mr. Wong arrived on a rusting bicycle. Bound to the rear fender were a half-dozen wire cages, each pre-loaded with a hunk of octopus tied to a trip wire. He placed several of the cages around the house, grinning toothlessly as he told J.W. that for every rat he had actually seen, there were twenty more in the walls and foundation. As Mr. Wong rode off, J.W. hid all the traps, save for one behind the kitchen door.

J.W. made dinner that night, warning Krista she wasn't allowed anywhere near the stove, that it was her night to relax after what she had been through, dealing with thieves at DeStahl Shipping. Khai was also in a foul temper over the loss of her first Asian friend. She screeched and flung her plate like a discus, spurring Krista's mad dash into the kitchen for paper towels. The hysterical screams drowned the thunder of the DC-10 blasting just feet overhead.

Though J.W. had planned to start his official study program that night, he convinced Krista to have a glass of *Mei Gui Lu*, rose petal wine. After three, she relaxed and spoke softly. "I guess there are some things here I'm going to have to get used to, like the wringer washing machine and the gecko lizards. There are a lot of them. Do you know if they bite? And there's the walls and the drapes stained with that oily jet fuel. My face is kind of oily, too. But the rat. I don't want rats around my baby."

"Everything's under control, my darling. Think about it. We caught the bastard, and I'll get rid of him tomorrow morning. I promise."

Krista nodded and began a fourth glass of wine, but there was a squeak followed by a guttural hiss from the kitchen. The cage banged and clanked, then shuffled in from the kitchen, self-propelled, the rat's legs squeezed through the wire mesh.

The creature's long-nailed feet tapped a static on the hardwood floor as it made its way toward Khai's room.

Krista jumped out of her chair and shrieked, "Hey, Rat Man, for every one you see, there's fourteen you don't. And I can't get the smell of octopus out of my nose. And now it's in my clothes 'cause you put all those goddamn cages in the closet. I can't take it. I'm going home."

CHAPTER SEVEN

At the hospital the next morning, J.W. and Dr. Flowers made rounds on Mrs. Shou. She wasn't in her bed. The sheets and pillowcases had been stripped. Her chart was gone.

"Not a good sign, Hoss. I put her on one of those new cephalosporins last night. Wild guess." He sighed and shuffled to the nurses' station, though no one was there, and he stood shaking his head.

J.W. inferred from his mentor's drooping face that Mrs. Shou had passed away during the night. He wondered if Dr. Flowers would blame himself, and if he would cancel surgery and sit at home, terrified it might happen again. Would he question his abilities and, more morosely, ask himself why he had ever drifted so far away from home? J.W. could not bear to look at him and turned away, facing the opposite hallway. There, hobbling slowly, was Mrs. Shou's entire extended family. At the head of the parade rolled the patient in a wheelchair, a toothpick connected by plastic tubes to an IV pole. When the family recognized the doctor and J.W., they rushed over and took their hands gratefully.

Dr. Flowers drawled in a whisper behind his hand, "Dodged the bullet, my friend. Tell me there isn't a God."

Mrs. Shou's husband and children had called J.W. "Doctor" when they thanked him, as if he had had a hand in the care of the matriarch of their boat clan. It had given him goose bumps, but he was embarrassed by his true feelings. When J.W. had first seen first Mrs. Shou, she had appeared as frail as a bamboo stick-figure. He could not understand the fuss when she had faded on the operating table. She had lived a long life and, like every spirit, would soon pass back into the mystery. He had seen so many of the elderly perish in Viet Nam—Mrs. Shou was just another nameless, faceless ghost.

Yet, from the respect her family seemed to afford her, it was apparent the world had somehow benefited from the woman's brief sojourn on the blue planet. It was also clear they didn't share J.W.'s fatalistic view of those older than fifty, and for a moment, J.W. believed that, perhaps, her life was not as disposable as he had come to believe.

Still, it was hard to understand why Dr. Flowers had worked so quietly, but furiously, to save her. He knew her time was short, no matter the outcome of that day's surgical heroics. It wasn't Harlan Flowers who had caused the disease in her kidney, who had put her on that sampan, who had ignored the symptoms for so long there was now little hope of cure. Yet, he took his charge seriously, seriously enough to have nearly had a stroke when a half-teaspoon of her piss went missing. J.W. asked under his breath, "What aren't you seeing?"

While Dr. Flowers claimed he had merely guessed at a treatment for Mrs. Shou, claiming to have practiced medicine by the seat of his pants, *he* had chosen the antibiotic, not Mr. Wong, or the head nurse, or J.W. *Dr. Flowers* was the one who had found out about the new class of medications, the cephalo-somethings, despite the fact it would have been far easier for him to practice the old medicine he had been taught in the Fifties. No one, certainly in Hong Kong, would have ever known the difference.

Some nights, when J.W. called Dr. Flowers, his wife, Stella, apologized that Harlan was busy with his books, studying for the coming day's surgery, preparing, no matter how many hundreds of times he'd done that procedure, no matter how routine it had all become. That made J.W. feel small, especially when his eye caught the pile of pre-med texts whose knowledge still lay locked within their virgin covers. And J.W. began thinking that perhaps doctors really were gifted creatures, capable of harder work and purer thoughts than he would ever attain.

With the rattraps gone, and with Krista's clothing back from the drycleaners, she calmed a bit and spent the days playing with Khai. The baby was beginning to walk, and the challenges of Asian life switched to avoiding the stark humidity of Hong Kong's spring. Assuming Dr. Flowers, a staunch Christian missionary, would surely take Easter Sunday off, the Weathersbys made plans to travel to an ancient fishing village in Kowloon, one reportedly founded hundreds of years before the inauguration of the Ming Dynasty. J.W. was excited at the prospect of finally witnessing the real Hong Kong and dining on the fresh steamed fish he had read about in the classical Chinese texts at the Sorbonne; when that was done, he'd start on a kilo of sweet grilled pork and finish with several bowls of traditional fried noodles. But at 5 A.M., Dr. Flowers called J.W. to the hospital for an emergency hemorrhoid operation.

After surgery, they had a second cup of tea.

"You okay?" J.W. joked. "You never drink more than one cup."

"Need something to keep me awake. Was up most of the night studying for the surgery boards. Never ends, J.W. Thought about you around 2 A.M. Wondered if you and I were the only ones in Hong Kong awake, beating the books. Even if it was just us, reckon I was in good company."

J.W. was silent, but that night, he took a rag and washed away the glaze of dust and spent jet fuel from his desk. He refilled the pen, opened the biology text to page one, and began his new life, once again. Thirty minutes later, however, he stuck his head in the bedroom. "My butt hurts."

"Why don't you take a rest. It doesn't have to be done it in a single night."

"Okay, but just for a few minutes.'

He awoke on top of the covers at dawn and sprinted up Waterloo Road to the hospital. Dr. Flowers was sipping his third cup of tea.

That night, J.W. pushed on for an hour before getting a cup of tea. He planned to sit back down, but nodded to himself that he had put himself through a mini mental marathon and closed the books.

In the morning, before leaving for the hospital, he stood over his desk and surveyed the progress—four pages. When Dr. Flowers asked, over a bowel resection, what subject J.W. was up to in his grand plan, J.W. couldn't remember if he had studied biology or physics the night before. That evening, J.W. outlined the pages he'd covered, just to have some record, the thinnest proof of the time he was investing. By the end of the week, though, just twenty pages of the biology text had ink stains—the other seven-hundred remained unblemished. All that remained in his head were the few facts he had carelessly scribbled in the spiral notebooks.

J.W. spent the next two nights at the desk, most of the time fretting. The third evening, he went to Krista as she was doing the dishes. "They were right."

"Who was right?"

"All of them. This is ridiculous. I'm too old to learn. My brain is a dry cow patty."

"So, we can go home? You get a job?"

He spent the weekend at his desk, squirming, reviewing his failures as an undergraduate. His new notebooks had an eerily similar cast to those he had thrown together at Sterling College, the writing as large and slapdash as everything academic he had done there, when nothing had mattered, and his grades had reflected it. The fat dean had spoken the painful truth; the studies in Paris had been in the humanities, just so much fluff, nowhere near as demanding as the rigors of hard science.

But who cared about notebooks? No one would ever see them, and so he went on over the weekend, making clumsy marks in the books. By Monday night, the end of J.W.'s first week of study, precious little pre-medical knowledge remained inside his head.

The Weathersbys went to dinner at the Flowers' that night. J.W., at his mentor's insistence, brought the spiral notebooks to show Stella, his wife. "She's got a PhD in biochemistry, ya know. Might be able to hep y'all out, Hoss. She's the smart one in the family."

Stella's face remained blank as she turned the pages. She looked up and smiled thinly. "J.W., may I make a few notes, perhaps in the margins? You know, expand on the concepts a little."

Her writing was orderly. She developed each idea with a painstakingly drawn diagram. With J.W. was sufficiently deflated, she excused herself. The room went deathly silent. When she returned, it was with an armful of spiral notebooks memorializing the sixteen hours per day she'd invested over four years as an undergraduate at MIT. She handed J.W. the first—his eyes crossed. The pages were covered, every inch, with hand-written chemical formulae as elegant as if they had been engraved professionally. Each was buttressed by a diagram of the molecules that formed the compounds. There were reams of lecture and lab notes, and in the margins, cartoon characters mixing chemicals and melting substances. She had also scratched portraits of difficult professors, complete with call out boxes and snotty little poems.

At home that night, J.W. tore the first pages from the notebooks and started over. This time, the writing was smaller and neater, but when he showed Stella the work a week later, she asked, "J.W., Harlan tells me you were a commando in the army, a Ranger. Is that right?"

"Yes, ma'am."

"'Do it better than the last time, and you'll do it over and over until it is.' You ever heard something like that?"

"Yes, ma'am."

"And I did as well at MIT. A woman at MIT in the 50s? The gall of showing up to study for a PhD—it was more narcissistic than a thirty-three-year-old thinking he can get into medical school."

At ten that night, J.W. ripped the pages out and started again. Now, each illustration met Stella's admonition: do it better than the last one, or do it over. At the end of the week, he rode his bicycle to the Flowers'. Stella, without expression or permission, took the spiral notebook and added a few chemistry comments in the margins, but offered not a word about the form and quality.

As the explanations and drawings became increasingly detailed, the spiral notebooks became ends in themselves, the material measure of the time and emotion spent in such large sums over those months. J.W. sought to cram more and more of the pale green pages with the proof of his future, of his state of grace, the fat dean be hanged.

At the end of each evening's study, J.W. reviewed the data and drafted questions for the next day. After surgery, over toast and increasing cups of tea, J.W. grilled Dr. Flowers about the biology and chemistry, the physics and math, he had covered the night before. Dr. Flowers answered slowly, less assuredly than when he was operating.

J.W. asked if Dr. Flowers knew Watson and Crick, the British biologists from Cambridge who met for tea each morning at the Eagle Pub. J.W. asked if he could explain how they finally uncovered the secret of the chromosome, the template that programmed all life. Dr. Flowers looked away. "Not sure I know about them." The Krebs cycle and the mapping of proteins, J.W.'s next volley of questions, were concepts barely seeing first light the day Dr. Flowers began operating on his second twenty-five thousand patients.

As J.W. peppered Harlan Flowers with questions about esoteric biochemical doctrines, the aging doctor became slower and more circumspect in his answers. While J.W. may have been dispirited by the unsatisfying answers, the fact remained the man was a medical doctor, and the space he occupied on this Earth was hallowed. His mind was, by definition, a bottomless font of knowledge. He was infallible, invincible.

After a month, J.W. was spending three hours a night at the books. The questions he concocted for Dr. Flowers became picayune, unrelated to the world of gall bladder removals, breast biopsies, and circumcisions. Harlan Flowers stopped drinking tea and eating toast after surgery, simply disappearing between cases. One morning, J.W. found him hiding in the men's room.

Krista finally asked J.W. over dinner, "Why are there fewer cases to assist on any more? You make him mad or something?" When they ran into Dr. Flowers in Hong Kong later that week, the doctor sputtered that things had been very slow, but that he had been thinking about him.

At dawn the next morning, J.W. rode the 7-A in the other direction, into New Territories, to the Hong Kong College of Natural Sciences. In the corner of the ten-foot-by-ten-foot biology department office, a dozen Chinese students milled about the secretary's desk, their eyes glued to a chubby, though handsome, Caucasian man with a typed list in his hand. J.W.'s entrance brought an immediate hush and a momentary shift away from the paper to the outsider.

J.W. took a deep breath and blurted, "I'm wondering, is there a graduate student willing to tutor chemistry? For compensation, of course."

There were whispers in animated Cantonese, and the man allowed the mass of students time to answer, but no one did, so he dropped the grade sheet on the secretary's desk and took a hurried step backwards. As the implosion built, he nodded for J.W. to join him in the hall.

In a heavy Eastern European accent, he asked, "Exam scores. A man could lose his life in the crush. I'm not a graduate student, as such, but what sort of tutoring are you seeking?"

"Well, you see, sir, I'm studying to become a doctor, but I have a problem. It's not that big a problem, but I don't have any of the prerequisite courses."

"I see. No prerequisites to become a doctor. And what sort of tutoring are you seeking?"

"Actually, I really don't know. I have to pass the MCATs in nine months. It's mostly questions about biology and chemistry. Haven't started the physics. Do you do chemistry and physics?"

J.W. used the open-mouthed pause to present the spiral notebooks. It was hard to sense from the canting of the man's head if he was impressed, or if he saw the tiny writing and diagrams an exercise in anal compulsive psychosis. With the unveiling of the notebooks, several of the graduate students crowded into the hallway and stood behind the two foreigners. They gawked, commenting in Cantonese about the elementary level of chemistry to which the stranger, an older man at that, had barely risen. Several more students trotted over, so the professor took J.W. by the arm and pulled him deeper into the corner.

"Did Klaudia put you up to this?"

"Klaudia, sir? No, sir. You see, I really want to become a doctor, but I need tutoring. The dean at Marimore Medical College encouraged me. So, it's in the realm of possibility. But I have to do well on the MCATs. I think I've got a decent chance if I can just..."

"My name is Piotr, Piotr Sówka" he interrupted. "Be at my offices promptly at 9 A.M. on Thursday." He nodded formally, keeled around, and was gone. The hall was silent until a swarthy, young Chinese man, his face covered in acne, lifted his nose and clucked in a false Eastern European, "Vat goes on?" J.W. about-faced to the muted cackles of the eighteen-year-olds.

⇥ ⇤

"That's great, J.W.," Dr. Flowers chimed when J.W. called him from a phone booth outside the chemistry department. "Y'all come and help me with a breast biopsy on Thursday morning."

"That's the morning I'm supposed to see Professor Sówka. I'll cancel with him for this week."

"Don't you dare! I'll move the case to the afternoon."

Piotr Sówka was a recent addition to the faculty of the Hong Kong College of Natural Sciences, having taught biology for years in Uganda, at the University of Kampala. That was until he and his wife, Klaudia, were taken hostage, bound, gagged, and pedaled into the jungle in a bicycle rickshaw. On the third night of captivity in a thatched cell, their guards were called to a Marxist-Leninist political meeting which was presaged by billows of thick, cloyingly sweet cigarette smoke and Bob Marley reggae music that blasted so loudly, the men could not help themselves and broke into dance. As the boogying became furiously animated, the Sówkas smashed the wall out of their ooze and straw prison and ran off, barefoot, through the red earth of Uganda. For two days, they walked by night and hid in the jungle during the sweltering days, until a police Land Rover passed them on the main dirt highway. So relieved to see the authorities, they fell together in the back seat and cried.

They were taken to a transfer station, another mud and thatch hut, and arrested when they could not produce their papers. Tied to a log in the rear of the hut, Piotr promised the guard a hundred pounds if he would let Klaudia relieve herself. The policeman untied her and followed her just outside the door where he stopped her and pointed to the ground. When she squatted, he dropped to his knees to get a better look, and soon began rubbing his crotch. Piotr turned a way for a moment, but when he forced his eyes back, the guard's hand was moving forward. Piotr sucked in a massive breath, lifted the log, waddled forward, and smashed the guard's head. Blood spurted on Klaudia, but she jumped to her feet, spit on the prostrate form, and untied Piotr. The police Rover was parked behind the hut, key in the ignition. It was the only vehicle and the only radio for miles.

At two hundred meters from the Polish Embassy in Kampala, Piotr stopped, put Klaudia in the back seat, cinched her seatbelt, and slammed through the embassy gates. They were on a plane home to Warsaw before sunset.

For a time, Professor Sówka taught at a private school near Cöslin, in Northwestern Poland, in the Pomeranian Region, where Klaudia had grown up. They settled into a cottage on the Baltic sea. The misty, cool days of the summer, however, soon became more than either could tolerate after their years in the tropics, and with winter only a few months off, they began the usually long search for work at a foreign university. It took Piotr, however, less than two weeks to be offered a position at The Hong Kong College of Natural Sciences, and six months later, he was appointed full professor and granted tenure.

It was he who brought up the matter of reimbursement at their first meeting, promising to issue a statement at the end of each month. While J.W. should have asked what a professor of his distinction commanded for private tutorials, he did not have the nerve, and they talked and talked, instead, about biology and medicine.

Professor Sówka did physics and chemistry, and he also did motor mechanics, inviting J.W. to help him replace the transmission in Klaudia's Morris Minor. Dr. Sówka also climbed Lion Rock Mountain early each Sunday morning to sit on the summit, play the African lute, and ponder what drove human endeavor, asking himself why some people spent so much energy on the thin gamble of success.

And he respected J.W.'s pleas for, "Just one more question, sir," often spending two, sometimes three, hours grinding away at the blackboard, laughing and sweating, gently jamming what must have seemed woefully rudimentary concepts into J.W.'s aging brain. At the end of their third session, he paused while shaking hands to say good-bye. "You really weren't sent by Klaudia, were you? It's far worse than that."

J.W. left the professor's barely air-conditioned office each Thursday morning drenched with sweat, smiling as he dove back into the steaming streets of Kowloon, excited to rush home to tell Krista of his discoveries. But often, only a brief note sat on the dining room floor when he arrived home, for Krista had discovered a klatch of European women who met each morning at the park near the great cemetery on the hill. Krista told J.W. defensively, "It's a chance for Khai to meet children that look like her."

At the end of the first month of Thursday tutorials, a letter came from Professor Sówka's office. J.W. braced himself, expecting a statement of nearly a thousand dollars, four years' salary, but inside was a note inviting them to his home for dinner. Piotr ended the letter noting that he had enjoyed their month together and looked forward to eight more. J.W. searched deeper in the tissue-thin envelope for a bill, but it was empty.

That night, J.W. created a formal study schedule, budgeting a minimum of three hours per day at the wicker desk. "That would mean," Krista calculated with her face contorted in mock thought, "if you really do it, you will have put in more time studying here in a month than you did in four years at Sterling College."

The writing in the notebooks became smaller and more terse. J.W. invented a shorthand language of Chinese characters, English symbols, and Vietnamese couplets. Harlan Flowers thought it amusing, Piotr Sówka, "curious".

J.W. pasted together a two-foot-long sheet of graph paper. He labeled every day until the MCATs, a string that went on for hundreds of graph boxes, as endless as a two-dimensional Great Wall of China. He pinned it over his desk. The chart was depressingly void of all but the promise of thousands of hours of study, so long and so empty, that after a couple of glasses of wine, J.W. crumpled it and lay down for a nap. But he could not rid his mind of the picture of a completed grid, a year's work, inscribed for eternity, a powerful charge for the medical school admissions cannon.

⟩⟨

J.W. spent five and six mornings a week in the OR with Dr. Flowers. The afternoons were consumed at the colony's factories and warehouses. He bought, for shipment to Viet Nam, hand tractors, powdered milk, medical supplies, globes for class-rooms, and musical instruments for war-battered high schools. Marc Banter occasionally telexed from CWR in Philadelphia, instructing the Weathersbys to fly to Tokyo, Singapore, or the Philippines, to purchase kilometers of fishnet for the people of the Vietnamese coast, or specially engineered wood screw mak-ing machines that had been adapted to allow operation by the war-wounded para and even quadriplegic teenagers of Xa Dan Street in Hanoi. Those machines, designed and built in Tokyo, were ingeniously created to permit workers devastated by the war to use their teeth, or the stubs of arms and legs, to work the heavy equipment and produce finished screws to rebuild Viet Nam. When J.W. asked the powers at Children's War Relief World Headquarters if purchasing the goods for Viet Nam was a violation of the U.S. Trading with the Enemy Act, CWR assured the Weathersbys the American government would never discover their purchases, and even if they did, it was all humanitarian aid and exempt from the rules.

On each trip out of Hong Kong, J.W. dutifully lugged along the texts, the spiral notebooks, and the resurrected graph. At midnight, he added a little red dot to mark the number of hours he had spent that day attached to rickety chairs in rickety hotel rooms throughout Asia. By late December, nearly four hours per day had passed with J.W.'s head in a pre-med book. There were no gaps, not a single day, until Christmas, when J.W. allowed himself a sabbath.

In surgery, J.W. had more questions about the procedures and less of a notion of what they were doing. It had all seemed so simple at first, months before, when J.W. took Dr. Flowers' word for where they would find each body part. But medicine was de-teriorating into a jumble of faces, syndromes, and internal or-gans that resembled only remotely the glossy prints in his biology book. The parts of the body they treated were diseased, altered, nearly non-functional, and to his untrained eyes, unrecognizable. He cringed when patients called him doctor.

The hospital seemed more and more broken into separate camps, the helter-skelter, anxious world of medical professionals staffing operating rooms, and the lethargic, apprehensive world of their patients. In J.W.'s sleep, he pictured the slow-moving ill, people who knew nothing of surgery or antibiotics. He thought back to the little man who had called Dr. Flowers at 3 A.M. a few weeks before, moaning that his hemorrhoids were on fire. That case finished at dawn, leaving time only to wash up and start the daily surgery schedule. The patient, a Mr. Wong, had thanked them warmly, appreciating their help so late at night. He allowed that the hemorrhoids had indeed been growing more painful for many months, but he had been so scared the cure would be worse than the disease, he could not present himself to the hospital. That night, however, he became frightened when blood began gushing from his behind.

J.W. saw Mr. Wong again a few weeks later in the man's print shop. J.W. was excited about their human connection. J.W. had sacrificed for him, given a night of his life to address a patient's pain, and now the patient would give him a break on business cards. But the man recognized J.W. only after J.W. reminded him of their night together in surgery, and all Mr. Wong said of the bloody affair and J.W.'s sacrifice was the Cantonese equivalent of, "Yeah, and that comes to fifty-four Hong Kong dollars."

When J.W. mentioned the episode to Dr. Flowers over surgery, he muttered, "Ah ha! The prostitute principle."

"Yeah, now I get it. He's a whore. That's how he got hemorrhoids." J.W. laughed sourly.

"No, he's not a whore, J.W, he's just a patient." Flowers paused and shook his head. "J.W., professional services are valued very highly until the service is delivered. Then, all of a sudden, you're not worth a plug nickel. See, we're catching these folks at their worst, scared, in pain, in no control whatsoever of their lives. Their mortality's been dumped in the hands of two short, squat, foreign devils. That's why we would do better to get paid up front. Godliness and all that, but it may be a good thing to remember over your next forty years."

A month later, on the morning they wheeled Mrs. Shou back into surgery, Harlan Flowers arrived late. He brushed past the door of the waiting room where her family squatted silently beside empty, padded chairs. In the OR, he uttered his usual prayer, but held her hand a bit longer and more gently, exhaling as he finally let go. The two Americans scrubbed, gowned, and nodded to the Nepalese anesthesiologist. She returned the gesture, commenting that Mrs. Shou had been drawn to a deep plane of sleep. Dr. Flowers took the scalpel in his right hand, let his eyes raise to the ceiling for a moment, and made the initial incision. He cut through the original scar and tugged at soft tissue that fell apart easily. J.W. clamped off the bleeders with hemostats; Dr. Flowers tied and cut.

"Too long," J.W. grunted after the first snip. Dr. Flowers' face lifted, and his eyes smiled over the mask. They went deeper into the morass of scarred muscle and facia. Her constitution was so frail, her powers of healing so compromised, the layers of tissue had not recognized even their own kind over the past months. What had been virgin membrane on their initial foray into her depths was now a thick carpet of half-cooked pancake batter.

Dr. Flowers picked at bits of what he recognized and peeled them to the sides, saving what was left for a last-ditch effort at healing. The anesthesiologist began her usual rustling, snatching bottles of chemicals off her cart, injecting greater and greater doses into the IV tubing, and admonishing, finally, in an urgent staccato, as if an angry parent, "Doctor!" She gasped, "Your patient's blood pressure!"

Harlan Flowers did not blink. He simply worked with greater self-control. "Dress me slowly mother, I'm in a hurry," he mumbled then looked up at J.W.'s confused eyes. "It's an old Cuban saying," he announced distantly.

Mrs. Shou's blood pressure crashed silently. He knew, for there was suddenly no more bleeding. "She's gone," he muttered in submission.

There were no heroics, no screaming, no committee of medical and religious personages to oversee her passing. It was very quiet, aside from the deep breath with which Dr. Flowers sought to clear his demons, the ones that had added Mrs. Shou to his private list of defeats.

The family listened without expression. They took his hand and thanked him, repeating the gesture with J.W., but this time, the coattail pride had worn through, and J.W. couldn't wait to get out of the hospital, to go home and do his real job, buying antibiotics for the refugees crowding the suffering cities of Viet Nam.

For J.W., the luster of facing families after surgery had suddenly lost its sheen. He no longer wanted to be responsible for people's lives, just like Harlan Flowers didn't want to take Mrs. Shou back to surgery. The principal difference was that Harlan Flowers had no choice, and all J.W. had to do that afternoon was crawl back to DeStahl Shipping and eat a thick slice of humble pie.

CHAPTER EIGHT

K rista thought a rest from the books might blunt the day's sadness, so J.W. guzzled a couple of San Miguel beers and sat back on the wicker couch, happy for the reprieve of another seven or eight years before lives would be credited to his watch. The real perspective came not from the alcohol, but from Khai, who had fallen asleep holding his legs in her tiny arms. J.W. understood that just as Mrs. Shou was passing, his daughter was emerging for her brief journey.

J.W. pulled himself off the sagging wicker, kissed Khai on the head, and carried her into the study cell. The intransigence of earlier that evening cost him six hours of compulsive, tiny, chemical equations and diagrams of woody stems and single-celled organisms. Khai lay sleeping on the rug behind him. J.W. wondered if Cervantes was right, that the journey was better than the inn.

At midnight, he picked Khai up and put her in the crib. Her scent was so enchanting, his eyes moistened. By anyone's standards, he understood he was blessed, but he didn't quite know why. J.W. sang to her for a few moments.

As he started out of her room, the phone rang. By instinct, he looked at the calendar and calculated how long the patient Dr. Flowers was calling about had been ill. His mind's eye could picture only a huge rosette of hemorrhoids, all night in the OR, and an ungrateful customer for life. The voice, however, was distant and only barely familiar. When J.W. was sure it wasn't Dr. Flowers or Professor Sówka, he blurted, "Yeah, what 'a ya need?"

The answer came with an unexpected warmth and a laugh. "Hello, China! It's Bernie!"

Bernie related flowing tales of how hard it had been to find the Weathersbys, the reason he hadn't called before. His voice faded in and out, an echo repeating several times that he and Bobbie Jo were coming to Hong Kong on business, and would they have time to see them for a chicken dinner? J.W. asked who was going to mind the store in the City, but Bernie had graduated from men's clothing and rededicated his life to a new end. "Can't wait to tell you."

━╣╠━

When Krista, Khai, and J.W. met them at Kai Tac airport, a procession of Chinese men followed immediately behind Bobbi Jo, commenting loudly in Cantonese, "My God. Look at her. *Ay ah*, you could get sucked in and lost if you tried to pillow *this* one."

J.W. turned to them and lectured that they were as rude as pigs, and a few took an aggressive step toward him, but most just asked each other, "What did I say wrong?"

Dr. Flowers invited Bernie to watch an appendectomy. Bernie stood in a corner of the operating room, hushed in wonder. Over tea and toast, he admitted that, as glamorous as his life seemed to those ensconced in Hong Kong, medicine really was special. Dr. Flowers nodded and put another slice in the toaster.

Bernie's entrepreneurial passion had matured to the vending of industrial packaging tape. His office took up most of the hall closet in their Manhattan apartment—his warehouse was a dump in Harlem. He allowed that the clothing business had been an adventure, but he'd discovered his employees, the ones he had sent to a special school to learn how to spot shoplifters, were pilfering more from the store than the unchecked hordes of kids who still walked out with three and four layers of shirts and sweaters.

"I tell you, Dr. Flowers, it broke my heart. I paid them double what Saks did. I bought 'em pizza for lunch. Any topping they wanted, pepperoni, sausage—it didn't matter, and still they screwed me. I didn't understand, and I tell ya, it bothered the hell outta me 'till I came up with the tape gig."

He laughed that he wouldn't shave for a few days and show up at a shipping company loading dock in dirty jeans and a tank top. He'd loiter for an hour, until he was a fixture on the landscape, then wander into the factory and befriend the minimum-wage guys packing cardboard cartons. He brought them smokes, beef jerky, and beer, and when the conversation lightened, he'd pull out his various pastel-colored tapes, especially the ones with the candy apple red lightning bolts repeating every few inches. He waited a day, shaved, wore a three-piece suit, and made an appointment with the shipping supervisor to apologize for his slovenly brother, Knute.

Bernie related the convoluted tale of Knute's birth and the tragedy of his affliction—water on the brain. Bernie would dip his head and mumble that he had been entrusted with Knute's welfare after their parents had died, coincidently, right near there. There followed tap dancing, the step choreographed by the location of the warehouse. If it was close to the East River, the Hudson, or the Battery, they perished in a boating accident. If it was in the Bronx, the deaths were a result of a cab accident or armed robbery on Bruckner Boulevard. The one thing Knute did know, though, was packaging, and that the factory was using inferior, yet over-priced, material.

Bernie proffered his wares, demonstrating the various grades of tape, color-coded to reflect strength. If most of the employees on the dock were black, that was the color of the strongest, and the most expensive, tape. If the workers were Irish, it was green. The Italians loved the multi-hued, green-white-red rolls.

Bernie chuckled, mostly to Dr. Flowers, "The tape's all the same—except for color and price." He also laughed when he described his retired parents, who happily lived in Florida and bragged about their only child having become a business tycoon in New York.

Dr. Flowers was speechless. This was not the stuff of success in Marian, Alabama. Though J.W. had prepared Harlan Flowers for the East Coast, the surgeon's jaw hung as if he had agreed to allow a Martian into surgery.

There had been some changes, however, in Bernie's world-view, and at the roast chicken dinner hosted by the Flowers that night, not only did Bernie confine his consumption to merely three-quarters of a bird, but he graciously presented his hosts with several rolls of tape. Stella was drawn to the chartreuse with the red lightning bolts; Harlan had no preference.

On the morning after Bobbie Jo and Bernie left the colony for Tokyo, Harlan Flowers looked up from the gall bladder he was teasing out of an old man's abdomen. With slightly befuddled eyes peering above his mask, he mused quietly, "Wasn't that was somethin', Hoss?"

⊷⊷ ⊶⊶

The graph of study hours filled bit by bit. The only days not marked with little red dots were Christmas and J.W.'s thirty-second birthday. On New Year's Eve, he turned the last page of the fourth spiral notebook, shaken out of his stupor by the click of the date window on his windup watch. He woke Krista, wished her a Happy New Year, kissed Khai in her sleep, and, settling for only four hours at the books that night, added a dot to the graph.

While Piotr Sówka and J.W. met twice a week as the MCATs approached, Dr. Flowers and the shipping offices saw less of J.W. He'd phone DeStahl with an item to be purchased, and they would arrange for it to be manufactured, delivered to the colony, and transshipped to Viet Nam. All J.W. saw of the order was the bill of lading and his cancelled check. There was no time to do anything other than sit ensconced in his study cell, nine and ten hours a day.

Two weeks before the MCATs, J.W. sweat in the little room, poring over, memorizing, rewriting, and fretting that there were still concepts he hadn't yet, nor would likely ever, fathom. By mid-afternoon, the growing heat of Hong Kong's early summer overwhelmed the air-conditioner. The cranking noises became earsplitting, and the scent of cooking mildew filled the house. Before he could unplug it, the off-on switch long since rotted out, acid electric smoke began gushing from the vents and the melting wall socket. There came an internal explosion, loud hissing, and a final burp of tepid, soaked air.

As he struggled to ram the smoldering corpse out the window, away from the house, his eyes caught an attractive, elegantly-dressed, ring-and-necklace-bedecked Chinese woman carrying parcels down Paris Road. He watched, a bit lasciviously, as the figurine swayed regally along the sidewalk. She noticed him watching through the hole in the house, and turned away, though subtly stretched her neck back, pooching her breasts forward. He smiled gently, eyes locked on the woman until a dark figure appeared from the ether to collide with the lithe form. She swirled abruptly then cried out in a piercing shriek as a bedraggled Chinese man threw his arms over her. Through the jumble of the man's filthy burlap clothing, J.W. caught the glint of an eight-inch dagger jabbing against the woman's neck. When she threw herself to the ground, the man straddled her, the dagger held high above his head, aimed at her heart. She jammed her purse at him, screaming "Take it, take it."

Instead, he kicked it away violently and yanked the jeweled necklaces from her throat. When they didn't come loose, he jabbed the knife under them and hacked madly until he sawed through the pure Asian gold. He snatched at the bracelets, but they were too tight, and he couldn't get the blade under them. He aimed his knife toward her wrist, but J.W. was, by now, through the window, howling madly. The blighter sprang to his feet and ran off, barefooted, along Paris Road toward the hospital.

J.W. stood over the woman and took her arm to help her up. "Don't touch me. You just get my jewelry back."

J.W. sprinted onto Waterloo Road, past the Flowers', head swinging wildly left and right, until he sighted the exhausted man turning into Mission Hospital's labyrinthine grounds. J.W. caught him at the great cement wall surrounding the parking lot. The felon whirled and pointed his knife menacingly at J.W.'s throat. J.W. threatened him with a deep feral growl, the one he had used to bully football opponents a decade before. He'd even overheard one receiver tell his teammates, "That's some kinda gotdamn animal? Stay the fuck away from him." And so, the roar had become his staple when frightened.

The Chinese man stood erect, his face frozen, the only movement a rapid twitching of the skin patched over a missing eye. He threw his knife across the parking lot, dropped submissively to the ground, and wept.

Within seconds of his surrender, orderlies, neighbors, and passers-by converged. A white-uniformed hospital worker rammed his way to the center and kicked viciously at the downed mugger's face. J.W. shoved him away and bellowed, "Hey, asshole, the man's down. Leave him alone!"

But the vigilante righted himself and flew back screaming, "Mother fucker," at J.W. in Cantonese, Mandarin, and finally English. As the man's dirty white bucks became misted with fresh blood, his rage only deepened, and J.W. tackled the man, driving him to the pavement.

J.W. looked down. "Orderly Wong?" he shouted. "You don't even know what the hell's going on, and you assault the bastard? Now it's your butt in the fire! Wait 'till the cops get here." J.W. turned away but hesitated long enough to call over his shoulder, "And I'm going to make sure your ass fries for dumping Mrs. Shou's water down the pneumo tube."

J.W. turned back to witness the corpus of onlookers shoving madly inward to get in a swipe or two on the quaking perpetrator. A nurse flew out of the hospital with three rolls of packing tape, and the assailant's mouth, hands, and feet were bound harshly, scarlet lightning bolts repeating on a background of chartreuse.

The arrival of the Hong Kong constabulary brought a renewed attack on the trussed prey, the assailants looking up into the cops' eyes with submissive pride. The police stood by admiring the tape for a moment but quickly moved into the swell, flinging people out of the way. They shoved the tethered man into the back of their Land Rover and were about to leave when J.W. demanded they arrest Orderly Wong. The officers consulted with the mob and decided to take J.W. to headquarters to sort out if he was a hero or an accomplice after the fact for having interfered with the first phase in the delivery of justice.

At the grubby police station, the thief was led into a little green room with sweaty walls. J.W. was led into another interrogation cell and cross-examined. J.W. was warned not to leave the Colony for the next two months, and he was handed a document, in Chinese, declaring him a material witness in a felony. "You part of crime now."

Three days later, a police Land Rover banged into the curb outside the Weathersbys' flat. Four officers exited. The only policeman with red-tabbed shoulder epaulettes, Hong Kong's official indicator of English language ability, was the driver. He stayed with the vehicle. J.W. was served a smudged carbon copy of a subpoena, in Chinese. He was to appear before a magistrate in eleven days, on the very Saturday of the MCATs. The police shrugged in unison when J.W. asked, in broken Cantonese, who he had to see to have the date changed.

Each official to whom J.W. made the pilgrimage shook his head in mock sorrow. "I sorry Mistah Wehdabay, you see no thing to be done."

Dr. Flowers and Professor Sówka fared no better.

The Weathersbys' barrister suggested J.W. was going about it unsuitably. He advised both Krista and J.W. make an appointment to see Mr. Wong, the Minister of Matrimony, and explain that they expected to be married the day of the hearing. J.W. was to whisper that Krista was pregnant, her cue to stroke her belly soothingly. When the official averted his eyes, J.W. was to finish the conversation with an imploring, "We have to, you know."

Three days before the MCATs, another gaggle of police appeared at the Weathersbys' flat. This time the paper was mottled so badly, J.W. was not sure it was written in Chinese. The police explained that his appearance before the magistrate had been canceled altogether. They mimed that the perpetrator had hung himself.

The MCATs were administered at only one location in South East Asia, the University of Hong Kong, and only once that year. The day before the test, J.W. rode the 7-A to the Star Ferry, across to Hong Kong Island, and up Pokfulam Road to Mid-Levels to visit the exam lecture hall. He was struck by the size of the cavern, but more so by the sheer numbers of humanity wedged into seats and aisles soaking up the wisdom of physics. Every scholar was right-handed, each furiously taking notes in identical notebooks. Every head sported jet-black hair, identical length and style for the men, identical length and style for the women. J.W. thought of an American lecture hall, with its myriad body shapes and sizes, and limitless skin shades and hair color. He wondered if he would find a seat on the day of the big exam, and if any of the other test-takers would be Western.

The morning of the MCATs, however, the hall was empty, save for three students nervously waiting at the door. The other two applicants were serious Chinese men in their early twenties, surprisingly old for so bold a venture as seeking admission to an American medical school. J.W. had to assume they'd prepared unfalteringly for that moment, that every student over the globe sitting for the MCATs that day had been as driven as he.

Ten Chinese examiners, University staff and professors, were stationed at points evenly spread over the room. As the three scholars entered the hall, the chief proctor announced that regulations required examinees be spread out as far as possible. J.W. was directed to front row center, ideal for a concert, perhaps, but he was now in the immediate line of sight of, and only inches from, the three monitors assigned to patrol the lectern area. J.W. protested that he had a need for a little personal space, but the chief proctor informed him haughtily that they had had trouble with foreign students cheating in the past. The other two scholars were placed in the very top row, their seats at opposite corners of the hall.

J.W. had saved a Mars Bar and a Snickers for almost a year, to get him through the day-long ordeal. Everyone did that in the States. The chief proctor, who now came close enough for J.W. to read her name tag, Mrs. Wong, stood above him and thrust a Chinese copy of the regulations in his face. She jabbed a fingernail at the booklet so rapidly, J.W. muttered, "You hear a woodpecker in here?"

Mrs. Wong tsooked and wrote a translation for J.W. "Test Of medical college Admission, student all no allow have something at table. Have pencil Number 2 and test ok. Other all not have." When J.W.'s eyes glanced up, the candy was snatched from his desk.

J.W. protested sarcastically, "I want to speak to my embassy."

The hue of the chief examiner's face neared the red of the lightning bolts on Bernie's tape. She was trembling as she went into deep consultation with her colleagues, made several hushed phone calls, marched back to his seat, and thrust the candy bars an inch from his nose. "You show me."

After J.W. opened both wrappers, making somewhat of a production of breaking the bars into gooey pieces, bits of chocolate shooting about, she turned around and took her seat at the desk. J.W. smiled and made smacking noises with his lips as he sucked strings of caramel off his fingers.

When her whistle sounded, J.W. took a deep breath and plunged into the candy bar. The initial questions were simple, but the fifth and sixth were on subjects about which J.W. had forgotten to lug books to Hong Kong—quadratic equations and

Cartesian coordinates. A wave of panic blinded him, and he could not seem to advance beyond those questions. He blackened one answer on the sheet, erased it, put down another, erased it, then snarled at Mrs. Wong, the last refuge as his thoughts became mired in science neutral. J.W.'s brainwaves degenerated into a closed loop of self-chastisement for his weakness at one pole, and accepting that medicine simply wasn't in the cards at the other. For seven precious, unrecoverable minutes, J.W. sat frozen in disbelief that it all had come down to blasting away a year's work in less than an hour.

He hyperventilated himself into oblivion, resurfacing only as the chief examiner announced there were three minutes remaining in the first section. The whistle blew. J.W. felt great happiness and terrible, gnawing pain all at once. As fast as his pencil could fly, he finished the answer sheet, marking, "B, C, B, C, B, C, B, C," for almost twenty questions—as much chance voting for those two responses as any. He smiled that he had been quite clever, not having had to move his pencil as far as if he had chosen A and D.

Five minutes later, when the chemistry section whistle sounded, J.W. ignored his candy, chewing instead on his pencil, commanding himself to breathe slowly as he concentrated on the image of his spiral notebooks, culling to life the tiny writing on the pages. The fog lifted at question four, and he was suddenly able to focus on the formulas and equations. He grinned at the proctor and tackled the problems, flipping mentally through the pages of his year's work. The rest of the day passed in a dream, and J.W. left the hall depleted.

CHAPTER NINE

The weeks that followed were the first J.W. had spent in nearly two years without the weight of the books hanging over his head, and he wasn't sure what to do with the time. He and Krista went to restaurants and kung fu movies, rode the Star Ferry until they puked during a typhoon, and took a trip to Laos, just for fun. They didn't stay long, not wanting to be away from Hong Kong when the call came—the results of the MCATs.

J.W.'s mother phoned several times from New York to ask if he had heard, but each time, he reminded her impatiently that he had used her home address for the results. She would know before he would know, so why was she calling and getting him excited? "Hey, mom, you gotta phone me immediately when the envelope comes. I don't care what time it is. Just call."

At the six-week mark, the point by which the testing agency had guaranteed the scores would be disseminated, there was still no word. His mother phoned the testing center in the Midwest and demanded to know what was taking so long. With threats of litigation, she extracted from the secretary that a foreign test was missing, and that until it was determined if foul play had been committed, none of the results from exams taken outside the U.S. would be released.

"Well, which country was involved?" his mother snapped.

"Can't tell you that, but it was in Asia, and not India."

"That doesn't leave a lot to the imagination, madam. That means my son's test is missing!"

A Snickers Bar had scuttled J.W.'s dream. He took a cab to the University of Hong Kong and petitioned for a conference with the chancellor. The latter was appalled, and promised to get back to J.W. in short order, though he assured that the whole notion of a dishonest official was preposterous, simply impossible.

Friday at midnight, after another week had slipped by without word, the phone rang. It was either Dr. Flowers announcing the arrival of the latest of the procrastinating hemorrhoid sufferers of the Colony, or it was the chancellor of the University of Hong Kong.

"No, Mom, haven't heard anything yet. You?"

J.W. could smell the scent of burning phone lines between her home and the testing agency.

At midnight on Saturday, the phone rang again. J.W. flew out of bed. "The answer, the answer," he called out, as his hand trembled lifting the receiver. A stranger's voice asked to speak to Mr. Weathersby. It was surely the testing center. "Yes, sir, how may I help you?"

"J.W., I'm Milt Aster, a friend of your parents. We met them on a trip. They said you lived in Hong Kong. We just got in. We're at the airport. They said you'd love to show us around the city. Do you have a car?"

"Show you around the city? Look, it's midnight."

"Sorry, it's noon for us. Yeah, well, we have no way to get around, and your mom said..." J.W. covered the phone, calling out to calm Khai, who had been startled by the phone and was screaming in a night terror.

Krista called from the bedroom, "What the hell's going on out there?"

J.W. tried to answer, but Khai howled louder. The neighbor's dog began to wail; lights snapped on all over Kowloon Tong. More of the mangy local hounds joined the cacophony, and Khai screamed more thunderously. Krista jumped out of bed. J.W. slammed the phone onto the receiver. It rang again.

"What the hell do you want, asshole?"

"This is your mother."

"Oh. Hi, Mom. Do you know a Milt Aster?"

"I hope he didn't bother you. That jerk. What did he squeeze out of you? You want to know about him? Let me tell you about the time..."

"Mom, why are you calling?"

"I have a telegram for you. Do you want me to open it?"

"Read it. Read it." He heard the envelope tearing. "Medical College Admission Test. Which section do you want to hear first?"

"Just read it!"

"Science Portion: 785. Is that good?"

When J.W. was silent for several seconds, she asked again, "Is that good?"

"It's about as high as you can get. It's unbelievable. Say it one more time."

Harlan and Piotr hailed him heartily, though asked if they could talk about it in the morning.

CHAPTER TEN

J.W.'s special delivery note to Dr. McNamara at Marimore University was answered by another administrator, a form letter advising that while they were happy J.W. was interested in Marimore Medical School, all communications were to be directed to the admissions department, not the dean. There was a small, handwritten sentence from the acting director of admissions, advising that Dr. McNamara was no longer the dean. He had stepped down for personal reasons.

J.W. phoned Marimore. The operator in Hong Kong demanded so much information before completing the call, the admissions office was closed for the weekend when the phone rang. Early Tuesday morning Hong Kong time, J.W. tried again. It was the same overseas operator.

"The city Pennisswalia in what state?" the operator demanded.

"No, sir, Pennisswalia is the state. And it's P-e-n-n-s-y-l-v-a-n-i-a. Philadelphia is the city I'm trying to call. I told you that last week!"

"I tell you now, Pennisswalia is city. You tell me state, or I no make connection."

"Look here, what is your name?"

"Wong."

"Listen, you little twit, I am the bloody Governor of this colony. You connect me to Philadelphia, or I'll have your slim ass condemned to prison as an enemy of the state and sent to China!"

"Dean McNamara," the receptionist intoned seriously a microsecond later, "died last night of cancer."

J.W. was instantly furious with McNamara, with Krista, with the gods, and even Khai. But later that night, after a couple of San Miguel beers, he thought back to the hours Dr. McNamara had invested in him. The Dean's words a year-and-a-half before had endowed J.W. with a powerful tool, one that would give currency to his plea anywhere in the world.

And who the hell was he to place his stupid admission to medical school above the life of a decent man, a man who gone the extra mile to give a student with feeble prerequisites two hours of his time, who had given J.W. hope, when, surely the man had some idea he was already seriously ill. For a few days, he did nothing but wonder just who he had become. It was not, he believed, what was supposed to be inside a doctor.

The Weathersbys spent much of the remaining CWR money over the phone as they packed to leave the Colony. The lion's share went toward antibiotics for children bombed out of their homes in Hanoi. The phone rang day and night with questions from the pharmaceutical companies, the banks, and DeStahl Shipping. One call was from Robert Ball, at DeStahl's Kowloon office. "I have some troubling news. The final shipment of penicillin from the Philippines went down on a ship that sank during a monsoon."

J.W. paused. "I didn't hear about that. Okay, so what do we do?"

"Well, for right now, we'll get with our supplier in Singapore. We'll need a cashier's check. And we'll need to move quickly. We only have one ship going to Viet Nam for the next five months. The money has to be here by tomorrow."

"What about the insurance? I just can't be writing checks for the same goods twice."

"Oh, that will come when it does. We can work directly with your home office when it arrives. But please understand, that often takes years and years. It is the nature of the insurance industry."

J.W. was quiet. He considered trying to put a call into CWR, but it was the middle of the night there. "Well, I'll just make the executive decision and guess at how much of the million we have left. I'm pretty sure there's enough. Okay, how do I get the money to you?"

Ball gasped, "A million? Is that US dollars or Hong Kong?"

"US. It was in the papers. *Your* Hong Kong office became aware of it and released it to the South China Morning Post."

"How does CWR raise that much money? Amazing. You must be very respected. I mean one person entrusted with so much."

J.W. shared CWR's vision and their yearly budget. He answered a dozen questions about their projects, and by the time the conversation drew to a close, Ball had drawn from J.W. a compilation of CWR's philanthropic work in the Third World, and J.W.'s history as a soldier.

Ball spoke warmly. "You'll be in medical school in no time. And it sounds as if you're going to be a hell of a physician. Look, why don't we do lunch tomorrow. You can pass the cashier's check, and we'll continue this fascinating conversation. Come up first and see my office in Kowloon. The most expensive floor space on Earth.

J.W. wore a white shirt and tie, both of which were drenched with malodorous sweat when he finally stopped searching and telephoned DeStahl's main office on the Hong Kong side. They denied vehemently the existence of an office in Kowloon, or that there was a Mr. Ball in their employ.

Marc Banter called that evening from Philadelphia, advising that the State Department was suddenly aware of their plans, and that the Weathersbys, along with CWR, were to be charged with violating the, "...Trading with the Enemy Act for providing unlicensed goods to Viet Nam."

"Let me be direct," Banter sighed. You're in deep Kim Chee. They're threatening a bunch of years of federal prison time and tens of thousands of dollars in fines. But don't worry. CWR'll, pay the fines."

"And how 'bout you doin' the time?" J.W. snapped, but Marc Banter complained the connection was fuzzy and hung up.

CWR's director telephoned the next morning and warned, "You might be arrested at immigration when you land in Hawaii on the trip home. We don't think so, and I'm even more involved than you are, and I'm not hiding. But be prepared. We'll have an attorney in Honolulu to meet your plane and represent you, but have your toothbrush in your back pocket, just in case. You know, you three could stay in Hong Kong and wait until things blow over."

"Hey, sir, I've got work to do. I'm goin' to medical school next year. We're coming home."

At midnight, eight hours before their flight home, the phone rang. Krista lifted the receiver, listened in silence, then covered it with her hand.

"Hemorrhoids!" J.W. screamed.

"It's CWR's executive director," she whispered.

The man's voice smiled "The matter of your federal violation apparently went all the way to Dr. Kissinger and, we think, President Ford. We have a man in the State Department. That's what he says. Guess your war record was examined, and our history considered. All of a sudden, we've been granted special shipping licenses, all pre-dated. Our humanitarian aid has been summarily approved after the fact."

J.W. asked, "So how do I account for the six Hong Kong dollars I spent on a new toothbrush?"

CHAPTER ELEVEN

Philadelphia had not changed dramatically. The Paris Inn's walls were a little sootier, and J.W.'s favorite deli, the one in which Khai had attained the rank of persona non grata at age six months, had closed its doors. Perhaps its clientele had stayed home, where they belonged.

The Weathersbys discovered a grand old home only five miles from Eastern State College, the only school that accepted J.W. for the mandatory pre-med courses. The others denied admission on the basis of the late application. J.W. undertoned to Krista, "Shit, I can't even get into a community college."

The third floor of the Victorian was for rent, and though they had to walk through the living room, up the stairs, and past the owners' second floor bedroom, the neighborhood was safe and quiet. The landlords of the drafty, nineteenth century mansion were a young, but vocally unhappy, interreligious couple—he, a Catholic from Southern Ireland, she, a Protestant from Belfast. The Mulligans had an infant daughter and one cooking. House rules were detailed, including instructions on when and how the Weathersby's would situate their garbage on the curb, where they could park, and how much electricity they were allocated to heat their rooms. The landlord's dog, Adolph, a dull-eyed pit bull, greeted the Weathersbys at the door each evening, teeth bared, hackles raised as high as his pointed ears. He howled at night when his masters fought, and so did Khai, which sent the Mulligan's baby into screaming rages.

With the first electric bill, Mr. Mulligan sat them down to reiterate the parameters of their power allowance. "You two's got three electric clocks, goin' twenty-four hours a day."

Mrs. Mulligan added over her shoulder from the kitchen, "Toss 'em out. They're wastin' my money."

Mr. Mulligan barked, "I'm handling this. *Póg mo thóin.*"

"What!?"

"You heard me, kiss my ass."

The Mulligans became involved in one of their more volatile discussions that afternoon. It continued into the evening, a marathon of spiritual stains, the final volley commencing while she was vacuuming the second floor landing at midnight. While they exchanged religious epithets, Adolph yowled, Khai shivered, the windows shook in concert with the baby's paroxysmal shrieking, and the vacuum cleaner whined on and on at the foot of the Weathersby's doorless third floor rooms.

At 3 A.M., J.W. stole down the stairs and approached the still-blowing Hoover. He reached to turn the switch and, almost by instinct, retracted his hand just as Adolph lunged from the Mulligan's bedroom. Mr. Mulligan followed. "Call the fuckin' cops. I caught the bastard. And just for that, the vacuum cleaner stays on."

Krista and J.W. spent the rest of the night packing. At 6 A.M., Krista and Khai stole off to search for a new home; J.W. left at seven to register at Eastern State. When she returned home that evening, Krista collapsed into a tattered lounge chair and began to cry. Khai grabbed her legs and squeezed. Krista lifted the two-year-old into her lap and buried her in her warmth.

"We looked at sixteen apartments. All trash. I will not live like that. And then I come home, and that asshole is strutting around the living room, naked, goose-stepping to military music. I will not live like this."

The Weathersbys disappeared early the next morning, entrusting their earthly belongings to cold storage. They drove back to the Paris Inn to beg for Room 360, drove to see the pediatrician for Khai's fever, bought the antibiotics for her ear infection, brought her back to the doctor for the rash that developed after the first dose, settled on an apartment seven miles from Eastern State, and bought books for J.W.'s pre-med courses. They'd managed to spend more in that one day than they had earned in the last three years. The largest expenditure was for a new brake line on the Buick. It was to replace the one that had ruptured when he jammed his foot on the pedal to avoid Adolph, who chased them as they left the Mulligan's for good. Actually, J.W. aimed at him on the last trip, but Khai protested, and he hit the brakes so violently, the line burst and the car rolled into the Mulligan's weed-choked rose garden.

─═╪ ╪═─

J.W.'s appearance for final registration the next morning was met with a hand-scribbled note on his computer card directing him to the office of the Dean for Undergraduate Affairs. Professor Bakalar was concerned that J.W. was attempting to squeeze two years of pre-med courses into one ten-week semester. "Twenty-eight hard science credits, my friend?" he asked sarcastically, "Three lab courses? You can't do that. Never been done in history."

J.W. answered, "Sir, I'm stuck between a rock and a hard place. I've got no choice. But I can handle anything you can drop on me. I'm a Viet Nam vet, you know."

Dean Bakalar snatched the schedule from J.W.'s hands and signed on the dotted line. "Classes begin tomorrow morning. Good luck, soldier."

As he entered the first lecture hall, he felt a sense of a déjà vu. In the front two rows were black-haired students, identical hair-styles and lengths for the men, identical hairstyles and lengths for the women. "Those are the Asian kids" a student sitting next to J.W. snickered. "That's how you know what your grade's gonna be. Take the number of Oriental kids, divide it by the total number of students, times one hundred, and if that's greater than ten, you're out in the cold, no chance for an A. They work hard, man, every day, all damn day, study, study, and compulsive fuckin' study. I can't do that shit. The only days they take off are like their birthdays and whatever their Christmas is."

The second class—physics—same score card. By the fourth hard science course that day, and with the mental fatigue from counting black-haired heads and dividing by ten, J.W. felt himself slipping back into the gray funk, yet another mountain with no downhill after the climb. But he righted himself in his seat and conjured ways to recapture the pluck that had driven him that far. His situation called for extraordinary measures, an infusion of wisdom.

Bernie and Bobbie Jo had deepened their relationship. Bernie was consumed with peddling his industrial tape, she with those who peddled VD.

"What a great life, eh?" Bernie laughed raucously into the phone, declaring, "It's deliciously simple."

"Deliciously, uh huh."

"Yes. Listen. If this number of yours is greater than ten, Dr. Einstein, take that course at night, when the working kids and factory people take classes. Spreads your day out, gives you some breathing room. And for Christ's sake, don't tell them why you're switching."

J.W. called Dean Bakalar's office early the next morning.

"Be here in an hour, soldier!"

"You were right, sir, should've listened to you. You really know your stuff. But I've already paid for the courses. Maybe I can try a couple of them at night. Would that be okay? Should've listened to you."

Dean Bakalar leaned back in the leather chair, rubbed his chin, then jutted forward to snatch the paper out of J.W.'s hand. He scratched a few official administrative phrases on the bottom alongside his signature and snapped, "Better luck this time, trooper."

The early weeks were easy—the same material J.W. had sweat blood over in Hong Kong. But the books from which he'd garnered his information for the MCATs had been published several years before the discovery of the concepts that were already old hat to the kids who had just come from the basic science courses. J.W. had an inkling of how Harlan Flowers had felt, always behind by a hair's breadth. J.W., though, had no place to hide.

Monday through Saturday at 7 A.M., J.W. was on his beater bicycle, El Buraq, which he'd named after Mohammed's flying white horse, the steed which had the face and breasts of a woman, the tail of peacock, and great wings. The mount flew Mohammed, the great sage, to the far-off al Aqsa Mosque, at the edge of Medina, just as the bicycle would lift J.W. to the great temple of medicine. He bounced down the cobblestones toward Eastern State, the first few miles weaving along colonial streets and past the patrician homes of Philadelphia's glorious past.

Most of those mansions had recently been purchased by Yuppies taking advantage of the rock-bottom prices to which real estate had tumbled during the energy crisis of the 1970s. The new owners, all young professionals, however, had forgotten to factor in the cost of heating the drafty, high-ceilinged, monstrously large homes, the very reason they had been relegated to the chopping block by the old wealth of Philadelphia. "For Sale" signs dotted every other lawn.

The next leg of the journey was the one that most riveted his attention. At the corner of Germantown Avenue and North Broad, he turned left to pedal south. That was the beginning of the miles of burned out, turn-of-the-century brownstones. Winos littered the corners, and curls of green glass from their shattered bottles often caught in the worn tread of his tires. Angry kids shook their fists at him—others were more direct and threw rocks. J.W. changed his route daily, especially on the nights he finished class at ten or eleven. On the trip home, screams often reverberated from the gutted buildings, and once, a man staggered out a doorless portal, a dagger sticking from his shoulder. J.W. stopped El Buraq to help, but the man's girlfriend, actually his ex-girlfriend, sprinted out of the same building wielding another blade.

The victim grunted painfully, "Run like hell, man. Bitch gonna stick yo ass. Muh fuckah be crazy."

At first, the woman howled at her former beau, and J.W. pushed El Buraq slowly into the darkness. But the woman caught J.W. out of the corner of her eye and sprinted toward him, closing the gap so quickly, he could not stop to mount El Buraq. When she was a dozen yards away, he wheeled around, bared his teeth, and began his hissing and spitting routine. He lifted El Buraq above his head, belching a deep guttural growl.

The woman stopped short. She glared at him before screeching, "You some kinda gotdamn animal, muh fucka?" J.W.

smiled—his act had worked once again, but the woman spat, "I'm gonna cut yo grinnin' muh fuckin' ass, muh fuckah."

He issued one more snarl, fired a hocker at her feet, swiped at her with the bike, and sprinted for Germantown Avenue. The woman followed, slashing at him until she nicked the back tire. There was a pop, a hiss, and the slap of feet beating the crumbled cement pavement as J.W. pushed the bicycle at a dead sprint for a mile. Safe on Germantown Avenue, J.W. called the police from a coin box.

"Yeah, we'll send a unit out."

"When?" J.W. demanded.

"Where'd you say that was again?"

"I already told you. Hey, you listen. I'm a goddamn taxpayer..." but the phone clicked and the dispatcher was gone before J.W. could finish his thought.

J.W.'s legs toughened from the months of biking all the way down Germantown Avenue, right on North Broad, through City Center, past City Hall, the right turn onto Market, past the Paris Inn, across the Schuylkill River, into West Philly, up Baltimore Avenue, and onto Eastern State's campus.

But his fatigue also grew with the never-ending cycle of exams and fights with Krista over his absence. By Thanksgiving, J.W. had devised a scheme of missing classes, a rotating schedule of skips, synchronized with the almost-daily quizzes and tests.

During the rare hours at home, Khai sat by him as he studied. She played with plastic models of atoms, molecules, and bones; she drew stick figures of the things on her mind, often taking great delight in presenting them to J.W. before the sun rose. As the pressure of grades deepened, however, Khai wouldn't let go of his legs, spending hours under his desk squeezing. Her drawings also became more urgent, often thrust in front of J.W.'s face while he tried to study.

Perhaps he was sweating over a simple physics or a math problem the night she repeatedly shoved J.W.'s book aside. "Khai, daddy's trying to study, damnit!" Krista stood at the door of the study closet watching silently. Khai showed him the drawing again. J.W. grabbed it out of her hands. It was a stick figure superimposed over the form of an animal.

Khai pointed to the paper and cried, "Daddy and Adooofff, bad doggie. Adooofff bite Daddy. Khai hit bad doggie Adooofff."

J.W. eyes reddened. He promised Krista and Khai it would only be a few more weeks, and the semester would be done. "When I'm a doctor, we're not gonna worry about money or that kinda crap anymore. It'll all be worth it. You'll see."

Krista put her arms around him for a moment, but a moment later, she was gone.

By December, the sleety, East Coast streets made the trip in and out of Center City worse than the ride through the crumbling neighborhoods. The cobblestones and potholes had taken their toll on his wheels; spokes snapped daily; nubbins of what was left of the sharp metal freely punctured his tires. After chem lab, anatomy lab, or physics lab, J.W. charged down Baltimore Avenue to the bicycle shop for parts. He'd park under an overhang, run to Mr. Papadimetriou's snack truck to warm his hands with a cup of coffee and a hot pretzel, then dash back to fix his tires. J.W. was spending as much time repairing El Buraq as he invested in his studies.

As J.W. bit down onto the crisp and doughy pretzel that dark, snowy noon, the flash of two familiar wheels whizzing by in the hands of a little kid caught his attention. The child moved with lightning speed, but his accomplice, an eight-year-old, was slower, and J.W. caught up with him on Baltimore and 46th. J.W. bullied him into spilling the ringleader's name, the one who had flashed by carrying El Buraq's wheels.

"It was Hardy Davis," the kid blubbered. J.W. hissed so loudly, the kid even gave him Hardy's phone number.

J.W. called that evening. "What? That boy's done found da wrench again? Wait a minute," his mother snapped as she dropped the receiver onto the table. She confirmed that the wrench was missing from its hiding place. "He ain't here. He playin' in da street," she announced disgustedly, but before she hissed another word, J.W. heard a loud cracking sound over the wire, and Hardy's mother cried into the phone, "Oh, my God! Not again."

The phone dropped a second time. The crack was followed by a volley of pistol shots that carried over the phone. "Lord have mercy," J.W. heard her cry from across the room, then the slam of a door.

The next day, J.W. had to take the bus into school. He called the police precinct for West Philly, but the desk sergeant consulted the log for the previous evening and declared, "Nothin' out of the ordinary on the night blotter."

On the first day of the semester, the anatomy lab instructor declared, with a wry smile, that the course would be a challenge, for only the gifted would pass his final exam, the naming of one-hundred internal parts of the cat, and not the easy ones like the substantia nigra and Ranvier's Nodes. Each of the thirty students was issued a cat cadaver, and every five days they investigated a new organ system. J.W.'s specimen was a tabby, which he named "Mao IV."

Maos I through III had been of Asian descent, rescued from various neighborhoods ranging from Kowloon City, next to the airport in Hong Kong, to Wan Chai, the Susie Wong District on

Hong Kong Island. Maos I and II meowed weakly at the bottom of rusted trash bins. They lay next to the remains of their deceased littermates. The two original Maos lasted only a few hours. Mao III screeched heartily when J.W. reached into the sewer to push the rotting vegetables and bones aside. He lifted the kicking, nipping waif by the scruff of its neck. The aggression went on for a day or two, but by the end of the week, he just lay by Khai's crib, breathing heavily and coughing. The Weathersbys spent most of their monthly twenty-five-dollar salary on medical bills at the only vet in Hong Kong, a Dr. Wong. Mao III died two weeks later of cat leukemia, leaving Krista and J.W. heavily in debt, and Khai believing that pets were, at best, evanescent creatures, whose life spans were measured in hours, like that of a fruit fly, but could be extended to fourteen days if a family's entire yearly salary was spent on health care.

Mao IV had been supplied to Eastern State College by a Mexican firm which wholesaled cat and dog cadavers to dissection labs. After dispatching the animal, the technicians south of the border drained the blood, then infused the vessels with latex—blue for veins, red into the arteries. The bodies were immersed in formaldehyde, shipped to the U.S. in clear plastic bags, and issued to students. J.W. picked through the pile, perusing each cadaver, until the instructor snapped at him to take the top specimen and go to his desk. As J.W. opened the bag, he was overcome immediately by the acrid, fetid waft of formaldehyde-pickled flesh. His eyes watered, and despite the mask of chemical stench, he could still smell death. He tightened, as if he had been thrown back into Viet Nam, and left for the men's room to splash cold water on his face.

When he came back to class, the rest of the students were following orders, prying open the mouths to scour out hardened wads of Kibbles and Bits. J.W. pulled Mao's jaws apart. The teeth were yellow and cracked. The animal's coat was patchy and covered with sores and scars.

Despite El Buraq's new wheels, as the snow deepened, J.W. began taking the bus more often, hauling the cat in a black garbage bag. He sat at the rear of the SEPTA bus, to protect his back, and to hide the reeking scent of formaldehyde. The other passengers were generally too stoned, or babbling too incoherently to themselves, to notice. One very snowy morning, as they neared Eastern State, J.W. picked his way through the plastic sacks cluttering the aisle. His foot caught the bag sitting at the feet of an old woman. She gasped, and J.W. expected a tongue lashing, but there were no words, just indignant quacking, like a duck being plucked alive. Suddenly, she locked her bloodshot eyes on the bag J.W. was toting over his shoulder. She pointed to it heatedly and then to herself.

"No, ma'am, I believe this is *my* bag, ma'am," J.W. nodded politely.

But the woman's ruddy, worn face took on a violet hue, and her squawking degenerated into a honking so vociferous, one of her fellow travelers grunted, "You swallow a fuckin' castrated goose or somethin'?"

The old lady pawed at J.W.'s bag, and he pulled back so hard, the plastic tore. There was a gush of noxious broth, followed by the body of the eviscerated feline pooling on the floor. It was as if they were witnessing the miracle of a birth on a city bus. The carcass slid two rows forward as the driver slammed on the brakes. He bristled down the aisle glaring at J.W., who was on a knee gathering up the body and as much formaldehyde he could slosh into cupped hands. The little name tags he had spent dozens of hours tying to Mao's countless organs and vessels were now a tangle of white thread reminiscent of the innards of Bernie's dust machine.

J.W. fled through the rear emergency exit. He sprinted down Baltimore Avenue, hooked a hard right, slipped, fell, crawled to his feet, and ducked into Eastern State's gate.

Later that week, Dean Bakalar paid a rare official visit to the anatomy lab. He asked, with wrinkled nose and red eyes, if any of the students were taking their cats off campus. No one raised a hand. He held up an article in the Philadelphia Enquirer about a riot on a bus when a madman, a pervert who tortured innocent animals, threw his latest victim at SEPTA passengers, bolted from the vehicle, and melted into Eastern State's Baltimore Avenue environs.

The dean wagged his finger. "Expulsion doesn't look good on medical school admission forms. Do I make himself clear?"

The final exam in anatomy was as advertised. The ten best dissections were tapped for the test. Mao was the first chosen. The only points J.W. lost on the dissection portion of the final were for the tiny white threads on the cat's organs. The lab was divided into ten stations—one cat under each numbered flag. Into each specimen were poked ten visceral toothpicks, glued to which were tiny, numbered, triangular flags. The answer sheet ran from one to one hundred. The students were allotted two hours.

Halfway through, J.W. went back to the cat with the flag numbered 63, to recheck some obscure nucleus in the brain. But flag number 63 was now poking out of the gall bladder. J.W. was sure it had not been in the gall bladder on his first go 'round, for he knew gall bladders. How many had he and Dr. Flowers extracted from the prehistoric citizens of Hong Kong. Fifty? Seventy-five? Even Khai knew the gall bladder. Why would J.W. have questioned that organ? He checked a few more of his answers on that cat. All were wrong.

J.W. appealed to the instructor. Someone, the little man agreed, had surreptitiously moved the flags, motivated by competition for grades and a place in medical school. The instructor called the professor of anatomy, who called the dean. Another threat of expulsion was proffered, and an oral exam summarily conducted. The poker-faced instructor, over whose shoulder

Dean Bakalar hovered during the three-hour oral final, refused J.W.'s request for some indication of how he had done.

In chemistry lab, the final exam was based on the use of known reagents to discover an unknown chemical. When the first student started the discovery process, he added a few drops from a bottle labeled Distilled Water. The mixture spit back, burning his face. The dean arrived and did a few tests, determining the "WATER" had been tainted with acid. The students were ordered to retake the test on the day before Christmas.

Marks were to be posted outside each classroom at the end of the year, but J.W. appealed to the dean for mercy, as he had to know earlier than that, moaning that he was already late in getting his pre-med grades into the medical schools.

"Yeah, you're late. By about eleven years, soldier."

During Christmas break, J.W. rode out to Eastern State several times searching for grades. Each time he went, he felt that same sour, gripping feeling deep in his stomach he'd suffered while shoving and pushing in Saigon to see the just-posted list of troops manifested on the next flight home out of the war.

When the grades were eventually published, at the close of business on New Year's Eve, J.W. had to kick through the snow between eight different buildings to gather his marks. The last three buildings were locked, and he had to beat on the door until a maintenance man let him in. With each list, his gut tightened a bit stiffer. Six A's, then seven. He saved anatomy for last, but none of the maintenance men answered his pounding. The campus patrol desk sergeant grunted and pulled a ring of keys off a rack. He walked slowly toward the anatomy building, grumbling that he hated the snow and hated the stink of science labs.

The eighth A was inscribed on a list pasted to the glass of the back door of the anatomy lab. J.W. peered inside. Mao's tabby tail poked from the middle of a pile of gray meat. The sergeant would not let him into the room to say good-bye.

J.W. stood outside the classroom, waiting quietly for something grand to happen, for a letter of congratulations to materialize from the heavens, for the prize offered to those who did in life what they had been told to do. But the procession of medical school deans did not coalesce from the ether; there were no somber men in a queue presenting offers of admission to paradise. There was only the huffing of the campus patrol sergeant, who finally snapped, "Say, buddy, found what you're looking for? I got a New Year's party to go to."

J.W. pedaled the seven frozen miles home on El Buraq. The snow packed on the cobblestones eased his ride and muffled his string of whoops. Only the closest passers-by looked up from their private worlds, though not one invested more than a second or two on the thirty-three-year-old man skidding along on the beaten Schwinn. A few of the kids, though, stared at the wheels.

J.W. stopped at the A&P for a dozen roses, and at the LCB store for a bottle of champagne. Krista was sitting by the window reading *Dr. Zhivago*, not very much farther than she had been when he left hours before. Khai was asleep next to her, the crib almost touching her chair.

"Congratulations," she offered quietly, even before J.W. kissed her. She remained seated and smiled. J.W. presented the roses and the bottle of champagne. "Now or later?"

She looked back at Khai. "Thank you. They're beautiful. Maybe later."

CHAPTER TWELVE

In early January, J.W. traveled to six medical schools for formal interviews. He was armed with eight A's, high MCATs, completed pre-med requirements, and a year as a surgical assistant. Before each interview, Khai inspected his pants to ensure he had remembered his belt.

Most of the interviewers scanned his file hastily—several advised he do more. "Register for another semester of hard sciences. Show us you can handle a medical education. It's not a cakewalk like college, you know. You need to be able to do more than dissect a cat."

J.W. listened politely, but inside he cringed at the thought of yet another headlong drive to an uncertain finish. He was so close, closer than any of the other people seeking admission, he was sure, but several deans regaled him with tales of scores of students with records stronger than his, kids with a full forty-year career ahead of them. There were no sure bets in this derby, he was warned over and over.

J.W. asked himself in bed each night as he tried to sleep, and in the hours long before dawn when he couldn't fall back to sleep, if there was a limit, when a goal deteriorated into an obsession. Perhaps it already had, but for J.W. there was no yardstick. He assumed they all knew how hard he had driven himself, but one early morning he realized no one knew, or gave a damn, about the endless days and nights he'd logged in pursuit of his dream. It was in his heart, but nowhere else. He thought of the children whose parents and brothers and sisters had been slaughtered in the Holocaust. Had anyone asked them how hard they had tried to go on living? Had anyone cared? It was in their hearts and nowhere else, and there it died.

At dawn, he crept to the phone. Bernie produced several remedies with lightning speed, offering them freely and smoothly. J.W. wondered from what distant planet this man had descended. A day later, J.W. registered at Eastern State for the next semester. He signed up for physical chemistry, quantum physics, thermodynamics, and differential equations. Dean Bakalar stared at the application. J.W. flashed his first semester grades. Bakalar looked up and mumbled, "I've already seen them."

He signed the card without a military remark. J.W. wrote immediately to the six interviewers with whom he had met, disclosing his plans for a daring semester. Then he sat back and waited.

Over the next four weeks, J.W. received acceptances from all six schools. He went back to Dean Bakalar and told him he had decided to take a break—to mend his family. The man nodded. "It's about time. I'll arrange for your tuition to be returned."

PART III

CHAPTER THIRTEEN

The first day at Boston's Brookline Union College of Medicine was peppered with welcoming speeches by ancient men who extolled the art of medicine. The fresh faces in the auditorium were warned of traps whose jaws lay wide open to ensnare unsuspecting or weak doctors: seduction by technology, seduction by money, and seduction by love-hungry patients.

They were also reassured that the major hurdles had been vaulted, and that the next four years, though challenging, were not crafted to weed them out. That process was over, for the investment made in them by the College, by the government, and by their teachers was to be so great, "…if a single one of you tries to quit, the effort we'll invest to change your mind will be greater than the effort you put in to get here in the first place.

"Exams will be graded on the pass/fail system, with a cream category of 'honors' for those of you so inclined. Some of you will take courses over the summer and Christmas holidays and graduate a year ahead of your contemporaries.

"By the fourth year of medical school, young doctors," the dean smiled warmly, "quitting is virtually unheard of."

To J.W.'s ears, these were echoes as foreign as Arabic. At Sterling College's freshman orientation, he had been told to, "Look to your left, now look to your right. In four years, one of the three of you will be gone." At the U.S. Army Ranger School, "...only one out of two of you will be here at the end." And when he was applying to medical school, the odds dropped to one out of three hundred applicants over thirty-years-old. To J.W., hearing the directors of a professional training program embrace the notion of success was incomprehensible.

If he could have picked any place to be on Earth, it would have been that lecture hall. Slowly, though, as he leaned back, the glow began to fade, replaced by the gnawing disquiet of old. He looked around at the class of the chosen. They were young, their minds unsullied by wars and mangled bodies and poisoned dreams, or by having begged for places in questionable medical schools, unblemished by having considered bribing corrupt deans. He was the wild card so venerable an institution as Union could afford. The price, however, was that J.W. would be watched more closely, and held to tighter standards, than his colleagues. It was a given.

J.W. searched again, looking for someone his age, but the oldest was twenty-four or twenty-five, if that. It was easy to see that the people with whom he was sitting had been groomed, mentored from elementary school to the last day of college, prepared to be in that hall, at that moment, swaddled in the radiance of their success. They had gone from high school to college, then the obligatory mommy-daddy-funded summer trip to Europe, and finally, to Union Medical School. J.W. slumped in his seat and stared at the ground.

J.W. wore his three-piece suit that first day in medicine, the one major expense of their stay in Hong Kong, aside from Mao III's vet bills. Hand-sewn by Tat Cheung Tailor in the

Hai Phong Mansion on Abraham Road, J.W. had paid eighty dollars, and because he had thanked the man in Cantonese, Mr. Cheung threw in three handmade white shirts. It was the pin-striped suit J.W. had worn to the medical school interviews, and with Dean McNamara's words ringing in his head, it seemed appropriate dress for his first step into the caste of American nobility. Of the one hundred new students, J.W. was the only one so attired. Another new student, who J.W. thought might actually be Paul Simon, was dressed in torn jeans and a stained tee-shirt. The man twisted his head to J.W., but Weathersby could not see his eyes through the Coke-bottle-bottom, rimless glasses. The man asked, "Are you a professor of medicine?"

"Nope."

"Then why are you dressed like that?"

"I'm just a medical student sittin' in the peanut gallery, like you. A dean told me to dress like this a long time ago. He's dead now. Hey, you know you look like Simon and Garfinkle, man."

"It's Gar*fun*kel; and I am Seltzer.

They both laughed, and J.W. stuck out his hand. "J.W. Weathersby. Seltzer what?"

"Marshall Seltzer. Hey…"

The speaker halted abruptly and cleared his throat as forcefully as if he was trying to clear a laryngeal tumor. Seltzer smiled and nodded for him to go on.

After the introductory lectures, J.W. mounted El Buraq and pedaled off campus. Seltzer was standing in the student parking lot next to a glistening Chevy Corvette convertible. He watched J.W. fold his suit jacket and vest, slide them into a plastic bag, and bungee cord the parcel to El Buraq's rear fender. J.W. smiled to himself, remembering that, less than a year before, he had hauled Mao IV on the very same fender.

Krista and Khai were at the door to greet him, but J.W. kissed them both hurriedly as he rushed by, off to his books. He thought of Seltzer and the others partying, celebrating their first night of medical school, just the next rung in their predestined station in life. They dressed casually and acted casually, not intimidated by the coming years. J.W., though, trembled. He was being watched.

⚔

Freshman year began the next morning. Classes met for eight hours in a single lecture hall. Labs were interspersed three or four times a day. There was no homework as such, just the expectation that medical students would always be prepared. One of the professors from the day before met them in the lecture hall and remarked, "You're already behind; and medical school doesn't start for ten minutes." Another stood and laughed. "Let me put that in the vernacular. Medical school is like the IHOP—in a sense. We serve you one hundred pancakes every day. First morning, you manage to get through them. Second day's a little harder. Third day, what you don't force down, those flapjacks go on the pile of a hundred the next day, and so on. Hope you're hungry."

Seltzer's wool slacks and madras shirt silently mocked J.W.'s jeans and torn Sterling College jersey as they were herded to their first class, Human Anatomy. Dissection lab convened in a seventy-year-old, faded, drafty fieldstone building. The familiar stench of formaldehyde greeted them fifty feet before they reached the grand wooden doors through which had passed thousands of the Twentieth Century's most respected physicians. Weathersby and Seltzer drifted toward one of twenty-five stainless steel tables. The cadaver they chose lay supine under a stained white sheet. Seltzer stared, as if waiting for movement.

132

J.W. considered reassuring him that he, too, had done the same thing in Viet Nam, in My Co, when he saw his first dead VC, but it was better to allow Seltzer absorb the lesson on his own.

A petite, young woman passed hesitatingly. She looked behind her, as if waiting for someone, but soon turned toward their table. The first thing J.W. noticed was her skin. It was perfect, the palest latte—and her eyes, the purest, deepest black he had ever seen. J.W. hoped she would stop at his table, and hoped she wouldn't. She caught him smiling, and he was sure she would keep walking. But she smiled back innocently and took a place opposite Seltzer. A young man walked up to her, and she touched his hand reassuringly. A fifth student drifted over and stared at her. She turned away, but he remained at the table.

The first lecture of medical school commenced with a tutorial on the appropriate behavior with which they would treat their cadavers. The professor of anatomy welcomed them. "The bodies in front of you," he began in a heavy Scottish brogue, "were actual people just like you. They were lives, only recently returned to the inscrutable. They have donated themselves for your education, not amusement."

He went on solemnly. "The face of the cadaver will be covered at all times in respect, unless you are working on that facet of anatomy. You will be assigned four to a cadaver, so please rearrange yourselves." The odd man at their table looked to the other four. J.W. drew closer to Seltzer, and the woman placed her shoulder against her friend. "Quickly, please." The interloper did not move. The professor remained expressionless as he put his hands on the man's shoulders from behind and steered him like a pushcart to a table with only three pupils.

The anatomist went on. "You will stay with your own group for the balance of this course. There will be no shifting around. Now, we move through the organ systems as a class, in a prescribed order. The lab is open twenty-four-hours-a-day, and you will be expected to do much of the work on your own, after formal classes." There wasn't a single groan.

"You will never remove any part of the cadaver from anatomy lab. Brookline Union College of Medicine is a distinguished institution that will not tolerate scandal. I'm sure you are aware of reported cases in which medical students have brought corpses off the campus, even onto public transport. Not very humorous at all. Doctors, uncover your cadaver's body, but not the face."

J.W. looked down at a chubby woman, skin wrinkled, probably in her late fifties. She was nude, yellowed, rigid, vulnerable. Her nails were long, chipped, and dirty, but there was a delicate curl to her fingers. A tiny flap of skin had been lifted from a faded area on her left ring finger where a wedding band had been cut away. J.W. was embarrassed by her nudity, but when he looked up, he realized everyone's eyes had avoided her genitals. To the right wrist was attached a white card inscribed with a long number.

Seltzer smiled. "We can call her '1436891', or we can call her 'Lily.' You be the judge." When no one answered, Seltzer looked across the table at the dark woman and asked, "Well, we know her name. What's yours?"

J.W. heard a softly accented, "Sharrazad Bakhtian."

J.W. blurted. "Okay. Where you from?"

"Here."

"Boston?"

She paused. "Why do you ask?"

J.W. averted his eyes and looked at the final partner. The bearded, scraggly-haired man mumbled angrily, "Arthur, if you must know." He turned away and stared out the oily, smudged windows. Seltzer looked at the young man for a moment before turning to J.W. and rolling his grandly magnified eyes.

When they uncovered the faces of their cadavers, the nervous chatter in the room ceased. It was hard to distinguish the lifeless forms from their own paralysis. Everyone stared except Arthur, whose eyes remained fixed on his greasy window.

A few silent moments passed in the lab, but whispers began again, and they quickly built to a fine chatter. Arthur, though, stiffened and slammed his fist on the stainless-steel dissection table. "That's it." He threw his rubber apron to the tiled floor. Sharrazad reached to grab his arm, though he pulled loose and stalked from the room. She started toward the door after him, but stopped, stood rigidly, exhaled with a sigh, and turned back to the table. When she saw Seltzer's sagging jaw, her eyes reddened.

The professor of anatomy described the coming months without missing a beat. There had never been an Arthur.

At lunch, Arthur emerged from the dean's office, gathered his belongings from his hallway locker, and stared at Sharrazad for a moment, though he left without a word.

In anatomy lab the next morning, a new student appeared at J.W.'s dissection table. His eyes were red, like Sharrazad's. He interjected, "I'm sorry. I must look like hell. I flew all night from Stanton to get here."

Jimmy Ray Grieman was from the Rockies. He was the first in his family, in the generations of loggers and dirt farmers, to graduate from college—in fact, the first to finish high school. He had been wait-listed at Union. Twenty-four hours before working at an anatomy table, he'd been working for minimum wage at North Star Mills, pulling twelve-thousand board-feet of construction-grade pine off the green chain every shift. "Two-fifty an hour," he laughed.

Seltzer smirked, "And now you're paying ten bucks an hour to be pulling guts outta a corpse. Makes sense."

When the dean had called Jimmy Ray's home the day before, Jimmy Ray's father called the yard supervisor at North Star and asked to have his son to call home ASAP. But the boss told Jimmy Ray he couldn't use the phone until his break. Jimmy Ray had a feeling, though, so he threw down his leather apron, rushed out of the mill, and drove his pickup along Route 22 to the first pay phone. He called home, and then Union, and didn't bother to go back to North Star for his last paycheck.

Sharrazad's face relaxed. She smiled for the first time and nodded as Jimmy Ray related his saga. Seltzer asked if their new partner lived in the wild mountains with the bear and elk. Jimmy Ray smiled distantly, allowing that he had grown up below the glaciers, along the Little Salmon River, just outside Black Granite.

J.W.'s ears perked, for he had heard of Black Granite, but could not remember where or when. The name, however, fostered a sour, heavy feeling in his belly, and he wrestled, wondering why a wash of heat had wrapped his face. When it came to him, he was even more troubled, for Black Granite was the home of a co-pilot with whom he'd flown with in Viet Nam. They had spent hours talking the night they were shot down, and the young pilot had spoken of the Rockies and the forests and rivers. As the flush in J.W.'s face deepened, he blurted, "Did you know a guy named Lieutenant White? Forget his first name. He was from Black Granite. Killed in May, '69. Shot down in a 'Loach.' I'm sorry man, I mean in Viet Nam."

The professor stopped in mid-sentence and stared at J.W.

"Nineteen-sixty-nine?" he whispered behind his hand when the lecturer began again. "I was only twelve. "Lotta guys from Black Granite died in Viet Nam. There's a memorial downtown. Don't know a White family, though."

Anatomy students were issued one pair of thin latex surgical gloves as samples, the professor suggesting they purchase a full box to keep their hands out of the formaldehyde. That was another eight-dollar expense, one that would have to wait. J.W.'s gloves tore as soon as he pulled them on. His hands were too big. Sharrazad's were too small. It hardly mattered. With or without protection, hands became marinated in the formaldehyde after the first hour—not a single student left the first session able to feel benumbed fingers.

The next morning, J.W.'s partners brought boxes of gloves. J.W. bummed a pair from Seltzer. They tore immediately, and Seltzer grudgingly tossed a second pair across the table. They lasted until J.W. ran his hand across a sharp, rock-hard lump in Lily's abdomen. The gloves tore away, along with a patch of skin at the tip of his index finger. He bled all over the viscera. The team of anatomists investigated the mass, and Sharrazad peeled away tissue exposing Lily's calcium-filled aorta.

Jimmy Ray muttered, "Don't smoke."

Seltzer added, "Don't smoke what?"

Sharrazad dropped her eyes.

By noon, their hands, gloves or not, were clubs at the ends of arms. It was the last morning J.W. would feel his fingers until Christmas. Others sneezed constantly, their lungs sensitive to the endless fumes wafting through the lab. Everyone's eyes reddened, and noses dripped clear fluid.

At the end of each afternoon, Sharrazad rushed from the back of the lecture hall to a peeling '61 Chevy. J.W. saw her once while he was pedaling home on El Buraq. She was standing in front of a grammar school. He waved, but she did not see him, her eyes squeezed shut as she hugged a little boy voraciously. J.W. asked her the next morning, before Jimmy Ray and Seltzer arrived, "Do you baby-sit for your sister or something? I saw you yesterday with a handsome little boy."

Sharrazad stared into Lily's innards and mumbled, "J'Aveed? No, he is my son."

"Your son? Jees, you look so young. How old are you?"

"Oh, I'm older than you think—in many ways. I'm ..." but their partners appeared, and she became very quiet.

Seltzer told them about a lady in New York who had put her cat in the microwave on defrost to dry him. The cat exploded. J.W. spoke of the dynasty of Maos the Cat, and how offensive he found feline jokes. Seltzer squeaked sheepishly, "I'm really sorry. I love animals. Cats especially."

"Nah, I'm just kidding, man," J.W. laughed and invited Seltzer and his live-in girlfriend, Natalie, home to meet Krista and Khai that night.

Natalie was a sylph-like creature, even smaller than Seltzer. Her hair was curly, but long, and it flowed softly when she nodded her greeting with pouted lips. Seltzer was quiet for a moment before apologizing, "I should have warned you. Nat doesn't really speak English. She's French."

J.W. looked at Krista and smiled. Krista blurted in French, "Why didn't he tell us?"

J.W. looked in Natalie's chocolate eyes and added, "We spent two years in Paris at the Sorbonne. I can't speak French worth a damn, but Krista's good. When we were in France, the Parisians used to ask her, 'What's a nice French girl like you doing with an American bum like him?'"

As Natalie's jaw lifted, she took Krista's hands and held them tightly. Her face relaxed and became even more lovely. J.W. was taken for a moment by her perfect features. Krista noticed.

Natalie laughed. "Oh, my God, I'm from Mons, in Belgium." She turned toward Seltzer and snapped, "I am not French, but I graduated from the Sorbonne. Oh, my God."

J.W. asked, "What school? Where did you live? Wait a minute, wait a minute, some wine for our guests."

Krista left the room, and Natalie went on. "The Academy of Fine Arts. My PhD was in the Dutch Masters. Especially Van Gogh. What a story!"

J.W. asked, "So what's a lovely French woman doing with a…a *medical student*?"

"The same thing as Krista."

They swashed quickly through three bottles of wine. Seltzer became pensive.

"I'm the wild card of the Class of '81. Just drifting around, a transient for the last few years. A waste, not like you Weathersby. The Sorbonne, huh."

Krista scrunched her eyes. "Can't imagine they admitted a hobo to the best medical school in the country."

"Well, I haven't done much since I dropped out." His voice trailed off.

Natalie cleared her throat, and Seltzer mused, nearly inaudibly, about a PhD program.

"My love, tell them the truth. I won't listen to you tear yourself down. Tell them."

He brightened for a moment. "You think I should? It's so boring."

"Tell them. We are going to know these people for a lot of years."

"Okay, you want to get bored out of your mind?"

Natalie grabbed his arm. "Stop it."

"Okay. I was on my way to Leningrad for the research portion of my thesis."

Krista interrupted gently. "Where were you going to school?"

"'Cross the river. Harvard. The PhD program in Soviet Studies."

Krista cleared her throat. "Harvard, a tramp, wild card? What am I missing here?"

Seltzer's spirits lightened as he spoke. "My premise was that Stalin had several mistresses tucked away all over the Soviet Union. He was scared of the one in Leningrad. Rumor was that he was AC-DC, and she had the goods on him. You guys know about Stalin?"

J.W. cracked, "Of course. He was my uncle."

Krista leaned forward and slapped J.W.'s knee. "Will you let the man talk, please?"

"So, during the German siege of Leningrad, '41 to '44, he purposely didn't send troops to break the blockade. He figured she wouldn't be able to get word out that way, and that she'd probably be killed by the locals who hated Stalin for abandoning them, or by the Nazis when they figured out she was Stalin's mistress. And, in fact, she died in '42, as far as we know, but Stalin didn't know, so he did nothing to save the city. At least that's what I was trying to prove."

J.W. asked seriously, "Please, why did you stop your research? That could have changed history."

Now Seltzer's eyes dropped to the floor. Before Natalie could prod him, he began again. "I was on my way to Russia on an Aeroflot jetliner. I didn't want to fly Deathoflot, but it was the cheapest fare. Wouldn't you know it, we ran out of gas over the Barents Sea. Something about a strong headwind. Had to land on a patch of ice on the far eastern coast of Russia. Nothing for miles. I don't know how, but no one was one killed—a few got injured. Lady broke her arm. She could walk, sort of, but her son got his leg broken when the stewardesses trampled him trying to get off the plane first. We all walked for two days. I splinted the kid's broken tibia. Didn't know that's what it was called at the time. Wound up carrying him on my back, along with the only copy of my thesis."

"Why didn't the pilots take turns with you?"

"You tell me. Anyway, we got to the village of Lumbovka. I was some sort of hero they said. The townspeople presented me with a Russian medal, Order of Friendship of Peoples or something. They got together and made it out of the top of a tin can and a little band of red ribbon they filched from the village *partkom* bureau secretary's daughter. It was her hairband. Locked her in a cold room until she stopped bitching. Can't wait to go back. Anyway, *partkom*, that's the village communist party committee, bureau chief's the top dog—Ivan. Good guy. We drank a lot of his vodka. I read part of my thesis to him. He knew a little English, so I left a section with him that night.

"When the KGB arrived a few days later, they found the papers on the chair next to his bed. They questioned him, and when they found out I spoke Russian, they started in on me. Must have been one of those rare days that Stalin's memory was back in favor. He was a god for twenty-four hours, then back to an enemy-of-the-people. They confiscated the thesis and arrested me. Took my damn medal then arrested Ivan as a subversive.

"They held me for ten days. KGB cocksuckers interrogated me twice a day, fed me vegetable soup—half a cabbage leaf floating in water next to a, you know, like a little sugar cube, a lump of animal fat.

"What I remember most was Ivan's shrieks. They'd come and get him, work him over for a few hours, then turn him loose. He got so weak in just two days. I wished I'd been a doctor so I could help him. All of a sudden, some Americans from our embassy roll into town in a ZIL. I begged the jerks to do something, but they just stuffed me into the back of the limousine and told me if I didn't shut up, they'd gag me." Seltzer smiled thinly. "So, now you know. Fuck the Soviet Union."

He talked about the months after he was released. "I told my PhD supervisor at Harvard, 'Fuck Russia.' He was Russian. So, I spent the next half-year reading electric meters in Florida. Any place just to stay warm. When summer came, I sweat through a few months on Reader's Digest loading docks, down in New York." He turned to Krista. "You watch. This winter, I'm going to set the human, twenty-four-hour, calorie-intake record. If the temperature gets below ten degrees Fahrenheit, I'm as good as in the Guinness."

At the end of the evening, Krista went to make coffee, and Natalie followed, but the kitchen was so small, Natalie stood in the doorway and spoke softly to Krista. "When we have had our coffee, I will show you some of my watercolors. Not very good, but they are of the Parisian streets. Maybe you will recognize the places. Probably too ugly to see."

When Krista came back into the room, Natalie opened a large folder. The images were breathtaking. Both Krista and J.W. remembered the streets she had painted. Each study was deeper than the last, and when she showed them her portraits and nudes, J.W. whispered, "Magnificent. How did you do this? These are sacred." She turned to him and blushed.

Krista asked J.W. to help serve dessert, but he did not hear her, nor the second time. Krista left the room but continued past the kitchen. When she didn't come back, J.W. found her, slipped under the covers in Khai's little room, staring at the ceiling. "Is there something wrong, Sweat Pea?" J.W. murmured and sat down on the end of the bed.

"Why? Should there be?"

"Krista, look, what's going on? I got friends out there. It's kind of embarrassing."

"I'm sorry I'm not as beautiful as Natalie. Or an artist. Or a PhD. She's so much better than me, huh?"

"Krista, don't"

"All of you wild cards are so good, aren't you?"

CHAPTER THIRTEEN

First year midterm grades were posted in the main lecture hall. A crowd of unusually alert, though mute, students jostled toward the list. One-hundred student ID numbers were arranged in order of results. J.W. stood looking over Seltzer's shoulder. He babbled in his friend's ear, "God, if you're up there watching, let me finish in the middle. I want to be mediocre, second-rate. Please, let me be buried in the middle."

A few of the students banged their way forward, breathing hard, shoving as if escaping a burning movie theatre. Ted Snelake lead the charge. He found his number, snapped, "Fuck," and punched the wall. Even the students who didn't know Ted remembered him from the first day in anatomy, when the professor removed him from J.W.'s table and physically steered him to a cadaver far from Sharrazad.

He was another "mature" student, a PhD in mechanical engineering from MIT. Early in the semester, J.W. had tried to befriend Ted and tell him about Stella Flowers in Hong Kong. "You would 'a loved her. She was one of the first post-doc woman in engineering at MIT. Great lady."

Ted sneered, "Yeah? Just look what she did. The place is crawling with girls now. They've dumbed down the whole place for 'em. They don't belong in the hard sciences. In fact, they don't belong at MIT. They're good for one thing, though."

When the first wave cleared, many steaming off spewing profanity, the next swell reached shore. Most of them erupted in sighs of relief. Weathersby's number was next to the number forty. He hugged Seltzer, who was a few slots higher. There were only two failures.

The anatomy practical was the last of the series of exams. His crew studied late almost every night for two weeks before the test, pouring over the scraps of what had been Lily. At midnight on the Friday before the final, J.W. dragged himself home, discovering the note Krista had left on the living room floor.

He called Bernie right away. "Bobbie Jo and I are commemorating our second anniversary. Are you and Krista free tomorrow night to celebrate our good fortune and yours? The tape business was sticky at first, J.W., but sky's the limit now." He laughed that he and Bobbie Jo had moved to a condo overlooking Manhattan, into a building with two doormen and manicured grounds. Their basement parking spots were three hundred dollars a month, each.

They rolled into Boston that Saturday in a custom BMW. Both were tanned, healthy, and calm. Bernie insisted on a French restaurant near Union, and at dinner, J.W. congratulated him on his choice of champagnes. "This would certainly have been my selection, but I would haven't stopped at eighty dollars a bottle. That's only ten boxes of surgical gloves."

"Just feel the crystal; it's so delicate," Krista gushed after three glasses of champagne, but J.W. could not even feel his fingers.

The escargots were delicate, the steak as soft as warm cream-ery butter. When they were done, Bernie ordered the finest cigar on the menu, handed it to J.W., pushed back, and filled his pipe. He puffed quickly through two bowlfuls of his private blend. After cognac, he drifted back to the conversation.

J.W. dragged them around the Union campus, finishing at the medical school. Bernie slurred, "I want to see the anatomy lab that you've been talking about." Bobbie Jo and Krista curled their noses and went off on their own.

An hour before midnight in the brusque wind of a Boston autumn, they opened the main doors to the anatomy lab. It was so starkly cold and bare, Bernie locked his eyes on J.W.'s back and coursed a straight line just inches behind.

They pushed through double doors into the cavernous lab. Dozens of overhead incandescent bulbs burned all night, radiating the only warmth for the silent, shrouded cadavers. J.W. whispered to Bernie that Lily and her brigade had heard them approaching, jumped back upon their frigid tables, covered themselves with the formaldehyde-rotted yellow sheets, and held their breaths. "I caught them once, dancin' around. You should'a seen their looks while they were hopping back on the tables. It was a hilarious."

"Why would they care, J.W.? Who do you figure they're afraid of?" He laughed nervously. "Think about it. Where they are, you don't have to give a damn what other people think. They're be-yond that bullshit, J.W. They have freedom from fear, right? Yeah, so who's better off?"

As J.W. went over the ground rules they followed in class, he noted the most delicate trace of Sharrazad's scent lingering about the table. It stopped him for a moment, but he uncovered Lily to see nothing had changed since he and Seltzer had left her two nights before. The organs and vessels lay as they had when they'd quizzed each other, over and over, faster each time, until they sped through every obscure structure in the abdomen in two minutes, forwards and backwards.

Bernie was nearly speechless. "It really is pretty damn final, isn't it?" he whispered.

J.W. demonstrated what he could of Lily's abdomen, though much had been removed as his class had investigated each organ system. J.W. wanted to cover her, but Bernie insisted they study more. He wanted to see and touch the heart. "What's behind the liver? Hey, one kidney's higher than the other. That the same in everybody?"

An hour passed exploring obscure corners of the body, and it seemed they could have gone on for days, but Bernie had passed his test. There was something more important to show him. J.W. interrupted his friend in the middle of a burning question. "Hey, you think this is good?" J.W. whispered. "I got something'll knock your putter straight. Wanna get freaked out?"

Bernie nodded quickly with an excited smile. "Wait 'till you see this shit. My partner and I were taking a break two nights ago and discovered it."

Bernie's expression became solemn as he followed J.W. through the dissection room's rear doors, into a century-old section of the building, and down two flights of narrow, worn, concave cement stairs. They halted at a musty room in the second subbasement. The hall lights were dim—several of the bulbs long since burned out, their blackened glass coated in formaldehyde grease speckled with layers of dust and cobwebs.

The air outside the heavy metal doors of Room 6 remained as cold and damp as when Seltzer and J.W. had ventured into the bowels of the medical school on Thursday night. The rusted hasp remained unlatched. J.W. opened the door and turned to Bernie. "Take a deep breath before we go in."

Inside, the formaldehyde fumes hung more thickly than in the lab. The dark room's only light came from the reflection of the wan hall bulb. It played on stainless steel racks from floor to ceiling. Plastic bags filled with six-foot long, three-foot wide, two-foot high manikins were piled three high on the shelves. Overflow bags were heaped haphazardly, one on top of the other, along the floor. J.W. felt along the wall for the light switch. When the solitary bare bulb lit the room, Bernie gasped. In each clear plastic bag lay a nude human, some prone, some supine, some with cloudy, opaque, staring eyes.

"Okay, next year's anatomy, I want you to meet Bernie. Say hello, everybody."

Bernie laughed weakly. "Hey, J.W., let's say we get back to Lily? I still got a lotta questions."

"Okay, but I got one more thing to show you." J.W. left the room turning in the opposite direction they'd come from. He stopped at a cubicle. Shadows played on the body of an elderly male on a dissecting table. He was connected to a humming machine pumping formaldehyde into his veins. The tag on his hand listed his name, next of kin, and date of passing. It had been but two days. Bernie pointed to the corner of the room where a pile of the clear plastic bags was stored, one pulled out waiting for the man on the table.

They climbed back to the main floor, Bernie in the lead. J.W. reexamined Lily's abdominal structures, discovering obscure plexes and anatomical detours, both men so engrossed in their work they did not hear stirring outside the main lab. Bernie looked up first, his face instantly as ashen as Lily's. By the swinging doors stood a terribly stooped, tiny old lady in a black head scarf. No hair was sticking out. The black cotton clothing continued from her neck to her toes, even her gloves. She was older than any of the cadavers, upstairs or down.

She pointed toward them. "Who are you?" she cackled slowly and painstakingly.

"I am Medical Student J.W. Weathersby, ma'am. I am working on my cadaver, ma'am."

"Well, then, who the hell is he?"

"He's my half-brother, ma'am."

"Is he a medical student?"

"No, ma'am, but he's applying this year, ma'am."

"Well, then, both of you, get the hell out of this lab. Immediately!"

Without quibbling, they pulled the sheet over Lily and wormed past the stick figure. She sneered as Bernie walked by.

Her suit was stained with bits of what looked like meat, the fabric reeking of formaldehyde. To leave the building, they had to pass a series of private research anatomy rooms, one of which glowed dimly under a swinging, bare, 40-watt bulb. An elderly man sat mesmerized in the corner of one of the rooms, staring at the light bulb.

Natalie and Seltzer joined the four of them for dinner at Boston's Durgin Park. The century-old restaurant was world-famous, not so much for its food, but for the abuse heaped upon the patrons by waitresses, bus boys, and even the employees who took your name at the door for seating. Presidents had waited in line to be escorted in, so Krista rolled her eyes when Bernie croaked, "Can't buck the line here, can you?" and promptly strolled up to an angry older woman standing guard at the door. He whispered a few words. The maître d' was called with a crook of the woman's head, and before Krista's eyes rolled back to neutral, the six of them were enjoying the finest of champagnes at the finest table.

During dinner, Natalie knocked over her champagne. A few minutes later, she dropped her knife, which clanged noisily to the floor. Seltzer shot her an impatient look and hissed something in broken French.

After dinner, they wandered through Boston's Farmers Market. Bernie started to ask anatomy questions again when they got to the butcher shop, and the three men looked in the window at a ham hock dangling in the darkened store. Seltzer asked, "My man, if that turns you on so much, why don't you apply to medical school? It's not too late. Look at Grandpa Weathersby over here."

Bernie was silent for an eternity but eventually laughed sadly and mumbled, "I'll be dead long before I could finish." Despite Bernie's forced grin, it was the only melancholy J.W. had ever seen in him.

CHAPTER FOURTEEN

Christmas brought a week's vacation. The class had remained intact through the first semester, except for Arthur. Sharrazad told them, at the Friday afternoon end-of-the-pain-for-a-week party, that Arthur had never wanted to be a doctor. He had despised pre-med at Harvard, but was afraid to tell his heart surgeon father. During interviews, he spoke of his ambivalence regarding medicine, but that uncertainty was construed as a sign of maturity. He was a musician, he declared, and wanted nothing more in life than to play the sax. The interviewers assured him medicine and music mixed beautifully. He hadn't been able to talk his way out of medical school, and it took months to build the defiance to quit. "The only saving grace," he had told Sharrazad, "is that Jimmy Ray got my place."

Jimmy Ray flew all the way home to Black Granite for Christmas week. He felt isolated at school—a logger's son with few clothes, no car, and no spending money. Jimmy Ray's tablemates worried he wouldn't show up for the second semester, but at registration, he was there in a string tie and cowboy boots.

J.W. asked him if he was going to a wedding. He laughed, and laughed again when they told him how relieved they were to see him.

"Hey, Union gave me a shot. I'm the class wild card. If I screw up, no redneck who grew up in double-wide'll ever see the inside of this place again, 'cept maybe as a cadaver."

Sharrazad smiled cautiously. "No, I'm the wild card, Jimmy Ray. You're a real American. I'm the one who doesn't belong here."

"So, that makes it unanimous," J.W. grinned. "Four wild cards."

"A bunch of also rans, lucky to still be around," Seltzer nodded, though his face tightened, as did those of Lily's three other wardens. "The only thing I don't understand is that all of us squeaked into the top quarter last semester, except for you, Ms. Sharrazad. You were like number four in the class, weren't you?"

She blushed at first, but that passed quickly, and a bitterness filled her eyes. "Yeah, a Baha. Grades don't mean anything, Marshall. They just measure how long you can sit in a chair. It's what's in your head from when you grew up that..." She stared at the floor for a moment then walked off.

⇥ ⇤

Winter semester began in the microbiology and physiology labs, the class broken into groups of thirty to investigate the effect of medications on living organisms. In micro, each student was issued six white mice, into which they would inject a slurry crawling with noxious staphylococcus bacteria. The mice were left to their own devices for a day after the inoculations, to let the infections fester. The next morning, the students got their first look and feel of what it meant for an organism to be toxic. Half the sick mice were injected with antibiotics and marked with a green

Magic Marker, the untreated with red. The patients who had been denied medication were as hard as rock the next morning, having departed during the night to their final reward.

J.W. wasn't surprised at the results of the experiment. Everybody knew staph kills, and antibiotics work. He asked Seltzer why each of them had been given nests of rats on which to practice their scientific art. They did the experiment several times with different antibiotics and different bacteria.

At the end of the week, J.W. sat in class and carped to Seltzer, "Six mice for the entire class would have done nicely, don't you think? I hate killing shit. Did enough of that in the army to last me a few lifetimes. These people call themselves doctors, caring human beings? Seltzer, we don't need to be murdering so many animals."

Seltzer squirmed in his seat and rolled his eyes, as if pointing.

"Hey, Seltzer, listen, I'm telling you, I'm really tired of killing things, man. This is bullshit."

Seltzer stammered, "Well, Dr. Chopra's standing right behind you. Why not express your concern to him?"

Dr. Bagwan Chopra, the Professor of Infectious Diseases, listened patiently before suggesting J.W. confer with the dean if he was dissatisfied with the content of the medical education for which he was paying a king's ransom. On Seltzer's advice, J.W. let it go.

Neurology lab commenced with a film of a live cat. "Hey, I know that guy, it's Mao V," J.W. whispered loudly to Seltzer.

The lab tech in the movie sawed out a square of bone from the cat's skull then poured a paste of irritating acid onto the creature's partially exposed brain. Almost immediately, the cat began a rhythmic twitching that culminated in a violent grand mal seizure; several more followed, each wracking the animal's body. J.W. would have taken their word that bad things happen to living creatures when their cerebral cortexes are painted by liquids with pH's in the two range, but when the lights were flipped back on, Maos VI through X were wheeled into the lab on cold, stainless steel carts. The organisms appeared to be asleep, fur matted with excrement, tongues hanging. A calico was delivered to their table. He was still breathing, though shallowly. A small portion of his skull had been cut away with a jig saw, exposing the pearly white dura mater, the protective "hard mother" tissue lying between the skull and the actual cells of the brain.

Phase I of the experiment commenced with the order to apply the same toxic paste used in the movie. Here, though, it was to be first slathered on the exposed dura mater, not directly on the brain. No seizure. In Phase II, they cut the dura mater away and applied the venom to the surface of the cerebrum itself. As in the movie, the cats flopped around in grand mal seizures, the students' reward for an experiment well done.

J.W. raised his hand. "Excuse me, ma'am, but why do we have to sacrifice a kennel's worth of cats to prove what we just saw in a movie? I mean, I believe you, okay?"

Dr. Zhang snapped bolt upright. Her mouth trembled, though only a few puffs of unformed words escaped. She marched out of the lab. The class was silent. Some of the women nodded to J.W.; most of the students, though, dropped their eyes into textbooks. An American professor walked through the door.

"I'm Doctor Sorg. If any of you want to discuss philosophy, you can do so after class. For right now, your job is to learn what it feels like to cut living tissue, to see what disease looks like, to touch it, smell it. Are there any questions?"

Ophthalmology lab was as shadowy as the local pub at midnight. On each table a tech carelessly dropped wire cages in which resided two twitchy bunnies, one with a blue collar, the other red. The object of the lesson was to allow Brookline's student experimenters to observe the effect of assorted substances on the cornea. When the instructor entered the room, J.W. dropped his head.

Doctor Sorg began without a greeting. "We use lagomorphs for this lab because their eyes are similar to those of humans. Now we will start by applying the chemical in the red bottle to the eyes of the red-ribboned rabbit." The drop had hardly touched Pete's eye before he lunged at Seltzer, locking teeth on his tormentor's middle finger. Seltzer danced around holding his bleeding finger aloft, demanding the animal be sacrificed and sent to a lab to test for rabies, but a call to Dr. Chopra calmed him. There had never been a case of rabbit rabies in recorded history.

J.W. whispered to Seltzer, "Why are we putting these animals through this? Show me a movie. I'll believe you. Okay?"

Sorg drew in a deep breath through his flared nostrils. "Look, I'm not a damn philosopher. I'm here to shove a medical education down your throat. You learn by seeing and by doing. It also gives you a chance to touch living things, learn how to handle them gently. We want you to see what happens when you stick needles and medicines into patients. And, let me try to understand this. You're willing to watch us torture animals on film, but not here in class? How 'bout you come by tomorrow and pick the animal for the next film? I'll see you at seven-thirty."

"It's a matter of degree, sir. We don't need to torture so many. That's all I'm saying."

"So, let's just kill one cat, and we'll have one cat film for all the medical students in the world. Come up with a better answer, and I'll take it to the dean. I don't savor killing things, either. I doubt any of us do, but like you yourself said, it's a matter of degree."

Cardiology Lab, where they investigated the use of medications on the exposed heart, was brightly lit. An anesthetized German Shepherd was wheeled in on a cart. His chest had been cracked and was held apart by surgical spreaders. The heart was lifted nearly to the surface by toweling wedged underneath it. J.W. left the room before the cart rolled to a stop.

At 5 P.M., J.W. watched through the library windows as his friends drifted across the street to the pub for a beer. They waved for him to join them, and after the second beer, Seltzer described the final experiment of the afternoon in vivid detail, especially the part where the dog was injected with a lethal dose of potassium, just like in prison death chambers. At the moment of the infusion, the students' attention was drawn to the chaotic, though strangely soothing, wave-like ventricular fibrillation as the dog expired. The kids sitting at the table drinking beer weren't happy, but they were excited about what they had learned, an important phenomenon in cardiology. They had witnessed the phenomenon with their own eyes. One woman said she'd never forget it.

When J.W. went back to pick up his books at the library, Jimmy Ray was engrossed in the micro text. He never went out with the group, having promised he'd never set foot in a bar, the curse of alcoholism so widespread in his family. Most of his friends and relatives, he had told his anatomy friends, had already poisoned their lives with ethanol.

J.W. sat down next to Jimmy Ray "You stay for the grand finale in dog lab?" J.W. asked sarcastically.

"Yeah, got no choice, man. I'm the long shot. Can't make waves. Kinda sick, though, the way some of them laughed when the thing went into V fib. That guy Snelake, what a prick. He said, 'Man, that is so cool. Let's do CPR, bring 'em back, and do it again.'"

Three days later, when the dean summoned him, J.W. blabbered several excuses for his behavior before the man uttered, "Have a seat, Mr. Weathersby."

"Sir, the reason I stomped out of the lab was because I don't like killing dogs or cats. I mean, I understand why we have animal labs, but one sacrifice is plenty. Don't you agree, sir?"

The dean listened patiently but appeared confused. "This is the first I'm hearing about your animal rights leanings. You are here, Mr. Weathersby, because you were in the anatomy lab late last Sunday night with your brother. Is that correct?"

"Actually, it was Saturday evening, sir."

"He wasn't your brother, was he?"

"Well, sir, we've been through a lot together."

"Level with me, please. What was going on in the lab Saturday night?"

"He's just a great friend who was interested, that's all. If it wasn't for him, I wouldn't be in medical school, and I sure as hell wouldn't be sitting here now getting my ass chewed."

"You're not getting your ass chewed. Do you know who that was?"

"Countess Dracula, sir?"

The dean couldn't suppress a smile. "No. That was Dr. Ranvier. Ranvier's Nodes?"

J.W. nodded and whistled. "Wow, my cat cadaver had one of those! So, now I can tell my grandchildren that Dr. Louise-Antoinette Ranvier knew my name."

The dean's lips tightened, but this time he chuckled. "I'm impressed, but it was Louis Antoine Ranvier, and this is the granddaughter, Dr. Vivian Ranvier. Have a nice day, Mr. Weathersby. And no one is forced to attend class, but every student is forced to know the material."

—⊰+⊱—

Seltzer did the experiments, and J.W. used his notes. Several months later, J.W. called and asked if he could drive over and get the data from the duckling lab massacre. Seltzer stammered, "Natalie's gone back to Chicago. We had a big fight. You don't want to come over. Place doesn't look so good."

J.W. asked, slack-jawed, "What the hell would you want to fight with her about? You outta your mind? She's perfect, fool."

"That's what everyone thinks," Seltzer slurred. "It's not so."

"What?"

"Look, all she does is paint or study. The place is a mess. She spills paint everywhere. She's getting sloppier. I don't have time to be a handmaiden. I'm busy."

J.W. found Seltzer's door ajar. He was asleep on the couch next to an ornate coffee table from which dripped a nearly empty half-gallon of Breyer's ice cream. Next to it were three Big Mac boxes; an empty, large, French fry container; a half-eaten package of Oreo cream cookies; and a bone-dry bottle of Thunderbird.

J.W. shook him, hoping he was sufficiently alive to direct him to the afternoon's notes. Seltzer stirred, his torso lifted, and in one fluid motion, his arm shot forward to the phone. His fingers flew across the touch-tone dial, completing the number in less than two seconds. Seltzer knew it so well, J.W. was sure it was Natalie's. Weathersby relaxed, waiting for his friend to beg for another chance. Or maybe he had dialed the emergency room to plead they come over and pump his stomach.

Seltzer rasped, "Cheese steak, one hot fry, no, make it two, a chocolate malted…" There was a pause followed by a rasped series of numbers, the first digits of his address. The phone dropped into the cradle, and Seltzer fell back into an uneasy sleep. The delivery boy flew into the apartment unannounced, snapped a ten off the dresser, left change, and held up a dollar bill toward his groggy patron, who barely lifted his index finger. The kid tiptoed out and shut the door gently.

Seltzer finally raised his head a bit and offered J.W. a single hot fry.

"J. Dub, this is the big one. I'm going for a personal best—not nine thousand calories, but ten thousand big ones in twelve hours. Can it be done?"

"I don't know, but I do know the standard caloric value of the meals on the psych ward, and I know the attending doctor's number up there, too. So make a choice, pal. It's either you call Natalie, or I call the 6th floor and have your ass admitted."

Seltzer took one large bite of the cheese steak, chewed twice, swallowed, grimaced in pain, then tossed the flapping sandwich roughly in the direction of the waste basket. It hit the wall, though, opened, and spilled on the living room floor. "Shit. Nothing's workin'. I never miss that shot. Okay, I'll call her, but you see right next to the cheese on the floor, all that paint? Now look at the rest of the rug. It's everywhere. Gotta buy a new rug. I'm not made of money." He sucked in a deep breath, pulled himself up on the couch, but fell back to sleep.

Krista was also asleep. There were no notes on the floor, but there was a curled-up dinner in the cold oven. J.W. cursed himself for not having purloined Seltzer's cheese steak.

Seltzer was in class the next morning, though even through his glasses it was clear just how dulled his spirit had become. He avoided J.W.'s stare. "You ate the goddamn cheese steak, didn't you?" J.W. demanded.

"And what if I did? I called Miss Natalie."

"Is she coming back?"

"She's thinking about it. But it'll just happen again."

"What'll happen again? The calorie extravaganza?"

"No, you turd, the fighting. I torment her, and she leaves. Who gives a shit about paint in every corner of my house? It's like I'm pushing her out, like I can't understand why she lies in bed with me and says, 'I love you.' I'm a Jew boy, a swarthy little bastard, and she's one of the chosen. Did you ever look at her?

She's fuckin' beautiful—inside and out. How can she love me? It don't make no sense."

"Good, so blow the best thing that ever happened to you on some kind of psychological mind fart. That's just more of your poor self-esteem percolating to the surface, pal. You earned the respect of a fuckin' village in the fuckin' Soviet tundra. You need more positive strokes? You're the best there is. You're at the top medical school in the country, near the top of the class. Lighten up."

CHAPTER FIFTEEN

The pharmacology final, the one that marked the conclu-
sion of freshman year, was two weeks off. J.W. could not find
Seltzer for days on end; Natalie had come back to Boston, but
left again. "One shove too many," she wept to Krista in French
on the phone.

J.W. was shocked when she'd called. Krista had never mentioned Natalie's name. Though the Weathersbys had continued
to see them occasionally, and Krista had been cordial, J.W. never sensed a warmth between them. On the Weathersbys' most
recent visit to Seltzer's apartment, Natalie had shown them her
latest effort. She had started experimenting in oils. One was a
self-portrait, nude. J.W. lingered on it.

On the drive home, Krista was very quiet.

"Something wrong?" J.W. asked, his voice cracking.

"Why? Should there be?"

"You sound like a broken record."

"You mean you've heard that before?"

"Look. Whatever it is, I'm not guilty."

"You think women are stupid, don't you? Bobbie Jo noticed it. She even asked me, 'Is he always like that?'"

"Is he always like what?" J.W. snapped.

Krista stared out the window at the passing slums of the Combat Zone. J.W. was about to defend himself and make her prove, as if in a deposition, that he had ogled Natalie's body, or that he had ever so much as thought about another woman. Instead, he rode home in silence.

Several days later, Natalie returned to Boston. She found a rose on her front stoop—it was from Krista. That night, the two women talked for hours.

⫸ ⫷

The pharmacology final was followed, not with a posted list, but just a notice that everyone had made it through the basic sciences. A few students had to take an exam or two over, but the class had survived. At the bottom of the message was an addendum that a memorial service for the cadavers was to be held in the lab complex.

Dr. Ranvier officiated, leading a prayer for those who had willed themselves to the doctors, nurses, and physical therapists of the future. Hundreds of students stood in silence. Seltzer turned to J.W. and choked, "My parents escaped the ovens. Treblinka. Grandparents, aunts and uncles? Never met 'em."

When the remains of the cadavers were cremated that afternoon, a pall of yellow, greasy smoke formed over the campus. Seltzer cracked one nervous, wrathful joke after another. At 4 o'clock, he sprinted to his Vette and squealed off campus.

CHAPTER SIXTEEN

A two-month summer break began for most of the class. Several students, in a great hurry for reasons Seltzer and J.W. could not untangle, took courses every July and August, earning enough credits to graduate a year early. Sharrazad was one of them. She sent J'Aveed back to New York to spend the summer with his grandma. Seltzer and Natalie flew to Belgium and then Holland. She wanted to expand her repertoire and embrace the work of Vincent Van Gogh. Jimmy Ray went back to Black Granite.

J.W. and Krista stayed in Boston. Khai attended day camp, Krista worked part-time, and J.W. did construction until he was invited by his foreman to find a different line of employment. J.W. threatened to go to the union, but the foreman spit back, "You're summer help. You ain't part 'a no union, asshole. I told you to scrape that paint off the sign over Throckmorton's Restaurant. I said scrape. I didn't say use a propane torch. That goddamn sign was as old as Boston. Now it's gone. Boss is pissed at me for hiring a college boy. Says I gotta pay for it. Like I said, get the fuck outta here before I have the boys toss your ass into the Charles." When he drove back to pick up his last check, the foreman spied him from fifty yards and came running. "You're about as smart as a pint of weasel piss that's half full. You'll get that check when fuckin' pigs fly."

J.W. put out the word in their neighborhood that he was a handyman, and available. He was enjoined to install plumbing, electric fixtures, and decks. He was soon running a thriving concern of his own.

As each of the private construction engagements began, J.W. listened assiduously to his customer's desires, took copious notes, then rushed to the hardware store and asked the clerk how the job was done. That worked well, and the summer was lucrative until the very end, when J.W. was commissioned to install a toilet at the Bizzacesso's townhouse on Comm Ave.

A very small miscalculation in the angle of descent of the downpipe eventually mired him in murky waters. J.W. answered a call from the family late on a Saturday night, a week after sophomore classes had commenced. Their top floor commode was backing up, effluent overflowing and drooling onto the second floor, then drizzling along the kitchen walls and into the hall closet where Dr. Bizzacesso, the County Coroner, kept his new camel hair overcoat and cameras. J.W. called Seltzer, promising to pay him union wages as a plumber's helper.

When the two walked in, Dr. Bizzacesso's fourteen-year-old daughter was pacing the floor, tufts of toilet paper stuffed in her nostrils. Seltzer eyed her, sniffed twice, gagged, and excused himself. At 2 A.M., seconds after J.W. had cleared a small channel in the pipe, he bound down the stairs, flew out the back door, and found his apprentice asleep in the backseat.

J.W. had left a note reassuring the family the problem was simply a matter of adding a degree-and-a-half to the fall of the pipe, and all would be well. He promised to sanitize the walls and pay for the dry cleaning.

The family rose before sunrise, convened a meeting in the backyard, and called J.W. at home. "Don't bother coming back. We'll get a hold of a real plumber." The phone slammed down just as J.W. began to laugh at the thought of a Boston plumber coming out on a Sunday. He also smirked when he got the bill from the guy. He told the man to kiss his butt. He wasn't about to relinquish half his summer's wages. The plumber threatened to let the city inspector know J.W. was working without a license. J.W. threatened to tell the police that he was being blackmailed. The plumber threatened to beat J.W.'s brains in with a pipe wrench.

Krista looked up from a tall glass of red wine. "What is it Bernie always says? Yeah, that's it, 'Think about it.' So, picture this, J.W. Headlines in the *Boston Globe*: 'Union Medical Student Found in Car Trunk—Multiple Skull Fractures—Mob Involvement Suspected."

J.W. paid in cash.

CHAPTER SEVENTEEN

B y third year, only one of their number had succumbed—Ted
Snelake. The penultimate insult occurred the night he was
told to examine a frail old lady on the cardiac care unit. In order to listen to her lungs, he instructed her to sit up in bed. She
wouldn't or couldn't, so he took her arm and yanked her upright.
Her shoulder dislocated.

The dean tried to give Snelake the benefit of the doubt, until
Ted explained his theory of patient care. "Look, if these people
are in our hospital, they have to play by our rules. You go to
court, the judge tells you what to do; you don't tell the judge, or
the bailiff. I didn't invite her here. She came to us to fix a mechanical problem, not to get married. You people give me exactly
twelve minutes to work-up a new patient. If I don't get it done,
you yell at me for getting behind. If you're not willing to run this
place like a machine, then don't ask me to act like one. It isn't a
kindergarten. That's my answer."

The Dean offered a solution. "Ted, we want you to get a CAT
scan of the brain, just to rule out organic pathology. If that's

normal, we'll have you chat with one of the psychiatrists. Would do all of us some good to speak to a mental health specialist once in a while. What 'a ya say?"

"Nah. I'll get the CAT scan. It's a machine. You can't program it to come up with the hospital line. It doesn't lie like one of your in-house shrinks."

"Okay, we'll find a psychiatrist elsewhere."

Two weeks later, Ted kicked in the door of his locker as he packed his things after seeing Dr. Gerstein out at St. Augie's, the psych hospital.

⊨⊨ ⊨⊨

Third year classes convened in the hospital. It was the students' first exposure to the hospital pecking order. Seltzer mumbled in J.W.'s ear the first morning, "Reminds me of a colony of baboons." Each junior medical student was assigned a senior medical student to trail, who trailed an intern, who trailed a resident, who trailed the chief resident, who trailed the attending physician. Interspersed were physical therapists, pulmonary therapists, social workers, nurses, nursing students, and often a 7th grader on career day. The lead elements were already finishing up in the next room as the tail paraded past the bed of the last patient. Seltzer snipped next, "It's like being a member of the Congolese Army Band."

At the end of a long day of observing residents render diagnoses and cures, medical students were sent home to read about what they had witnessed. The interns, on the other hand, modern-day galley slaves, the lowest organism in the medical hierarchy, and perhaps on Earth, stayed all night and all the next day, and sometimes the next night. Watching them die a little each shift, observing their psychoses deepen from lack of sleep, lack of food, and lack of positive human companionship, gave J.W.

pause; but he tormented them anyway, as one social class always abuses the next lower.

There were medical students who became so engrossed in the day's work, they remained after-hours, unable to satiate themselves with the drama and potent adrenaline of the hospital. For Seltzer and J.W., that phase began during their general surgery rotation. At first, they did intern scut, like retrieving lab results and pushing patients down to radiology.

Every so often, the medical student was tossed a learning experience. J.W.'s inaugural human medical procedure was to draw blood from Mr. Jenks, an older citizen whose cardiac difficulties had commenced in 1954, when he was sixty.

The house phlebotomist, a Miss Wong from Hong Kong, had been unable to locate a single vein from which to draw blood, so she paged the intern and barked over the phone, "You draw blood now." The intern, though, was busy showering and changing scrub suits several floors and two wings over after his most recent admission, a drunk who had vomited blood on him in the emergency room. He passed the call to the senior medical student, who passed the call to the junior medical student. "Weathersby, go take blood. Don't worry, the guy's gorked out."

"I've never done that before."

The senior student reassured him, "See one, do one, teach one. You must have seen someone drawing blood somewhere. Yes? So you're already on step number two. Just do it."

Seltzer came along, excited at their first responsible act as medical professionals. "Seltzer, promise me you're not gonna run out to your car if he farts while I draw his vital juices."

Mr. Jenks, who'd passed his prime in the mid-1930s, was asleep in Bed B. When they knocked on the door, the man in Bed A, a much younger patient, though he didn't appear any more robust than Jenks, looked up from a trance and asked

Seltzer to hand him a beer, "And make it cold." Seltzer looked at the man's food tray for a six-pack but found only an empty cup of Ensure. On the floor beside the bed was a slab of congealed hospital meatloaf. The man eyed Seltzer scraping the load off the linoleum. "And that food is shit. Let's see you eat it, Doctor." Seltzer closed the sheets around Mr. Jenks' bed and helped J.W. roust their sleeping patient.

"We need to take some blood. It's for a test, sir, okay?" J.W. yelled in Mr. Jenks' ear.

The man in Bed A answered. "You don't need my goddamn blood. Just gimme a beer. I already told ya."

Seltzer opened the sheets and apologized. "Sorry, but we're talking to your roommate."

Patient A burped, passed gas, a loud one, and lunged at Seltzer, who laughed because the man's arms and legs were restrained. He fell back onto the mattress and howled, "I wanna fuckin' beer."

Seltzer closed the room door.

Mr. Jenks' veins were as described by Phlebotomist Wong— shrunken to microscopic dimensions decades before. J.W., though, found a sliver of a vessel on the back of Mr. Jenks' hand. He mumbled as he cleaned the skin with an alcohol swab, "I saw on St. Elsewhere, where they couldn't get blood on some guy, so they used a butterfly needle. I'm going to try that."

The man in Bed A hollered, "I can smell you drinkin' in there."

J.W. took the tiny device from the IV tray and shouted to Mr. Jenks, "There's going to be a little poke, sir, okay?" The patient remained insensate.

From Bed A, the unhappy man screamed, "Don't stab me! Don't stab me! Just gimme a beer!"

J.W. slid the needle under Mr. Jenks' parchment skin, inching it at a snail's pace toward the hair-like vein. His eyes grew to half-dollars as dew drops of not particularly ruby liquid dribbled into the syringe. J.W. looked up at Seltzer with a smug grin, but as the last cc of blood was sucked into the tube, Mr. Jenks slapped J.W.'s hand away. The needle popped out, and a puddle of blood formed on the sheet. Seltzer handed him a towel, and J.W. sopped it up. While he worked on the sheet, a grape-sized lump of blood coagulated under the point J.W. had inserted the needle. When J.W. saw it, he barked, "Shit!"

The man in Bed A screamed.

Seltzer nudged J.W. "That guy's suffering more than your pal over here."

J.W. placed a bulky bandage to hide the hematoma, and the two junior surgeons left the room. J.W. showed the vial to Miss Wong, who curled her nose and hissed, "Yeah, but you use butterfly."

⊱ ⊰

J.W. watched Khai reading silently in her bed that night, the same bed in which he had grown up. He ached to think she could ever be even a fraction as unhappy as he had been thirty years ago as a child. Standing at the crack in the door, J.W. wondered what he could do at that moment to circumvent the nights of sleepless worry over threats from teachers, principals, uncles, aunts, friends' parents, crossing guards, the safety patrol, and even the local merchants.

His childhood had been squandered just one transgression away from the dreaded call to his parents. J.W. shivered, remembering lying in that bed one spring Sunday morning, after the call from Mr. Doyle, the owner of the corner candy store.

"Mrs. Weathersby, he comes in here every Wednesday after school with a dollar bill in his hand and buys candy for him and George. That's twenty candy bars. What those two don't eat, they throws away in the gutter."

His mother called him away from the TV. "J.W., show me your bankbook from the school savings plan."

"They didn't give it back yet."

"Your sister got hers. Where's yours?"

His parents watched him search under the covers, on his bookshelf, under the rug, and outside the window, but his mother sighed impatiently, walked to his dresser, opened the top drawer, and plucked the book from under the socks. "Not well-hidden at all. Hubbie, look at this: ninety-five dollars! J.W., your sister is two years younger than you, and she's got over a hundred. Where's the rest?"

"I donno."

His father repeated the question.

"I donno. I think they give you a new book each year."

"Your sister doesn't have a new book. Where's the money?"

"I donno."

His sister had been hiding right outside the door, pressed to the wall. With the final "I donno," she stuck her head into the room.

"Mom, I think you should ask George, because J.W.'s always buying candy for him on Wednesday afternoon. If there's any left over, they won't share with me. They throw it away."

His father, jaw set, hissed, "Come with me, J.W. We're going for a ride."

As they walked through the living room, his sister pirouetted a few orbits and dropped in front of the TV, humming the haunting melody from "Victory at Sea". J.W. lived all week for that cherished hour. Unlike school mornings, on Sunday, he was out of bed early; there were no complaints of stomach aches or sore throats. He'd sit transfixed for an hour as navy pilots vaulted off World War II carriers. *Those* men never blinked in fear. When they landed on deck, it was to cheers, not rebukes. No one told *them* they were second-rate or inadequate. No one threatened *them*. They were heroes, aces, revered. All week, every week, J.W. dreamed about growing up, going to the Naval Academy, maybe even dying for his country in a P-40 Warhawk.

But not this Sunday. His dad ordered him into the De Soto. J.W.'s sister turned up the volume on the "Victory at Sea" theme and opened the window as the car pulled away.

They drove silently along deserted streets, J.W. staring straight ahead, no hint of their destination until his father turned into Police Precinct 11. "Come on," his father ordered, "we have business inside. I always figured you'd wind up here."

J.W. followed through the red-brick façade into the jurisdiction of Booking Sergeant Patrick Delanoy, who sat above it all on a platform behind thick glass. J.W.'s father approached the officer slowly, head ever so slightly bowed. He spoke behind his hand.

"Park yourself on that bench until we call you, young man," the sergeant growled. The hardwood seat to which J.W. had been banished was worn smooth by more than sixty years of criminals, and it was bloody cold. Sergeant Delanoy rose slowly, and with a crook of his index finger, ordered J.W. to follow. He pulled a ring of giant, cast-iron keys off a rusted nail and unlocked the bars to the holding pen. "This kid stole," he proclaimed to the disheveled, bewhiskered occupant. The old man shook his head in disgust and spit on the cell floor.

"You don't want to land up here, do you?" the sergeant demanded.

"No, sir."

"Then don't steal!" he shrieked, his face as bright red as a stoplight.

The last few notes of "Victory at Sea" were pounding as J.W. passed through the living room to spend the rest of the day, and week, in his room. The silent treatment lasted even longer. Ten years later, the night before the ROTC cadets were to choose a service at Sterling College, the naval officers drove through campus playing the "Victory at Sea Suite" over loudspeakers. J.W. chose the army.

Looking at Khai in her room that night, J.W. longed for his daughter to be spared the sad, fear-filled nights he'd passed on that bed decades before. She looked up at him. "I love you, Daddy. Would you lay down with me?" As she fell off to sleep, he embraced her so tightly, he was afraid he'd hurt her.

CHAPTER EIGHTEEN

A fter four weeks on the surgery rotation, J.W. was assigned to otorhinolaryngology. It took several rounds of asking before J.W. discovered that meant ear, nose, and throat. The attending physician, Dr. Ronald MacDonald, met with them for an orientation meeting. "Only the spelling of the last name has been changed to protect the restaurant chain."

Despite his preeminence, he welcomed them to the course with an offer to be at their disposal, day or night. He afforded them carte blanche in his clinic, and left them alone until they asked for help. Yet, he treated them as if they made a difference. It was the second time in medical school J.W. felt happier to be there than any other place on Earth.

Sharrazad was among the students who sat with J.W. in classes for hours in the morning, and in ORL clinic for the rest of the day. The first lesson taught them which end of the otoscope was placed in the ear and which side the doctor looked in. It was a lecture Bob Hecock had apparently slept through, for despite the hour of instruction, he got it backwards on his first patient. With a smile, Dr. MacDonald went over the concept of the tools of his trade once again.

He taught them how to approach sick children, how to involve kids in the exam, and how to place the scope so gently in a child's ear, the patient never felt the coned speculum. He demonstrated the head mirror, and how to use it to visualize the vocal cords without gagging the patient to the point of vomiting.

He suggested they watch Sharrazad. "Miss Bakhtian's hands are gentle. You need that when you're around kids. She has grace. Watch her. Learn from her. Learn from each other."

J.W. looked at Sharrazad, at her hands, at her high cheekbones, at the silkiness of her coal black hair. Her gentle beauty unsettled him. Eyes that had been just deep onyx now sparkled. Her skin was flawless. His chest tightened.

Sharrazad was the image of a peasant girl he'd known in Viet Nam, a woman he realized he had never gotten over. The last time he'd seen her was the day he left the countryside, the earrings he'd bought her in Saigon sparkling in the ferocious tropical sun. A wave of guilt, followed by a swell of loneliness, passed over him.

He watched Sharrazad for a bit, until she looked up from her patient. Their eyes locked. For a trice, the loneliness vanished.

In late October, on a magnificent autumn afternoon, Sharrazad and J.W. sat alone on the patio outside the clinic break room. They sipped tea and talked about growing up in New York. J.W. learned that Sharrazad had lived in Manhattan when she had first come from Iran. When he leaned back and smiled, her shoulders relaxed, and J.W. commented, "Hey, young lady, I heard you speaking to that Puerto Rican patient in Spanish. It flowed, like your English. Huh, so that's," J.W. counted on his fingers, "Farsi, English, and Spanish. Any others?"

"Not that hard. We lived next to Spanish Harlem when we moved to New York. Half the kids in school didn't speak English. I had to learn both. No one knew what Farsi was. They thought Iran was an Arab country, so they got some guy from a Middle-Eastern bakery to speak to me in Arabic. Besides the words from the Koran, Farsi is as different from Arabic as it is from English. Didn't go well. So, I learned English and Spanish. I was only 15. No big deal when you're young. Couldn't do it now."

"Not at your advanced age—no way." He asked her if she wanted to hear a story about when he was a kid, and he saw his first Latin beauty. "It's a little strange, but it's really true."

"Please, tell me."

"Okay, but don't get mad at me. I mean it's about foreign kids in New York."

"Don't worry. I won't take umbrage. Please, go ahead."

"I was barely eight-years-old. I could hardly spell my own name. It was at my school playground in the Bronx, on a Sunday. The kids from the Puerto Rican street came to the yard to hang out. There was this one time they came with this beautiful girl. I had never seen anyone that gorgeous. I mean she looked like you."

"You stop." She lifted her hand to tap him but pulled it back before her finger touched him.

"The boys were teenagers, I guess. One of them was carrying a metal chain, like to lock up your bike. He started yelling at the girl and made her turn around. He whipped her and whipped her until she begged for him to stop. I wanted to stop him, but he was cursing at her in English, the f-word, the c-word. I mean, I had heard the words before, but I didn't know they could have such power.

"She was crying so hard. I would have attacked him, but I was too scared. I wanted to be a hero, maybe make her love me, I guess, if a kid at that age even knows what it means. You getting mad at me?"

"Don't be silly. What happened?"

"Anyway, I guess I ran away. Next morning in school, I was in third grade—that's important for the story. I wrote the words on a note and sent them across the back of the room to Sally. She sat at the end of the fifth row, I was at the end of the first row."

"You were at the back of the class? I don't believe it."

"May I continue?" She waved the back of her hand at him and laughed. "Thank you. So, little Miss Sally gets all hot and bothered and marches right up to the teacher, hands her the note, and points at me. I had no idea what my newfound vocabulary meant, other than it was the only English spoken by the Spanish kids from across Kingsbridge Road. It had to be important, because the girl didn't run away. God, she was beautiful. The way I saw it, it was the words that had the power over her. And I had to be the most powerless kid in New York. My mother didn't, shall we say, share control well with others.

"So, Sally runs up to Miss Claire, waving the paper, sobbing, 'Help me, save me!' So now she was using the words to control me. I must have been as pale as our Lily. Miss Claire graduated from teaching college in the 20s, maybe earlier. She had to be a hundred-and-ten, and was a spinster. The principal, Miss Boris—that one was the pedagogical product of the Nineteenth Century, I'm tellin' ya. So, here's what they did. I was supposed to take the note home and have my mother sign it. Yeah, right. These people grew up before the Bill of Rights or something, before there was such a thing as cruel and unusual punishment. Am I boring you?"

She clucked her tongue and hissed, "Will you please..."

"Okay, okay, so next morning, I sneak out of the apartment early and hide in the cloakroom. I sign my mother's name. It was Judith, but I signed it Judth. Teacher went crazy. Has me stand in a corner facing the wall out in the hallway, then she gets Mrs. Fiori, the second-grade teacher, and they have this like security council meeting. I get sent back to second grade until the note gets signed.

Mrs. Fiori puts me in the first row, behind Dirty Joseph. I don't know, the kid was from Ethiopia or something—lost tribe of Jews. Skin was dark, but there were no black kids in our school, so everybody just thought if he wore a yamaka and had dark skin, it had to be dirt—even the teachers. And he couldn't speak English. She told all the kids not to talk to me. Said it right out loud.

"Soooo, next morning, third grade teacher has me appear before the class. 'You got that note signed?'"

"No."

"Back to second grade with you. And that's where you'll stay until it gets signed."

"Next morning, same drill. Finally, on Friday morning, she has me in front of the class. 'No, I don't have it signed.'"

"Huh. I want to speak to your mother. Where is she?"

"She's in Washington, D.C."

"And what is she doing *there*, young man?"

"Meeting the President."

"That's it!" she screamed. "You go back to Mrs. Fiori's room and stay there for the rest of your schooling!"

"On Sunday evening, my mother returns from D.C. Her boss was making some kinda presentation to Truman. She sat outside the Oval Office while the boss was inside. When they were done, president walks her boss to the door, steps out, and shakes my mother's hand.

"My father, me, and my sister meet her at Grand Central Station. In the car, she's telling us about the White House, about shaking hands, and my sister starts teasing me. She's like singing, 'J's in second grade, J's in second grade.'"

"My father says, 'No, Sweetheart, J.W.'s in third grade, and you're in first.

"But Daddy, Dirty Joseph told me he's in second grade."

"'He doesn't even speak English,' I pipe up from the back seat.

"So, my father looks in the rearview mirror. He stops the car and stares at me. He knew. When we get home, he calls Miss Claire. I still remember how he was making twisting motions with his mouth as he was listening to the tale unfold. He kept nodding to my mother, cupping his hand over the mouthpiece, whispering, 'It's true.'

"I went back to third grade next day, but I had to carry a behavior book for the rest of the year. Sharrazad, I would lay in bed during those years, feeling small as a bug, caged by a concrete world. Always trouble hanging over my head. It was so thick, I couldn't see the truth or the hypocrisy. Not back then. I'm a little better now.

"The funniest part was when my father stopped the car and looked in my eyes. He knew. Parent always knows. You know that with J'Aveed."

Sharrazad suddenly jumped up and moaned, "*Al hum de le la*! It's Wednesday." She ran to the phone. "I forgot again. Every late minute's two dollars at the day care." When her call was answered, she apologized in a whisper, over and over. "Please? It won't happen again. Thank you. I love you." She collapsed on the couch and began to cry.

"J'Aveed is my life, and I'm even blowing that. I've forgotten my own son. What is happening to me?"

"Sharrazad, I know I'm out of line, but..."

"It's okay. He's nine, I'm twenty-four. I'm sure you can do the math. He was born right before we escaped from Iran. The trip was a nightmare, but it was better than being beaten any more by my husband."

"I didn't know about any of this. I'm sorry."

She leaned back, though remained silent, as if drawing the loose ends together for herself. As she began again, the tears ran freely. "When we got here, my mother watched him while I finished junior high and high school. One of the teachers wouldn't pass me in chemistry unless I applied to college. I asked him if he wanted to baby sit J'Aveed while I studied, but he just told me that he wasn't going to rescue me. He said I belonged in college, but how I managed it was my own responsibility."

J.W. felt a guilty uneasiness in his belly as he began to lift his hand to touch hers. He stopped, fearful of frightening her.

"So, I wound up in a small Catholic girls' college in Manhattan. A Baha'i girl learning the Rosary, going to confession."

"No. You wound up at Brookline Union College of Medicine, Sweet Pea, to become a doctor. See, you thought, no, you believed, you were the wild card, not as good as the Americans. But you were better. Even the nuns at Mother Maria's Catholic Academy of the Rosary Bead, or whatever, made you come here, didn't they? Same as high school, right? You have that effect on good, bright people, don't you? You got accepted at *ten* schools, didn't you?"

She stared at J.W., and her cheeks reddened, "How did you know that?"

"J'Aveed told me, at one of the class parties, Sharrazad."

"What else did he tell you?" She smiled embarrassedly as she picked up her books and started for the door. She turned back. "And to you, I am not Sharrazad anymore. My name is Sharra, but please J.W., just between us," and she ran from the room.

The next morning, a twelve-year-old girl was brought to the clinic by her mother. Rachelle's breath had been so awful for the past year, no one could be in the same room with her, especially when the windows were closed. Winter was coming, and the family was growing edgy. Last December, the odor had been so overwhelming, the family had had to build a ceiling-high partition in the corner of the bedroom. Rachelle slept in it with the window wide open.

J.W.'s first impulse was to tell the woman that if the child brushed her teeth occasionally and ate properly, and maybe went to the dentist every couple of years, she wouldn't have the problem. J.W. paused and laughed to himself about an incident in Viet Nam when he had smelled so bad, no one would get near him. So, he stepped off his high horse—halfway. "Glad you rushed right down to see us."

"We've been to a lot of doctors, dentists, too," Rachelle's mother growled, pursing her lips. "Nobody knows a damn thing. Why can't you help us? We pay our bills." She went on to name the slew of doctors they'd visited. The last suggested she try the University, where Dr. MacDonald practiced. "They said he was the best in the world."

"He is."

"Well, then, I want him to see my baby."

"Ma'am, I have to explain how things work here. It's a teaching hospital, so first, Rachelle has to be seen by the intern, then a resident, then other regular doctors. If they can't figure it out, they'll call Dr. MacDonald."

"It'll have to be one for the books," the intern snapped when J.W. told him about the little girl. "How many cases a day do you think Dr. MacDonald can handle? Let *me* take a look," he added with distaste. It was his considered medical opinion that the little girl should pay more attention to oral hygiene.

"You mean brush her teeth?" the mom huffed. "We've had her to six dentists. Her teeth are perfect. Come on darling, let's go! These people don't know nothin'."

She took the child by the hand and left, but J.W. called her house that evening to apologize for the intern, and to ask them to return in the morning to see Dr. MacDonald. J.W. had unexpectedly run into him and presented the case of the little girl with the big problem. "Well, let's take a look at her," he offered with a bit of excitement. "Is she here?"

"No, sir, but she will be first thing in the morning."

And she was. J.W. read about halitosis that evening, in Dr. MacDonald's textbook, and thought about it all night. In the morning, J.W. ordered x-rays of her head and throat, as the book prescribed, then presented the package, child and all, at 8 A.M. Dr. MacDonald took a brief look at the films, uttered, "For God's sake," took Rachelle by the hand, and laughed, "Come on, sweetheart. You're so pretty, I want to get some more pictures of you." He pointed out to the mom, Rachelle, and J.W. that the x-rays showed a metallic foreign body in her nasal pharynx, deep inside her nose. It had been pushed so far back, it wasn't' visible from the nostril.

Surgery was scheduled for the next dawn, and as the late autumn sun crested, Dr. MacDonald turned to J.W. with the Coca-Cola bottle cap he had extracted from Rachelle's nose. "Good. We're done. Man, that thing stinks!"

The operating room staff swooned as Dr. MacDonald ordered pictures of the offensive foreign body, and the photographer had to be helped from the room. J.W. was glad Seltzer wasn't there. The scrub nurse dropped the cap into a specimen bottle, shut the lid tightly, and drew a skull and crossbones on the jar. Dr. MacDonald asked J.W. to inform the family of their success. "You earned it," he smiled, giving J.W.'s shoulder a tap.

Rachelle's parents shook his hand and thanked him warmly. In their eyes, J.W. saw two worlds coalesce, but just for an instant. The four soon stood with little else to share, just as in Hong Kong after Mrs. Shou's family had thanked him. Here, too, the gulf had been bridged, but after the shaking of hands, there was nothing left to bind them. J.W. felt the abyss reopen.

J.W. thanked them for thanking him, and that sentiment marked the termination of their relationship. The senior resident was standing in the hall. She overheard the conversation and said to J.W., "When they thank you, and you don't thank them, *that's* when you've gotten there."

J.W. didn't see Rachelle or her family again, and it didn't matter. The child was better, one of the rare times he would witness the system working as intended. It had been a good week.

The month on ORL rotation passed in a mist of chattering with Sharra long after the day was over, and guilt for his growing thoughts about her. J.W. wanted to confide in Seltzer, but feared his friend would eventually sink into a well of alcohol and tell Natalie, so J.W. kept his own counsel. Better to hang on for a few more days, until the end of the course, and quietly start the pediatrics rotation. By Monday next, he knew it would be months before he saw her again, for Sharra was scheduled to do internal medicine, two hospitals away.

And anyway, it was J.W.'s private fantasy. He had never mentioned a word to Sharra, never even hinting that she had become much of what he spent his time dreaming about. It was all just fantasy, a truth that deepened when he passed her in the hall a couple of days later and noticed the diamond engagement ring.

"It's Arthur," she spoke faintly. You remember. He was at our anatomy table the first day." Sharra's eyes closed for a moment, and she added almost inaudibly, "I hadn't seen him in two years, and then he showed up with the ring. He's such a nice man. He doesn't beat me or my mother." She turned away and whispered, "I'm sorry."

On the final day of the rotation, Dr. MacDonald hosted a party for the departing students and the intern who was still not talking to J.W. Sharra didn't attend.

⊱⊰

J.W.'s first patient on the pediatrics rotation was Bennie Stevenson, a five-year-old towhead with a tummy ache. He had cried and refused to go to kindergarten that morning. Because Bennie never cried, his mom took him to their private medical doctor, who examined the child for less than thirty seconds before ordering him transported by ambulance to Children's Hospital.

Bennie had a large mass in his groin, about the size of a dwarf pea, and a big lump in the area of his spleen. J.W. could not feel either, though the pediatric intern assured him that with time, J.W.'s clinical skills would mature. Bennie was scheduled for a CAT scan, and while the family waited for a slot in the only scanner in Boston, the lab techs came and drained Bennie of generous aliquots of blood. His mother and father waited, then waited and waited some more. When the CAT scan results came back to the floor, the attending physician gasped. The mass in Bennie's belly was huge. He had cancer.

Bennie vomited that evening. The surgeons left the room within five minutes, poker-faced, pushing their small charge on a gurney to the operating room. Bennie's parents followed obediently, holding hands, fingers ghost-white.

"He's going to be fine," J.W. reassured. "You know about the new medicines, don't you? The ones for can..." J.W. caught himself and went on quickly, "All sorts of tricks these guys've come up with. You'll see."

183

Despite Dr. Weathersby's considered prognostication, Mrs. Stevenson cried as she stared out a window blankly into the cheerless Boston night. Bennie's dad, who had taken the call while at work, was still in his Massachusetts Highway Patrol uniform. Sitting bent forward, head in his hands, made him look small and frail. He nodded politely to J.W., in control of his manners if not his heart.

J.W. thought back to the ticket he had been given on the turnpike a year before, and of how he had hated the trooper, and wanted to get back somehow, to punish him. J.W., fresh out of medical reassurance, related the story of the summons to Trooper Stevenson. "Three over the limit? I'll bet that was Bob Slimmer. He gave his own mother a ticket. The guy's by the book. Can't tell him anything. Hey, Doc, when Bennie's home, maybe you'd like to ride along with me on a shift."

Bennie's Wilms tumor was still below the diaphragm. That was good. The surgeon removed what he felt was the entire cancer, sent part of it to the lab for tissue analysis, and sent Bennie back to the floor, where he awoke a few hours later in pain. He didn't cry. Bennie never cried. The nurse injected a medicine J.W. had never heard of into the IV, and the child calmed, but soon the medicine's effects wore thin, and the child tossed and tossed, begging his mother for water.

After an hour, J.W. asked the nurse if it was okay to give the child something to drink. She stiffened as if J.W. had pinched her butt. "Can't you read?" she upbraided indignantly, pointing to a handwritten sign on the head of Bennie's bed. "He's NPO!"

J.W. asked the senior medical student what NPO meant, but she was appalled by his ignorance. J.W. did not bother asking the intern, because if the intern had known at some time in his medical career, he was too tired to remember. J.W. found the second-year resident, who handed him a pocket medical diction- ary. "Look it up."

"Non per oral," nothing by mouth.

J.W. returned to Bennie's ward and watched him beg his mother for water. When Bennie's eyes produced a single tear, J.W. slipped him a few slivers of ice, sat back, and felt useful. Mrs. Stevenson took J.W.'s hand and thanked him, her tears flow- ing freely. In thirty seconds, Bennie vomited. The nurse was in- censed. "Has this child had anything to drink?"

J.W. thought to himself, eat, drink, two different things. Bennie ate the ice. That's not drinking.

"No, Ma'am," J.W. said as confidently as Bernie would have, "Nothing to drink."

"Well, he better not have."

An hour passed. The surgeon stuck his head in the room. "Bennie's got a long road to go, but we'll make him more com- fortable. How 'bout some ice chips, partner? Let's have the nurse give you some."

The nurse brought a cupful and forced them on Bennie, two and three at a time. After a few mouthfuls, he gagged up what was left in his gut, but she persisted until the surgeon came by and suggested gently, "Nurse, what'a you say we give our cowboy a few more minutes before any more?"

⚔ ⚔

As J.W.'s pediatric rotation neared completion, an infant with Down's syndrome was admitted for vomiting. The diagnosis was duodenal atresia: no food passed beyond the stricture immedi- ately after his stomach. His parents were young, healthy profes- sionals with nothing in their medical histories to suggest they might produce a Down's syndrome child, save the slim odds that it could happen to anybody. The couple was distraught, and though they were counseled by several factions of the nascent right-to-life movement, they chose to refuse surgery for their devastated son. The infant would be given an IV to provide fluids, but without an operation to remove the blockage, he would starve in a few days.

Several of the pediatric intensive care unit nurses refused to become involved in carrying out the death sentence on the damaged infant, so the patient was transferred to the corner of a lesser ward. More nurses protested, and meetings were arranged for all medical personnel involved in the infant's care. J.W. hadn't been gone from Viet Nam long enough to fully accept the death of a child, for whatever divine reason, and most certainly not as an act of human reckoning. It was especially hard to let the child die when his only crime had been a conception that included an extra, submicroscopic strand of atoms called a chromosome. This was, however, one situation in which J.W. would only sit and listen. There was nothing a junior medical student could add. This was hospital policy.

On the night the condemned infant was transferred to the corner of a forgotten pediatric ward, J.W. was walking the tranquil halls searching for bread to make toast. A gargantuan man in a blue hospital blazer stomped past J.W., fire in his eyes. J.W. felt the floor stop rumbling when the man stopped, turned toward him, and called back, "You on the pediatric service?"

"Yes, sir."

"Do you know about the child with Down's syndrome?"

"Yes, sir."

"I need some help. Some of us here in the hospital aren't going to let him die because the parents don't want him. The surgeons are ready, and they want me to bring him to the operating suite."

The man's face tightened as he bristled, "That infant is healthy. If they fix the problem, he'll do fine. Down's syndrome?

Do you know some of these kids have normal intelligence? That's more than I can say for his parents and half the administrators around here. Come with me."

"Sir, I can't do that, sir."

J.W. did not believe those words leaked from his mouth, but he had judged very quickly that the man was asking him to obey a prohibited order. Even in the army, it was the soldier's duty to disobey a command he knew was patently illegal. J.W. had disobeyed one in Viet Nam, the night he was ordered to fly into a monsoon. The general insisted J.W. crank the HUEY's turbine engine, load his crew, and get him back to Saigon and his air-conditioned, dry apartment.

"No, sir. The weather's too ugly, sir. It's unsafe, sir."

"I am giving you a direct order, Lieutenant! Fly this chopper to Bien Hoa, now, or I'll have your commanding officer rip the wings off that flight suit. Do you understand me?"

"Sir, the crew, my crew and my passengers and my aircraft, are my responsibility, sir. I am the pilot in command. I respectfully submit that I have made the decision it is not safe to fly tonight, sir."

Lieutenant White, his co-pilot, marched to J.W.'s side, and the crew fell into formation behind them. Closest was Thunder Chicken, the crew chief, with his beak held high, nostrils flared, like a hound on the scent. Next came Pecos from Hell's Kitchen, another working-class stiff with nothing to gain by taking sides in so one-sided a fight.

The general fumed for forty-five minutes, as do all bullies when their bluff is called, but he backed down, and by the end of the week the crew and J.W. had forgotten the incident, at least they weren't swanking about anymore. At the P.M. briefing on Friday, J.W.'s commanding officer tossed him a letter from Saigon Command. Charges of insubordination had been brought against him and his crew. J.W. crumpled the letter, tossed it on the ground, and pretended to spit on it.

The CO growled, "Very impressive. We'll put you in for an Oscar. Meantime, pick it up and read the rest of it."

In the next sentence, the III Corps commander, himself, ordered that the charges be dropped and that the crew be cited for having acted with courage and fixed purpose in the face of adversity.

Thunder Chicken broke out the beer, though bitched, "I'm a fortified wine man, myself, sir." The colonel agreed to give them the night off, eight full hours on terra firma. He accepted, with gentlemanly aplomb befitting his Southern heritage, the bottle of cheap Vietnamese wine Co-pilot Lieutenant White had stashed in his flight bag. The colonel placed the gift under a towel and strode single-mindedly to his hooch.

Now, years later, standing before a hospital official, J.W. felt himself in the same mire. He wondered if the civilian world was buttressed by the strains of justice that ordered the military.

The security guard blustered with moral and religious pronouncements as J.W. stood at attention, watching his medical career flush itself away. He forced his neck back to search the man's brilliant red face. The bellowing demanding J.W.'s compliance rose a dozen decibels. J.W. pictured instead Pecos, his door gunner, and tried to imagine what had become of his friend from the Puerto Rican barrio in Lower Manhattan. J.W. wondered if Pecos' eyes had ever met Sharra's, at the border between their lives, and if he had ever made love to a woman as beautiful. What would Pecos have said to her in Spanish as he reached his climax? What would she have whispered?

J.W. touched the image of Sharra's face, heard her soft voice, and remembered the engagement ring. "It's better this way," he whispered to himself, "J'Aveed needs a father, and so does Khai. It's better this way."

When the haze in J.W.'s head cleared, the man grunted angrily, spun around, and loped off in a rage. He bashed open the doors of the ward on which the marred little boy lay starving. He swept the child from the bassinet, passed J.W. without a word, and strode toward the operating room. His eyes were glazed, scared, though driven. The night charge nurse followed into the hall and called, "Mr. Kennedy, please stop!"

But he kept marching resolutely, cradling the infant. "You must stop, Mr. Kennedy!" she yelled frantically while running back to the ward to phone security. In their wrinkled blue blazers, the two gray-haired hospital guards on graveyard blocked the OR doors. Their colleague stood at attention, seething at his co-workers, but he walked back to the ward. He silently handed the child, not gently, to a student nurse and stalked out. When the infant died the next morning, there was no fanfare, and no recrimination, though many questions lay in the wake of the baby's short life. By the end of the week, the matter had faded, "… as do most things in four days," Seltzer suggested.

J.W. was gone from the pediatric service before Bennie left the hospital. The boy's dad called and invited J.W. to ride a shift. He gave J.W. the radar gun and told him to choose the next few victims. "Give 'em ten over," Trooper Stevenson suggested. "That's what most of us do."

"Not that guy, Slimmer."

"He's a piece of work."

J.W.'s first stop was for sixty-seven miles per hour in a fifty-five. They pursued for only a quarter mile before the driver, an elderly woman, pulled over. "Little old lady, probably just confused some. I don't know. Something smells wrong, though," Trooper Stevenson mumbled as he sat in the patrol car waiting for the dispatcher to check the woman's license. Bennie's dad presented the summons, which left J.W. cheerless, until, twenty minutes later, with siren screaming, they arrived at a fatality accident. The woman they had stopped had rolled her car off the side of the turnpike. Fire had consumed her overturned prison. Witnesses said she was driving like a madman, her face contorted in anger as she passed car after car.

J.W.'s next stop was for sixty-one. "That's the law," J.W. growled. "If the public doesn't like it, too damn bad. Vote and get it changed." Bennie's dad called him Trooper Slimmer, Jr. It was the only time J.W. ever saw the man laugh.

⇌ ⇋

J.W. met Seltzer for lunch in the hospital cafeteria later that week. Sharra sat alone in a corner. It was hard to see her hands, and though he could not make out the sparkle of an engagement ring, J.W. was sure his mind was playing tricks on his heart. Seltzer asked what J.W. was staring at.

CHAPTER NINETEEN

The Premature Infant Intensive Care Unit, the PICU, the next rotation on J.W.'s menu, was a realm of blood vessels more fragile and harder to pierce than Mr. Jenks'. A long, thin room in another remote corner of the hospital was filled with cramped rows of isolettes, each an intrauterine environment of warmth created by overhead lamps. Two and three-pound infants barely able to move their fingers lay within, their eyes protected from the light with little black masks—so many Lone Rangers and Zorros. J.W.'s pinkie boasted greater girth than the preemies' arms, his index finger bulkier than their legs. Most of the diminutive patients were intubated with straw-sized, crinkled, plastic tubes that reached far into their lungs.

Khai asked if the preemies cried, but when J.W. thought about it, he realized the only sound in the ward was the round-the-clock, incessant hissing of the mechanical respirators, and the rapid-fire, two-thousand bleeps per minute of the banks of cardiac monitors keeping watch over the twenty miniature patients. A rare preemie had only one IV line; most prickled with three or four. Adults needed one-hundred-twenty-five ccs of fluid an hour from an IV to survive; these kids got 5cc's an hour, a teaspoon's worth of saline, and even that tiny amount of fluid often puffed them up like over-hydrated sponges.

All the preemies had problems breathing. That was where the research money was going, and Union was a major recipient of those funds. It was because of Dr. Bagwan Chopra's landmark work on preemie respiratory disease. Dr. Chopra, J.W.'s first-year mouse lab professor, had discovered that baby lambs' lungs were similar to those of the preemie. All the students taking the intensive care rotation were privy to his personal teaching in the form of daily mini-lectures. In the middle of one of those classes, Dr. Chopra suddenly stopped and stared, recognizing J.W. as the student who had been unhappy exploiting mice two years before. He crooked his head, as if he was surprised J.W. was still a member of the class, but said nothing and went on to describe lambs as easy to keep, gentle, and nice creatures.

J.W. whispered to Seltzer, "Also makes a hell of a kebab."

Just before Christmas vacation, Dr. Chopra returned to the intensive care unit to present his final lecture on breathing problems in preemies, extolling again the nobility of the lamb. Looking straight at J.W., he presented the students an opportunity to further the cause of animal rights by challenging the committed amongst them to take home seven of his little darlings for the holidays, while he was in India.

Dr. Chopra's stare was not the only one J.W. felt, and he slowly raised his hand and muttered, "I'll take one home, sir, but not the herd."

"Oh, this is very good! Von vill be fine. It is unfortunate that it is only for two veeks."

Khai knew nothing of farm animals, only of evanescent cats. J.W. envisioned Khai as the envy of every child in their tightly packed, inner city neighborhood, and he pointed to a woolly creature that Dr. Chopra's experienced hands plucked from the cage.

When Dr. Chopra placed it with great care into J.W.'s arms, he added, "Oh, you must be very careful. Yes, you must alvays vatch here." He pointed to a three-inch wide, foot-long bald patch on the side of the lamb's chest, along the center of which ran an industrial strength zipper.

"Dr. Chopra, excuse me, sir, but why does this sheep have a zipper in its side?"

"Oh, Doctor. Dis is an excellent question. You see, dis vay, ve have free access to animal's lung, to experiment and determine vhich medicines do vat tings to lungs. But you mustn't open it. It vould cause pneumothorax, a packet of trouble."

J.W. loaded Mao into the wicker basket on El Buraq and tied him down with a bungee cord. Krista seemed amused, but only initially. The first topic of concern raised by J.W.'s wife, as she backed another step away, was where to keep it. They debated Krista's recommendation to leave him in the frigid Boston winter, out in the postage stamp-sized backyard. "He's got a wool coat, for God's sakes. He stays outside."

J.W. cajoled with a cold smile, "This one's a house pet. Never been outside. He'll die if he stays in this cold. This is a gentle creature. He's dedicated his life to saving premature human beings."

Krista shook her head no. "This is not a barnyard."

"It's a sheep. It's not like it's going to attack anyone. How much damage could it do?"

In fact, Mao didn't purposely do any damage. The diarrhea, squirted in small deposits throughout their very tiny home, was a product of the thirty or so pills J.W. was to shove down its throat twice a day. Within hours, the new carpet was deeply stained, as were the pine floors, Khai's bed, her mattress, their bed, their mattress, the kitchen linoleum, and the outside welcome mat, the latter when Khai opened the door to show her friends. That was when he escaped.

J.W. searched the neighborhood for nearly two hours and finally spotted him hopping up and down, moving mostly backward in the slush on Comm Ave. Actually, J.W. heard him first, coughing. Mao's nose froze as J.W. carried him the half-mile home.

Krista banished Mao to a cardboard box in the laundry room. He ate the carton. The diarrhea worsened. That night he bleated for eight hours. The neighbors, with whom they shared a brick wall, banged their fists. In the morning, any other husband would have been presented with an ultimatum. Krista, however, fed Mao. Khai played with him, and J.W. patrolled behind with a bucket and rags. Khai recommended they place him in Huggies. He ate the diaper. J.W. put Tabasco sauce on the next nappy, but he ate that, too. His diarrhea turned red, and there were bleats of pain each time he squirted. They finally took the washer out of the laundry cubicle and sacrificed what was left of the room. Mao worked his way behind the dryer and nibbled through the exhaust pipe, an insult about which they were unaware until Krista dried the load of rags and towels they had used to clean up after him.

J.W. took Mao back to the lab that afternoon. The pack of lambs was intact, screeching, pooping, and coughing. No one else, apparently, had acquiesced to Dr. Chopra's invitation. As J.W. pushed Mao's butt into the cage, the lamb squirted a stream of liquid scarlet at his boots and squawked in pain, but finally lay back down with his mates on the straw and fell asleep.

CHAPTER TWENTY

Toward the end of neonatology, lists for the next rotation were posted. J.W. noticed Sharra's name before he saw his own. They had both been assigned to anesthesia. His first thought was of the long hours in the hospital, the gentle time between cases, the relaxed atmosphere, the scrubs. It was a gift, but one J.W. didn't know what to do with. He supposed he was being tested.

Washing dishes that night, J.W. was so deep in anticipation and worry, he dropped a teapot they had carried home from Hong Kong. Khai and Krista were sitting at the table and looked up as J.W. threw the jagged pieces angrily at the trash can.

"Troubles, Bubbles?" Krista chuckled.

"Goddamn crap made in Hong Kong," J.W. grumbled as he left the room and went for a run. When he got back, the sink was empty. Khai was asleep and Krista was drinking a Rolling Rock and reading *Dr. Zhivago*.

"You still reading that? Man, that's years."

"It's a good story. Lot to learn from it, just like your medical books."

J.W. went to his desk and stared at the anesthesia text, but the image of Sharra's face clouded every page. He was confused. He had requested thoracic surgery as a next rotation, never even listing anesthesia as an elective, for he had no interest in learning the fine art of passing gas. In third year, though, you took what was offered and said thank you—it could have been gerontology. J.W. peered over the massive anesthesia textbook to his bulletin board, at the two purple hearts pinned to the cork. He scrutinized the gold medals he had been awarded for being wounded in combat. They had been his refuge each time he had come to a crossroads since Viet Nam. He often stared at them, as if they held the wisdom that had kept him alive in the war, but when he was being honest with himself, he allowed that they were just a place to hide.

The first Purple Heart was for the shrapnel that had blown into the back of his left calf. That was outside a primeval village in which they had landed to check the helicopter for damage. They had been circling, waiting for a lull in the fighting to drop in and rescue a downed, Australian helicopter crew. Thunder Chicken, J.W.'s crew chief from St. Louis, loved the Aussies, not so much culturally or linguistically, but for their Vegemite. Chicken worried he'd never find Vegemite in a Missouri ghetto, and he implored J.W. to dash in and save the crew from down under, for surely, they would gift him a lifetime supply of their bitter, salty, brown syrup.

"Sir, we gonna be great, sir. Heroes. Can you dig it?" he chortled over the intercom from his machine gun position at the left rear door. "Now, sir, I'm gonna buy your share of the Vegemite, no sweat, sir. I got money." He jabbered on and on, but became all business on his M-60 as bits of the Plexiglas started snapping out of the helicopter canopy into the co-pilot's face. J.W. spotted an open field and dropped in to assess the breakage.

On the ground, they found only a few bullet strikes to the windshield, and no structural damage. They laughed with fictitious bravado, lit cigarettes, and took a break. When Thunder Chicken grumbled that the Aussies were still in danger, and that they should get back on station, J.W. agreed, but first ran into the bush to take a whiz. As he was buttoning up, a crude, Viet Cong, 50-millimeter Sky Horse mortar round dropped from the torpid air, crashed through the trees, and came to rest in the mud just feet from his boots. J.W. saw the tailfin sticking out of the muck, and for a moment thought it was a dud. So many of the home-made enemy rounds were. Wisps of steam curled up from the miniature bomb as it cooled in the wet earth. J.W. tiptoed away, laughing aloud at these primitive children who would be their enemy, but a great cracking explosion erupted from behind, blowing him toward the ship. His calf caught fire as if drenched in blazing JP-4 fuel from the helicopter. Thunder Chicken grabbed J.W. and pulled him to the ship and tied an oily rag around his leg to stop the very superficial bleeding. They flew to a hospital near Saigon, talked a pretty nurse into washing J.W.'s leg, then cajoled her into putting him in for the Purple Heart. They flew away a few minutes later to search for the Aussies, but they had long since been rescued. Thunder Chicken would not talk to J.W. for the rest of the afternoon.

The second Purple Heart came months later flying a D-model, assigned to circle and support a firefight against North Vietnamese Army regulars concentrated over the Cu Chi tunnels. At first, the air force bombed and napalmed the forest until J.W.'s helicopter swooped in, firing its M-60 machine guns at burning enemy soldiers pouring from tunnels. Those underground passages had appeared first during the struggle against the French in the 1950s, and then resurrected twenty years later against the

Americans. As hard as the U.S. airmen sought to breach the earthen quarters with five-hundred-pound bombs dropped from B-52s, and Gatling gunfire from heliborne cannons, the enemy kept popping out of the rubble. They stood in the open, fearless, committed, tiny men firing into the sky with nothing more than rifles, fully aware how little was left of their lives or of their dreams.

After the bomber strikes, the Americans waited a day before sending the infantry in to sweep the area for BDA, bomb damage assessment. It was usually a safe, but awful, mission, with the carcasses of fallen soldiers littering the bomb craters, at least those who had not been eaten by the tigers who had learned that loud explosions often meant a free meal. This time, however, the NVA regulars were waiting for them, good soldiers, well-disciplined, well-equipped, a thousand miles from their families, aware they were never to return home—their only retreat, the mortifying steel of the American armaments.

As J.W. circled in the helicopter, exposing the NVA positions by drawing their fire, he felt the ship suddenly lighten. Lt. White pointed his Nomex-gloved index finger wildly at their fuel gauges as a radio call came from the boss circling a thousand feet above.

"Three Six, you're pissin' fuel!"

"I got eyes, sir!"

The HUEY burned three-hundred-and-fifty pounds of JP-4 an hour, but that was only when the fuel tanks weren't riddled with 50-caliber slugs. They were now losing that amount of gas every thirty seconds, and as the little fuel gauge needles neared the end of their ride, so did J.W. and the crew. The twenty-minute fuel warning siren whooped, followed by the piercing five-minute fuel warning an instant later, until J.W. pulled the circuit breaker on the warning siren so they wouldn't have to listen to it as they died.

When J.W. looked down from the overhead circuit board panel, they were in a dive toward the bomb craters. By instinct, J.W.

jammed the collective to the floor and searched the triple canopy jungle for a soft, green place to end their lives. J.W. shouted to his co-pilot, "Lieutenant, both hands on the collective, *now*! You pull like hell when I tell you, and not a goddamn second sooner. You got that, boy?" When they were eighty feet above the ground, J.W. would have him pull as hard as he could to lift the lever that no longer had hydraulic boost from their fuel-starved engine. The plan was to autorotate into a run-on landing, walk away with their lives, and face the barrage of inquests and paperwork to explain away the loss of a half-a-million dollars in twisted aluminum.

"Stare at the collective. Don't look out of this ship. If you pull collective too soon, you'll use it all up. We only got one shot at this," J.W. ordered a last time.

Lieutenant White obeyed, but for only briefly. When he couldn't stand it for one more second, he raised his head to see the ground coming up at a couple of thousand feet per minute. Reflexively, he wrenched the collective, squandering what momentum the main rotor had gathered. They fluttered like a maple seed into one of their own stinking bomb craters.

The HUEY hit with less of a burst than J.W. had feared, and for a flash, he believed they'd discovered a new way to autorotate. But that was before J.W. noticed himself flying through the Plexiglas canopy. His inertial seatbelt had failed, and he tumbled forward over his feet, landing at the bottom of a rain-filled crater. J.W. gulped for air, sucking in the disgusting water that burned his eyes and skin, water that had gone into chemical conspiracy with the cordite, the spent explosive of yesterday's American, five-hundred-pound bombs.

J.W. was blind. The putrid liquid ate at his clothes and his lips. He smelled so bad, his crew wouldn't come near. Thunder Chicken crawled off to find another crater in which to pass the time until the rescue chopper skidded in. He mumbled prayers it would be the Australians. The only trooper who stayed with J.W. was Lieutenant White, the co-pilot. He babbled apologies until midnight, when he calmed enough to speak of his home, a small town west of Cedar Springs. J.W. had never heard of Black Granite, and all he knew of the Rockies was snow. But Lieutenant White spoke longingly, poetically, of the primitive rivers, the spawning salmon, and the soaring granite peaks. He talked even faster when the rescue ship was shot down, never leaving J.W.'s side, ignoring his commander's zoo-like odor, and the blood that dripped from his nose.

"Hey, sir," he whispered around 2 A.M., "you ought to come up there to Black Granite some time. Stay with my family. You'll never leave."

J.W. promised he would.

At dawn, they sprinted from exploded hole to exploded hole, playing bomb crater bingo with a squad of VC who had come for parts from the downed helicopter. Over the portable radio, J.W. was ordered by the next rescue ship to pop yellow smoke to distinguish them from the bad guys. They tossed the first grenade, but the thick smoke of three other markers puffed yellow gas over the mile-long strike zone. "Someone's listening," the commander radioed to from above. That was followed by laughter on the speaker, but it wasn't in an American accent.

The CO ordered the crew to destroy the helicopter, but not go aboard, as the enemy might have booby-trapped the hull during the night. They crawled back toward the aircraft and, from a distance, threw three thermite grenades into the wrecked shell. The ship melted into a little ball of rare metals, stinking plastic, and the scent of Thunder Chicken's last bottle of Vegemite. Pecos had to restrain his distraught crew chief from running into the silver-white flames.

One of the B-52 bombs had unearthed a section of enemy tunnel, a hole just large enough to crawl through. Lt. White was the first to discover it. "Hey, sir, look at this. What have these people gone through? Man, they must really hate us foreigners." The two officers uncovered pitifully dank sleeping quarters, and each took a black silk hammock from its posts. J.W. stuffed his into the pocket of his flight suit and started to crawl out to the whap of a HUEY on a fast, wild, sideways approach. Thunder Chicken reached into the tunnel, grabbed J.W.'s arm, and while making gagging sounds, led him to the rescue ship.

They flew to the same hospital in which J.W. had been treated for his leg. The same cute triage nurse twisted J.W.'s broken nose, and a Donut Dolly came to take the information for Purple Heart Number Two. When the crew picked him up the next day, Thunder Chicken stared at the bandages over his nose and the cotton pledgets protruding from his nostrils. "Hey, sir, man, you look better than you used to, sir."

"Thunder Chick, that is insubordination, my man," J.W. warned. "You are off this crew. Report to the NCO club in Bien Hoa for your last days in this shithole."

"I'm short, sir, got everything to lose, but I still got a week 'fore I ETS. Be back in the 'hood in seven days, but I ain't goin' today, sir. You is stuck with me 'til a hour 'fore I leave."

Pecos also stayed to the end of his tour. Lieutenant White went home early, though. He had been promoted to pilot in command of a LOH, a tiny observation helicopter, a slot he held for just a week before he was shot down flying too low and too slow. The bits of his remains that were recovered were sent to Black Granite in a body bag. J.W. assured himself he would someday call the Whites and tell them their son had been a good man, a damn good pilot, a hero.

While the Purple Hearts were from a different epoch, J.W. kept them over his desk. How tied together those years and these had become. J.W. wondered if there was an escape from the war, then or now. Each battle followed the last, upstream, downstream, with the flow, against it. It was never clear which was the right way to be headed.

⊨⊣ ⊢⊨

J.W. left the house for a jog. Perhaps that would clear his head. The only problem was that the Purple Hearts, and the books, and the next rotation, and Sharra's image were there when he got back, and still there the next morning when the phone rang before 6 A.M. It was the dean of scheduling offering no apology for calling so early. The man said only, "Good morning. Do you want to switch your next rotation from anesthesia to thoracic surgery?"

"Sir, can I think about it for a while, sir?"

"Yes." He waited three seconds and added, "Time's up."

The gods were testing him more intensely. Two paths had opened, upstream, downstream. The fates had chiseled a spot in the surgery course and then leaned back to watch and laugh as J.W. struggled and sweat through the alternatives. He tried to stall, but the dean's impatient breathing became louder. J.W. also heard Krista breathing, lying by his side. "I'll take the surgery, thanks."

"You start today at eight. Good day."

CHAPTER TWENTY-ONE

In every profession, the sub-specialties are staffed by cadres whose personalities, and even physiognomies, suit that field.

In medicine, family practitioners are the common man, and perhaps a bit more generous around the waist than the cardiologists, who are often stick-like intellectuals. But vascular surgeons, like neurosurgeons, are a different breed altogether. These are technicians possessed with Biblical patience, and the facility to concentrate for hours on end without looking up from magnifying glasses, unaware that a shift of nurses has come and gone, and that day has hemorrhaged into night. Years of meticulously sewing tiny vessels and thread-like nerves fosters a fortress mentality. Others seldom enter their world, not even colleagues. In their very human hands, they possess the futures of fingers and limbs and sight and consciousness. Magnificent reputations flow into sewers, and brilliant careers are crushed under the weight of multimillion-dollar malpractice suits, because for thirty seconds a man thought about his impending divorce or his teenaged son's DUI—for thirty seconds of a thirty-year career.

Dr. Laird Van Noy had just been elevated to Chief of Vascular Surgery at County Hospital, a cog in Brookline Union's medical empire. J.W. had heard tales of his prowess to cut with both the scalpel and words. J.W. met him for the first time that morning at 8 A.M.

"Where the hell you been?"

"Sir, the dean just assigned me to surgery an hour ago."

"Ah, bullshit. This isn't kindergarten anymore," he grumbled.

J.W. scrubbed, gowned, and took his place alongside the operating table, conditioned by the time in Hong Kong across from Dr. Flowers.

"Who the hell invited you? Step back until I'm ready for observers from the peanut gallery."

J.W. thought perhaps Dr. Van Noy wanted a moment alone with the patient, to quietly reassure her, to ask God for strength to do right, but there was no holding of hands, no prayer for guidance. He just dipped his head and began.

Dr. Van Noy had grown up in New York City on the East Side, under the Williamsburg Bridge, only child of the founder of The Mounted Elk Hotel. A flophouse, The Elk had exposed young Laird to folks who had taken less care of themselves than might have been prudent. A fair amount of liquid refreshment was consumed on the premises, and Laird's father, an exceptionally large, powerful man, imbibed along with his clients, often to a savage degree. Though the boy was admonished to stay clear of the place when outbursts of alcoholic exuberance rocked the crumbling edifice, he was, nonetheless, drawn daily to a corner of the lobby to witness the various sideshows, fascinated and yet repulsed by the temper of poverty.

Laird Van Noy had accomplished more in school than anyone in his family, more, in fact, than all who had ever frequented The Elk combined. Laird was a neighborhood celebrity, touted by his father as "The East Side Einstein," until he was selected for a special high school that took him across the City on several bus and subway lines. By the time he arrived home at dusk, it was far too late to do the dog work around the hotel that had been his charge for all the years of his childhood.

His father finally withdrew Laird from the special school, opening a wide gulf, and Laird sassed him publicly as the reins tightened. They fought every day. The patrons sat in the tattered living room and took bets on who would manage the last word. After a while, it wasn't oaths that ended the confrontations; it was usually the back of his father's hand. That was until a late Saturday night, when the old man took a mighty swing at his intellectual, though mouthy, son, and collapsed on the floor of the lobby grasping his chest. He survived, but in a wheelchair, and never again spoke to Laird.

Through medical school and surgical residency, Laird developed great hands, a gut, a punitive streak, and the belief that one lived by the chronicle of his mistakes, not his triumphs. If you screwed up once, there was no way to redeem yourself, and he turned away from you forever.

He was hot as a pistol during surgery J.W.'s first morning. The circulating nurse, who was responsible for keeping canisters of oxygen open and ready in the operating rooms, had walked off for a break. Dr. Van Noy was doing a difficult arterial repair on a young woman, one of twins. Both had been injured in an automobile accident. While another team was at work fixing the first girl's relatively minor torn arteries, Van Noy was engrossed in the sister, who was fighting for her life.

The anesthesiologist warned Dr. Van Noy that they were low on oxygen. "Okay, I've got a great idea. Open another tank. If you're confused, they're the green ones."

"We don't have the wrench, doctor."

"Where the hell is it?"

Someone squeaked nervously that Nurse Jackson had been wearing it around her neck when last seen, and she was down in the cafeteria on break.

"Well, go down there and get it, goddamnit." Not a flicker of movement. "What the hell is wrong with you people?"

"If you say anything to that girl, she'll curse at you and maybe slap you in the face. And the administration won't do anything."

Van Noy threw down his scissors, growled, "Son of a bitch," and tore out of the operating room. He ran along the hall screaming obscenities through his surgical mask, all the way down the stairs into the hospital dining room. The tech looked up at him with a fury and hatred that would have floored a lesser man, but Laird Van Noy wagged a finger in her face and hissed, "Your ass is going to pay." He snatched the wrench from around her neck and stomped back to the OR to rescrub and regown. While it was only a few minutes before the oxygen was flowing freely, it was quite a time before the dust settled. The tech came back to the floor but decided to retire for the balance of her shift, though not before calling her unemployed fiancée, who thundered into the hospital and challenged the doctor out of the operating room into the hall for a fight.

The security officer arrived and placed his hand between the boyfriend and the OR door. This was at the precise moment the patient's family chose to spill out of the waiting room into the operating suite, riled by the screaming.

"Yes, ladies and gentlemen, there have been some raised voices. But don't you fret," the guard reassured, "everything's under control." The family, though shaking their heads suspiciously, dribbled back into the waiting room.

One of the nurses explained to the guard, "They're gypsies who just landed in the U.S. yesterday. Apparently, the father didn't know how to drive, but he bought this van anyway. They weren't a mile away from the dock before he flipped it off the

Harvard Bridge. Had to pull them up from the bottom of the Charles."

With no insurance and all their funds invested in a submerged vehicle, the twins were brought to County Hospital, where Dr. Van Noy was consulted and apprised there was little chance he'd be paid if he undertook the family's care. They had not been in the U.S. long enough to apply for welfare. While he agreed to accept them as patients, for to have refused would have touched off World War III with the hospital administration, he could not have dreamed his peace treaty with the CEO would be annulled by the wrath of a dozen landed immigrants, six furious operating room nurses, a hospital security officer stuck between a rock and a hard place, and a medical student who had shown up late on his first day, to say nothing of the desperately sick patient still on the operating table.

Aside from his foray to the cafeteria, and the break while the angry boyfriend was escorted from the hospital, and the return of the family to the waiting room, Dr. Van Noy had remained steadfastly at the operating table, now closing in on eight hours without so much as a sip of water. Finally coming to the end of the procedure, he took a deep breath and mentioned to the third anesthesiologist that day to take a place at the end of the table, "We'll be done in less than five minutes. Let me just take one last look around—make sure I didn't leave my watch inside this young thing."

Van Noy instructed the scrub nurse to put a retractor in the wound and afford him a broader field of vision. The exhausted woman, though, let the instrument catch one of the arteries he had painstakingly sewn. Bright scarlet spurted onto Dr. Van Noy's chest, his face, and into his eyes.

"Cocksucker!" he screamed, as he snapped a hemostat on the scrub nurse's index finger. She pulled her hand away so forcefully, the retractor flew out of the wound, arched across the room,

and clanged to the floor. It slid to rest next to the stand-by cir-
culator, a terrified, second-year nursing student who had been
urged to lie down in a corner of the OR to compose herself.

"Get me another scrub nurse, a real one this time!" Dr. Van
Noy demanded, "And what the hell are you doing on the floor?"

A female voice answered soothingly from the corner, "She's
not feeling well, Doctor."

"Well, why don't we all just lay down and rest? What the hell,
it's been a full day."

At the end of the procedure, Dr. Van Noy looked up and noticed J.W. in the corner to which he had been banished several
episodes before. "Go out into the waiting room and tell them
we've done everything in our power to help their daughter.
Something like, 'And while she's done well in surgery, there are
no guarantees,' or some such thing."

Dr. Van Noy escaped the OR through an ancient rear pas-
sageway just as J.W. was approaching the Roma family. They
stared at J.W as he spoke, were quiet when he finished, and quiet
when J.W. turned to leave. No one had responded to his offer to
answer as many questions as they had, and no one thanked him
or shook his hand.

At dinner, the overhead pager was a flurry of stat pleas for the intern
on Dr. Van Noy's service to report to the twins' room. J.W. had yet
to meet the intern, and drifted up to the floor to observe the care
of their surgical patient, but as J.W. entered the room, the entire
family, who had surrounded the bed, parted to allow him through.

"Thank God you're here. Are you the attending?" asked a
nurse emerging from the morass.

J.W. did not answer as he made his way through, sure he
would discover a real doctor somewhere in the crowd. He was,
though, the supreme medical authority of Room 203 South as

the girl's chest shuddered its last breath. The family started to vibrate in concert, an incensed, formerly powerless, now powerful mass, moving from the room into the hall. Three of the men tore away from the main body, screaming, throwing books, dinner trays, charts, and chairs. They wailed through the halls, unchecked, until the Mayor Kevin's riot police arrived with weapons unsheathed and visors in place. The show of force quieted the men, but that was apparently the cue for the women to take over. They screamed at the police in a language J.W. had never heard. An attractive, redheaded police officer, one of the SWAT team foot soldiers, removed her riot helmet, marched between the factions, raised her hand for order, and replied to the cries of the gypsy women, speaking in the same tongue in which they railed at her.

The chief of the gypsy distaff side, a woman with the blackest of jet-black hair and the blackest of jet-black eyes, stepped forward, not at all surprised the officer had spoken in her language. She, too, raised her hand to demand silence. The officer took another step forward and uttered an incantation. The gypsy women raised their arms and flailed about until the dark-haired woman lifted her hand higher. Arms thrashed again, but less vituperatively. The officer nodded to her fellow policemen, who moved forward to manacle the men.

The women accepted this quietly, until the police turned to lead their prisoners out of the hospital. As the screaming began again, a hospital administrator rushed from the elevator, offering in a conciliatory tone, "We are very sad your daughter died. Please forgive us for not saving her. Can't you see how hard we worked to help her, and all of you? We did our best."

The officer translated. There was muttering, but no screaming or arm-flailing. The administrator met with the police, who grudgingly released their captives. The officer and the dark-haired woman kissed each other's cheeks. Several of the men returned to the room, scooped up the living twin, and left the hospital.

Dr. Van Noy arrived an hour later, accepting without emotion the ream of forms thrust under his nose by the charge nurse. When she was out of earshot, he grumbled to J.W., "There's a lesson here, Doctor. I don't know why I can't learn it. I've gotten nipped in the ass enough times now. What is given away for free has no value, but what people have to sweat for, when they have to pay, that changes everything.

"I went to a medical conference in Rome last year. One of my Italian colleagues asked me to remove a neuroma from his foot. A stupid goddamn neuroma; I was glad to do it. Took a few minutes. Was fun to operate in another language. When we were done, he asked me about my fee.

"'Nonsense,' I told him. 'You are my counterpart, my colleague. I could never charge you.' He handed me a 25 lira coin, worth a penny or something, and told me, 'We in Italy believe that there is nothing for free. We must pay the doctor something; we must pay or the cure won't work.'

"The guy was right. It's the way of the world."

Dr. Van Noy sent two-dozen roses to the scrub nurse for his impropriety with the clamp. She sent them back, the cellophane still taped to the vase, filed an assault complaint, a rider to the one filed by the oxygen-wrench tech, and the sexual harassment complaint filed by the reposing student nurse, who had been incensed by the doctor's comment about all lying down together.

By the time Dr. Van Noy returned from a sudden vacation, the course in surgery was over, and J.W. had moved on to psychiatry.

CHAPTER TWENTY-TWO

Psychiatry was offered at both the inpatient asylum in the hospital, and the inpatient asylum at Saint Augustine's Institute. J.W. chose the latter, seeking relief from the faded, redbrick edifice of a hospital that had been his home for three years. The worst cases in the county were at St. Augie's, another attraction. J.W. had begun to question his own sanity, and desperately sought reassurance that he was not that bad off. Seltzer had chosen St. Augustine's as well.

The course began in the depths of winter. J.W. arrived at St. Augie's long before the sun, and left for home long hours after darkness had enshrouded the icy Boston roads. The silver lining was that, for weeks at a time, J.W. would not see the rust accumulating on the aging El Buraq.

J.W. chained his bike to the bumper of Seltzer's Corvette that first morning and gathered with his classmates around the lecture room table, joking nervously about the psychiatric shipwrecks with whom they would soon share the hour. As J.W. was busy scrutinizing Caaren Norberg's tee shirt, Seltzer grasped

J.W.'s forearm and muttered into his ear, "Medical school's a friggen Fellini movie! Jesus H. Christ, will you look at this!"

In the doorway stood a withered, elderly man hunched so far forward, the students at the table were gazing directly at the age spots on the top of his hairless head. The man forced his neck and eyes up to scrutinize, silently, the nest of innocent faces that stared back. A part of his scraggly white beard pointed at them, a portion at the floor, and a tuft of a dozen or so whiskers at the ceiling when he dropped into a Lazy Boy recliner at the head of the table. The man struggled with the lever until the chair snapped full forward. He exhaled a huff of frustration, and another as he pulled harder on the lever and pushed back on the seat. J.W. wondered why the mentally ill always wore their diseases on their sleeves.

It was 8 A.M., the hour all psychiatry students met for the daily lecture, to observe a real psychiatrist doing a real psychiatric evaluation on a certifiable nut. It was never clear why those tortured souls consented to allow their psychoses to be paraded before the squad of neophytes, but each morning, the students were promised a disheveled creature with an authentically atrocious disease from which they would never emerge.

From behind the Lazy Boy another figure appeared, an untidy woman in her thirties—greasy hair, greasy Birkenstocks, and a tattered, knitted book sack over her shoulder. Seltzer whispered, "Sixties, Pentagon anti-war riots."

J.W. mumbled, "Never had the pleasure. I was on the other side of the lines bayonetting hippies."

"You didn't miss much."

The woman fished a sheet of paper from her bag which the man took, but dropped when he groped around in his jacket pocket for glasses. He nodded to a straight-backed wooden chair when she rose from retrieving the paper. She sat stiffly, deferentially, waiting for the bony-faced man to speak. "I am Friedrich Gerstein, Director of Psychiatry, und zis is Choan. Ve begin."

"Ladies und gentlemen, you ah velcomed to zis psychiatry course. Ven you leaf here, you vil be conwersant in ze diseases of deprezzion, schizophrenia, und perzonality dizorder."

Seltzer caught J.W.'s smirk, and what J.W. thought was a reasonably subtle pointing of his index finger in Seltzer's direction at the mention of problematic personalities. Seltzer, however, kept a straight face as their professor commenced a diatribe outlining the appropriate behavior in his course.

"Zis is not a yoke!" he snarled at J.W.

The edges of Seltzer's mouth curled up uncontrollably, but when pierced by Dr. Gerstein's stone face, his lips sagged into a naughty dog's frown. "Ve ah faced here vis human beinks zufferink, vis pain deeper, more pwofoundt, zan canzer. Zey do not die of zeeze diseases. Zey lif a lonk time und zuffer und zuffer. It is our lifz vurk to addrezz zis pain."

He nodded to Joan, who read from a prepared text, assigning each of the students a personal patient to examine.

Dr. Gerstein's neck tightened but gave way, and his head dropped, though he went on speaking, staring into his lap. Seltzer scribbled on the corner of a spiral notebook, "Which is the inmate? You can't tell without a program."

Dr. Gerstein cleared his throat. He told them that diagnoses in psychiatry were to be made with the doctor's eyes and ears, for in the science of the mind, there were no mega-technological tests behind which to hide, and none in the pipeline. This was not surgery, or otorhinolaryngology, where x-rays revealed bottle caps stuck up kids' noses, hard signs and symptoms of illness. They were to be taught to listen to the patient, to what was said and what wasn't.

At 9 A.M., J.W. was introduced to Patricia Alverez, a thirty-five-year-old Mexican woman who had frequented psych units from Brownsville, Texas, to Bar Harbor, Maine, all within the past couple of years. She was entering day ten at St. Augie's, undergoing almost hourly counseling, waiting the three weeks for the antidepressant medication to drag her back to the world of the living. Despite the talk therapy, her disease had only deepened, and later that morning, she was scheduled to be treated with electro-shock therapy.

J.W. was appalled. That treatment was archaic, brutish, and dangerous. J.W. knew that. Everyone knew that. Why would Dr. Gerstein give the order to torture a patient while professing such compassion? J.W. wanted to warn Mrs. Alverez, to urge her to call a friend, to sign out AMA, Against Medical Advice. Though he had known her for only three minutes, J.W. considered rescuing her himself, refusing to be part of the barbaric medical malfeasance, perhaps even calling the dean at the medical school to seek help. But at the same time, J.W. realized that if he intervened, it would be the last act of his medical career. His orders were to take a history on Mrs. Alverez, not to assume her legal guardianship.

When she finally lifted her face, J.W. saw black, deeply beautiful eyes. But they were clouded with suspicion. He thought of the wariness in Sharra's, and his mind drifted as they began to speak. When J.W. drew himself back to the hospital room, he started on the standard psychiatric exam, but was barely able to hear what he managed to draw out of her. Her head hung for most of the hour, hands clasped tightly.

By her bed were Aztec sketches, though the edges of the meticulously drawn figures drooped as if they were human mouths curled down in despair, their withered forms all leaning to the right, headed downhill. They were colored with pencils in blues and blacks as deep as her eyes, exquisite forms, so intense in their sadness they exposed the depth of her disease. Mrs. Alvarez nodded subtly as J.W. looked at the drawings, and he took that as permission to thumb through the dozen sketches. In the center of each drawing was the abstract form of a human child, exceedingly emaciated, but with the same deep, black eyes of the artist.

"Did you do these drawings? They're beautiful."

When her head bobbed, he looked at a few more, smiled in appreciation, and placed the pile very gently back on the side table. He gathered his courage and asked if they could continue, though her answers remained barely perceptible. The consultation proceeded so slowly and painfully, J.W. wanted to jump up, run from the room, and leave her be. After a few more questions, he understood that rather than drinking from the waters of his cure, she was simply enduring him. Who was torturing her now? A real doctor should have been questioning her, not a novice.

Finally, after forty-five minutes and barely three lines of notes on his pad, J.W. stood uneasily, thanked Mrs. Alvarez, and escaped. He rushed past the cubicle in which Seltzer was deep in discussion with a huge man who sat restrained in a chair. Seltzer's patient also hung his head, not a word of his whisper audible. Seltzer looked up from the notes he was madly scribbling and rolled his eyes. His curled lip made J.W. chuckle; but it also embarrassed him to watch Seltzer at work, doing his job, when he, too, had little idea why he was there.

J.W. puffed out a huge breath, walked back to Mrs. Alvarez' room, knocked twice on the doorframe, and sat back down in front of his patient. She looked up at him as if he should be the one answering questions. Over the next hour, J.W. discovered she and her husband had come north from Mexico three years before for field work, domestic work, any work, something to do to feed their baby. She stayed behind in Boston while her husband traveled with bands of illegal immigrants searching for jobs. He sent his meager wages back to her, even after the baby died of meningitis. In a whisper, she told the wall how she had carried her son on her back, next to the tanks of pesticide, sweating across the fields of Mississippi. Her eyes remained dry.

J.W.'s training in psychiatry had come over the television, not from board certified learning courses, but from soap operas, watching actors portraying shrinks gently penetrating their patients' broken minds. TV patients, nearly always middle-class housewives, predictably collapsed in tears just seconds after the onset of the psychiatric probing. That was the cue for the psychiatrist to begin his treatment. J.W. remembered and delivered the next television line: "Was that hard for you?"

Mrs. Alvarez mumbled toward the wall, folded her hands on her lap, and sat there for an hour, until an orderly zoomed into the room, lifted her onto a gurney, and brushed past J.W. as if he were a chair. J.W. followed, a tail-wagging puppy, as his patient was rolled toward the treatment room. As he passed Dr. Gerstein's office, J.W. deserted the procession and knocked. The old man was trying to lift his head to stare out the window into the manicured grounds of the hospital he had founded and nurtured for thirty years. "Sit in front of me," he instructed as he pushed the buttons on this Lazy Boy, allowing the chair into a nearly flat recline. "How may I help you, Doctour?"

"Dr. Gerstein, I didn't think we did shock treatments any more. What's going on here?"

"Ah ha! You haf met Mrs. Alverez."

"Yeah, and anyone would be depressed if they had happen what happened to her."

"Zer is no ahgument vis zis." He paused. "Zo, zat means ve shut do nosing? Leaf her alone, Doctour?"

"Yes, no, I mean..."

"Vat do you mean?"

"I mean, there's got to be a better way. Let me talk to her some more. Let me try. She was beginning to open up. She told me about the baby and the pesticides."

Dr. Gerstein picked up the phone slowly and deliberately. He asked that Mrs. Alverez be brought back to her room. "If you got zat much out of her in vun session, you haf done your vurk vell. Please try. Oh, und Doctour, please no bizycles chained to motor carz in ze parkink lot. It makes ze patients excited ven zer ah crazy tinks goink on. Zey vant to know vich vard zat perzon is on."

J.W. spent two more hours with Mrs. Alverez. When her eyes reddened and her face dropped, he thought of Sharra. When the flicker of a smile finally crossed her lips, he thought of Sharra. J.W. wanted to leave for lunch with Seltzer, but he pretended he was sitting with Sharra and stayed. Sorrowfully, she repeated over and over, "It is the Lord's punishment. I must not steal. I carry the insectacida. I must not steal."

J.W. snuck into an open office and called Sharra that night. He told her of the Hispanic woman with eyes almost as magnificent as hers. "I want to try and tell her in Spanish, 'You only have the present moment and the future. The past is gone.'"

Sharra giggled, "You told *me* that once. So, now you want to be a Hispanic philosopher? Okay, here's how you say it…"

Her laugh turned a switch in his chest, and he blurted, "Sharra, I want to see you. I have to see you!"

She paused for so long, J.W. asked, "Sharra, are you still there?"

"I can't do that," she whispered. "I think I better go now."

The next morning, Mrs. Alverez listened politely and nodded at J.W.'s Spanish, but moaned over and over, "I must not steal. I carry the insectacida. I must not steal."

J.W. went back to Dr. Gerstein, who nodded toward the same chair. "Vat haf ve lernt?" he asked with a gentle smile.

"I don't know what she's talking about. She's perseverating about stealing and poison. She didn't kill her child. She didn't have a damn thing to do with it. Why can't you talk to her and explain that in terms she can understand?"

"Doctour, it doesn't matter vat caused it. Vat matters is zat she hazn't control of her mood. You zee, she is depressed. She cannot help it, no more zan a diabetic can lif mit oat inzulin. May ve 'ave your permizzion to restore ze chemicals in her brain now?"

Mrs. Alverez traveled the dull green halls back to the treatment room. J.W. was invited because she asked that he be present, but he conjured an excuse about having to report to the dean. Instead, he went home and told Krista.

"Look what you did. If the doctor said that's what she needed, who the hell were you to keep treatment from her for an extra day?"

"Yeah, you're right. I made a mess of things, including my grade in the course, didn't I? Do you think I blew it?"

J.W. waited for Krista's answer, but she left for the kitchen, and J.W. headed for the bedroom to escape in sleep. All he could imagine, however, was the long pause Sharra had made him suffer, an eternity, a game played with his heart. He lay in bed annoyed, then incensed, but he finally convinced himself his anger was over the way she did it, not the rejection.

At the hospital the next morning, J.W. stopped to see Mrs. Alverez first. She was out of bed, her hair combed. Her face had changed. She greeted him with the most subtle smile; her eyes had a trace of Sharra's sparkle. It made his chest tighten, and it made him sad. A stern voice came from the room across the hall. "Vel, Doctour, vat haf ve lernt?" J.W. turned to answer Dr. Gerstein, but he had shuffled off to the next patient.

After rounds, the third-year students gathered in the conference room. Next to Seltzer, drifting closer to him each day, was Caaren Norberg, the statuesque blond with crystal clear, azure eyes—the fantasy not one of them would ever consummate.

A handsome man with piercing, wild, emerald eyes was led into the conference room and seated at the head of the table. Other than his faraway stare, he was expressionless until he caught sight of Caaren. His eyes fixed on her golden hair, refusing to look away when Dr. Gerstein dropped into his chair. The professor introduced their patient and began taking a standard psychiatric history. "Vell, Issac, you are velcomed to our class. Sank you very much. Vhy are you in zis hospital?"

No answer.

"Vell, zen, plees tell us vhy ze polize brought you 'ere."

No answer. The doctor asked a third time, but Issac's attention remained riveted on Caaren, on her hair. Suddenly, he jumped out of his seat. "I have a statement to make to the press." Seltzer's magnified eyes rolled like plums behind the thick glass. Caaren's lips pursed, and she looked away. There were muffled giggles. Dr. Gerstein's eyes tightened as he glared at his neophytes—sudden silence.

"Blond pussy, man, that's what I want to say to the press. It be da bess." He looked at Seltzer and pointed. "You ever try it, muh fuckah? Y'all should before you roll yoh gotdamn eyes, mutha fuckah."

Issac paused and returned his stare to Caaren. "You know about blond pussy, don't cha? What them dudes say when they is doin' you? You know. They say blond pussy be the bess."

The students' lips curled up helplessly at the corners, but fell back to neutral when Dr. Gerstein lifted his head a few degrees. "Vell, ve shut get bahk to ze qvestion at hant, sir. Ven did first you come to ze hospital?" Dr. Gerstein asked as calmly as if he wished to know if the man took cream and sugar in his coffee.

"See, man," Issac leered, "it's the blond pussy like you that got me here," he muttered through gritted teeth, pointing at Caaren, whose face now flushed vermilion. In an instant, though, she straightened herself in her chair and stared back at him until he turned away.

During the questioning, Issac suddenly lifted his head and turned abruptly toward the window as if someone had called to him. He bellowed toward the window, "Man, my sister's wedding! Shit, just got to get to Texas, man. Can you understand that? Now get the fuck outta here 'for I cut yo damn throat."

He made a move toward the window, listened again, slapped his leg, and finally growled at the voices to which he, alone, was privy. But suddenly, he calmed, retook his seat, and stared off without uttering another word. Occasionally, his ears perked, an expression of terror his locking his face, as if he was propelled through a universe that moved Seltzer to whisper, "Shit, I'd rather be dyin' of *canzer*."

Most medical school rotations become the specialty to which students consider devoting a career—for a time. Each discipline had its own art and science, each specialty concentrating on a fascinating organ, a tiny body part to which a doctor's life energy might be devoted. As medical school progressed, students discovered that each organ held the capacity to fall victim to a fascinating array of diseases, any one of which could consume a millennium of study. At least that had been J.W.'s experience for the past three years, until that morning, when he realized for the first time just how committed one would have to be to science, to work, to the suffering of our fellow travelers, to take an oath to practice the discipline of psychiatry.

Sharra's voice was cautious when J.W. called that evening and told her about Mrs. Alverez. "I'm sorry I embarrassed you," J.W. sighed. "I couldn't help myself. It won't happen again. I promise. I'm sorry. It was unprofessional." She was silent. J.W. felt empty, hoping she would tell him what he wanted to hear, and frightened she might.

"It's okay. I'm glad your patient's better," she said softly.

Though J.W. had promised himself it was time to forget about her, he drove past her apartment that night, circling the block many times before he lost his nerve and went home. He called Seltzer early the next morning. His friend listened patiently and promised he would keep it to himself, but added, "Who did you think you've been hiding this from, anyway?"

J.W.'s heart sank in remorse before rebounding into his mouth in dread. It was, though, strangely, a very pleasant permutation of emotions, J.W. told Seltzer. He felt alive again, for the first time in many years. "What should I do?" J.W. asked.

"What do you want to do?"

"You sound like you're taking a fuckin' history from a patient at St. Auggie's. I don't know what I want to do. If anything happens with Sharra, I'll die of guilt when it's over. I know I will. But if it doesn't happen, am I'm going to feel empty like this forever? I don't know what the hell to do. I'm a hurtin pup, Seltzer."

"You're playing with fire, J.W. She wants to see you, too. She doesn't know what to do, either."

"How do you know that?"

"She told Natalie."

"Oh, shit. Why the hell didn't you tell me?"

"'Cause Natalie saw it in your eyes, and she wasn't about to get in the middle of you and Krista, the two nicest people she knows. My advice? Drop it. Forget about 'er. You got a lot to lose."

A great weight lifted from J.W.'s chest. Sharra's rejection was no longer so biting a heartache; no longer the quest she had been minutes before. J.W. could look at her and know she cared—it might even be their silent secret. There was a flicker of relief, but just for a moment before the wave of loneliness swept back over him, and it hurt all over again. J.W. wanted to call her even more.

The next morning, Sharra was waiting in the cafeteria at St. Augie's. She asked, nearly inaudibly, for J.W. to join her, but stiffened and blurted before he sat down. "I'm leaving Union."

"Why? Do you just want to me to leave you alone? Just say so, Sharra, and I promise I will. I never meant…"

"Of course not. And I will tell you why I have to, but if you tell anyone, Marshall, Natalie, anyone, it will cost me my life."

"What!?"

"J'Aveed's father is one of the madmen who have taken over Tehran. He threatened to have my aunt and her children murdered if she didn't tell him where I was. She wouldn't talk, so he had her gang raped. Then the muftis, you know, the ayatollahs, convicted her of sex out of wedlock and threw her in jail for ten years. After that, the others were happy to talk. So, now he knows where I am. He will come here and take J'Aveed back to Iran. I've got enough credits to graduate. I am going to live…I can't tell you where."

"Please tell me."

"I can't. If I tell you, and they find out you know, they will hurt Khai until you tell them."

"Khai?"

"To them, your child has no value on Earth except as an instrument to punish blasphemy. The ayatollahs are behind it, scratching to gain control of the culture. Nothing matters in Iranian politics except moral control over the population. They do it with Sharia—Islamic Law. Death of an infidel, and a female to boot, has no meaning. It is not even a death, because it was never a consecrated life. My husband's mosque in Teheran will even pay for his trip to the U.S. and back, and for their agents here in America to kidnap J'Aveed, drug him so his father can take him back to Iran."

"What?"

"J.W., listen to me. According to the Koran, J'Aveed is his property, his chattel, as am I. When I am found and J'Aveed is under his control, his father will give the order for the agents to beat me to death, or maybe even stone me. To those who do the stoning, it is not an illegal act. It is an act of godliness demanded by the Koran. I defied the Koran by taking his son. Since the Koran says *everything* must be done to maintain social order, and Sharia tells us how to do it, anyone who challenges the Koran, defiles the social order, and that condemns them as enemies of peace. Execution by hanging or firing squad is too good for them. The stone is God's will."

J.W. was speechless. "But why you?"

"I'm sure you've heard it thousand times. We were Baha'i, and I married a Muslim, into a wealthy family, the Bakhtian. I was fourteen. It was for financial reasons. My father had been a business man in Turkey, and his family wanted to expand and open shoe stores in Istanbul."

"You were fourteen?"

"Just. It's the way it is there. And they made me get pregnant right away to sanctify the marriage, *and* the business contracts. With J'Aveed born into the father's family, I was forever their property. He beat me, my mother, and even touched my sister. There is no such thing as a protection order. When my father disappeared, my mother sold everything in the house for pennies. You should have seen the eyes on the vultures, old ladies in burkas, running through the house, pulling paintings off the walls, throwing a few rials at the infidel, Baha'i bitch—less than the cost of a slice of bread. But we got enough for passage over the mountains into Turkey. We went to the American Embassy in Ankara and applied for political asylum."

"Your father disappeared?"

"He knew the Shah, Pahlavi, from the time they were children. They hated each other. Too complicated to explain. The Savak, the Shah's secret police, came in the middle of the night. We never saw him again.

"Look, J.W., all you have to know is that they are looking for me. We are going to another city to hide. Your government is helping us."

J.W. rubbed his forehead and tried to say something, but it came out as a sigh.

"I just wanted to say goodbye. You are the gentlest man I ever met. I love talking to you. I could do it forever. I only wish it had been in a different time, but that is our fate."

"What about Arthur? Is he going with you? I'm sorry. That's none of my bee's wax."

"We're not seeing each other anymore. His parents were not thrilled with his choice of... Anyway, there are a lot of things about him you don't know. And I'm the one who should be apologizing. I'm sorry." She jumped up and ran from the cafeteria.

In his pigeonhole that afternoon, J.W. found a white envelope of thick, creamy paper. A note from Sharra wished him luck and told him he would laugh about the whole thing someday. She signed it, "Fondly." There was a P.S.: "I won't laugh." At the very bottom was a tiny, barely legible, telephone number. The area code was LA. J.W. recognized it from the number the dean had given him in the Philippines to contact Mr. Maldonado. There were also a few letters written in the tiniest script—*Ayşe.*

The last week at St. Augie's dragged interminably. J.W. did night duty on purpose, to keep from going home, to keep from spilling his heart and destroying what was left of his marriage. The medical students did physicals on the patients the police brought in and tossed into padded rooms. Seltzer thought J.W. was particularly suited to deal with the criminally insane. In fact, J.W. got along very well with them, right up until his last night. A young woman in restraints was hauled in and placed on a bare cot in the holding room. She had long, wavy, blond hair held by a red bandanna. She wore just a bit of makeup, her teeth were white and as straight as his, and she was dressed in pressed slacks and a crisp beige blouse. J.W. stared at the smudges on her shirt and on her knees.

"The police dragged me," she accused defensively.

J.W. was assigned to evaluate her. There were no chairs, so J.W. sat on the padded floor. It was hard to write notes in the subdued light.

"Doctor, this is an outrage. I am being incarcerated for no reason. Do you have children?" She continued before he could answer, "A disgusting man in our neighborhood, Brookline of all places, exposed himself in front of my four-year-old daughter. I must have called the cops a hundred times about the asshole. I heard Heather scream, so I ran out. I saw him. Right there in front of my baby, his ugly goddamn thing hanging out. I picked up a stick to beat the shit outta the son-of-a-bitch. I had every right to wallop him. I mean, he was exposed. The police even saw him. He walks, and I'm held here? My daughter is alone. Someone has got to listen. Please help me."

Brookline? That was the most fashionable area of Boston, home of the better attorneys, doctors, and the Kennedys. "You're getting railroaded. I've heard stories about injustice like this. Sometimes a doctor has to make choices, even if they aren't popular. It's called integrity. You wait here for a minute. Let me see what I can do."

J.W. left the room to search for the staff psychiatrist, but he had left the hospital for dinner, leaving J.W. the ranking medical professional in the facility. He, though, was at ease, having been in this position, in control, many times in the army, as a company commander. He returned to the padded cell, untied the patient, and escorted her to the admitting office, where he promised they would make the necessary calls to get her right home. As they left the secured area, passing through the last of the locked doors, she screamed, "Doctor!"

J.W. turned to her. She kneed kicked him in the groin, pushed him backwards against the wall, screeched, and ran past the admitting desk, middle finger wagging over her head. She was around the corner and through the one unlocked door in the entire hospital before J.W. managed to pull his hands from his groin. Admitting called the cops, and J.W. was interrogated for an hour. When the police left to search for the escaped prisoner, J.W. was banished to the on-call room to wait for the staff psychiatrist.

J.W. was treated well. In a calm voice, the psychiatrist queried, "Are you aware tomorrow morning is the end of this course? Are you aware that is when your grade will be announced?"

J.W. cared not a lick about his grade, only being done with St. Augie's. The major problem J.W. saw in his present situation was, if he had really failed psych, one of the core courses, he would have to take it over again. But he relaxed as he calculated that he had already earned honors in all of his clinical courses. One flunk, he laughed to himself, didn't amount to a hill of beans.

As the sun rose over the Charles River, J.W. crept down to admitting and checked to see if his little fugitive had been recaptured. Back she was, but had been transferred, in irons, to a locked ward at the main hospital. At 9 A.M., the psychiatrist's assistant called the class to the conference room. One by one, they were directed to Dr. Gerstein's office to learn their fate.

J.W. was first. The old man was hunched in his Lazy Boy. The back of the chair suddenly lurched forward, squashing him. He spat, "Oy vey, not again." He turned his head toward J.W. "Und it's you. It should be you in zis chair suffocating."

J.W. dropped to his knees in front of the chair. "No, no! You ah out uff order! You must not beg!"

J.W. poked through the mass of circuits and gears, saw a hanging wire, plugged it back in, and the jaws opened. Dr. Gerstein leaned nearly all the way back so he could look J.W. in the eye. "You ah committink zuizide, Doctour, you know! Now you get in ze chair, und *I* pull ze wire." He smiled. "Zo, vat haf ve lernt?" He paused. "You zee, ve must be objectif. You must get ze facts in medicine, alvays bos sides, ze art und ze zience. It vas right to look into zis woman's complaint last night, but Doctour, you sink ze polize are arresting people for zer fun? I tell you not."

Dr. Gerstein wriggled to take off his suit coat, and rolled up his sleeve. On his forearm was a tattooed number. "Compliment uff Dachau," he muttered with less irritation in his voice than if he had been disciplining a wayward psychiatry student.

J.W.'s first thought was to tell him about Seltzer's family, but he realized Dr. Gerstein was speaking to him, not to the rest of the class. A man of his depth and position. "You know, I shoot hate ze polize. I remember zem from ze time ve ver beink round-ed up in Berlin. I hated ze ausority ze had to take my life, und my mutti und fatti und sent us to Austria to ze campz. Ve knew vat vas ahead. Ve all knew. Zer vas no ezcape. Zey ver omnipotent. But in ze campz, I lernt zey ver only as almighty as ve let zem be. Hat ve fought back, only if ve hat fought back. Ah, but zat is gone now. Ze put me into a vice und…a crazy man experimented…to see how much can bend ze human spine. But zat is zen, und now I haf zis chair, und a friend to fix it. I am lucky. Ve vil mizz you, Doctour Veathersby. Oh, und you haf ernt honors in zis course. Try und remember vat you haf lernt in zis time. And maybe you vill like to become a psychiatrist?"

CHAPTER TWENTY-THREE

That summer J.W. spent a few days each week on his own in the hospital, trailing attending physicians, enjoying the relaxed atmosphere, and even the nurses, who occasionally helped him treat patients. J.W. spent as much time back on neonatology as he could steal away from home, learning to perform lumbar punctures and to place arterial lines into three-pound preemies. The pressure of exams and grades had withered, and now there was medicine to be learned. He began to love the hospital, even at night. He looked forward to seeing his patients; they looked forward to seeing him. Pearls of clinical wisdom were offered generously, those informal days of August, by attending physicians too busy to allow themselves any teaching during the year. J.W. observed brain surgery and heart surgery, and he helped deliver babies. His eyes always clouded with mist as a new life embarked on its voyage, a habit he couldn't seem to break from the night Khai had come into his life. The obstetrical nurses and the OB doctors found that behavior peculiar, and it wasn't long before the dean had him in. "You okay, J.W.?"

"Never been better, sir."

"You getting along okay on OB?"

"Yes, sir. Never been better."

"Good, good. I guess one of the doctors was concerned that you seemed sad, or upset, that you were crying or something. You okay? Look, medical school's a challenge. It's a tough life. Maybe you've never been pushed this hard before. It's okay. The only reason I mention it is that nurses can be judgmental sometimes. It can make it hard to work in the hospital if they think you're weak. I don't mean you are weak. Just...just take it easy, okay?"

"Yes, sir. I think I understand. I mean my eyes got red. I didn't break down bawling or anything. I wasn't sniveling. I never said a word other than, maybe, 'Wow, what a miracle.' I didn't even say it out loud, really. Just to myself."

"Like I said, there's two camps out there. Doctors and nurses. Doctors are in charge, no matter all the hooey about working in teams. Nurses know it. Life's not a team, regardless of what Human Resources babbles. He who has the power must protect it, or it vaporizes. You look weak, that challenges the whole class of doctors—their authority. Gives the nurses something to hang their hats on. But see, the nurses are too scared to jump in until they get a whole gang together. Safety in numbers. Then it's a team all right, a platoon, unhappy at home, scratching for some-thing to make the doctors look bad, snatch some of that dominion for themselves. Remember, doctoring isn't miraculous diagnoses and brilliant cures. It's more about surviving in a society that's floating on a ship whose rudder has come loose. I'm not looking forward to the next few decades. Anyway, just take it easy, okay?"

⊷⊶

The first rotation of autumn was neurology at County Hospital. Dr. Van Noy saw him in the halls and bought him a cup of coffee in the cafeteria. The doctor's father had just died. "Cirrhosis," he said softly, shaking his head sadly. "He was a character, that one.

I wish he would have come here, just once, to see that his son had done good. I was his only link with eternity, the poor bastard. He escaped from Bergen Belsen with nothing, and he died with nothing."

J.W.'s jaw dropped. Before medical school, J.W. had never known anyone who knew anyone who had survived the Holocaust, yet Dr. Van Noy was the third person J.W. had met in the past two years with an umbilical link to those darkest days. "Excuse me, sir, I don't mean to be presumptuous, but I think you're a good man. I'm sorry you take so much crap."

"Well, Doctor, I've brought most of it on myself, and to be frank, it's been worth the pain. I told you once that I made a mistake by giving care away for free, that it always spits back in your face. I should never have said that to you. You just do it, and worry about the cost later. If you want to bitch about it, that's fine; it's a good way to blow off steam. Just never turn anyone away because they're poor."

J.W. had heard that same entreaty before, in the army, in Ranger School, from a fellow soldier, a Native American whose baby brother had suffered permanent brain damaged because no one would see him. It was a federal holiday and the reservation clinic was closed—the private doctors in town all turned him away.

But J.W. had been pinching pennies for so long, it was hard to drag himself out of the mindset of poverty, to believe he would ever be in a position to work for no pay at all.

Van Noy saw the confusion in his eyes. "Soon, you'll have more goddamn money than you ever dreamed of, Doctor. You'll have earned it, and you'll go on earning it, but it still won't be enough. So, you don't need to squeeze the last drop of blood out of a turnip. It isn't natural."

Neurology was an exact science. Nerves did what they had been destined to do, and there was no arguing with the objective signs they left in their wake when acting badly. Their impulses were measurable, their distribution standard. The harder one worked in that rotation, the more a student learned. He could not get enough, often spending the evenings sauntering the halls with his neurology team, the intern and junior resident, before rushing home to sleep, avoid Krista, and fly back on his bicycle at five or six in the morning.

When he allowed himself the luxury of thinking about a subject other than medicine, it was knee jerk guilt over spending so much time in the hospital. Medicine had weaseled itself into his life, a mistress into whose clutches J.W. had happily fallen. Sharra was gone, and the healing power of time and of loving his work softened the pain of waiting for the call that never came. J.W. laughed at the span of time, the years on curving roads it had taken to unearth his passion. As hard as he tried to find balance, he was moving faster and faster along a path that led away from the utopia he had promised Krista.

~=++=~

Krista, Khai, and J.W. drove south to New York to see Bobbie Jo and Bernie for New Year's. J.W. felt guilty basking in the warmth of his exhilaration as the miles slipped past on the Turnpike. There was reward for effort, for the belief that if you held on for one more minute, then for another, and one more, it would happen. It was authentic; dreams were not idle, misdirected, wasted, neurologic impulses—his were being realized.

Bobbie Jo and Bernie had moved to the center of New York, to an apartment in the shadow of the Empire State Building, its mass looming outside their bedroom window. The Stanford White brownstone had the same charm that had been incorporated in the Tiffany Building and the Washington Arch, White's Early-Twentieth-Century architectural masterpieces. The building was aged, but built with a care and artistry long since abandoned in the City.

Their flat was on the sixth floor. The carved mahogany trimming and the vaulted ceilings had been painted with cheap white paint years before, but Bobbie Jo had stripped and stained it deftly. It reminded J.W. of his Eighteenth-Century rooms at the Sorbonne.

The Weathersbys had been invited to stay in the apartment over the holidays while Bobbie Jo and Bernie went off to Mallorca. Bernie laughed that he had gotten rich again, having expanded the tape business to include cardboard boxes to which he had assigned various levels of merit. He presided over two warehouses, both stocked to the rafters with boxes and boxes of tape, and boxes and boxes of boxes.

Before leaving on their trip, Bernie drove J.W. to the docks to survey his inventory. Though the dust was overwhelming, Bernie sucked deep breaths of the air, as if he were an escaped prisoner tasting his first lungfuls of freedom. He was in wonderland. He walked softly and smoothly through the skinny aisles, oblivious to the carcasses of long-ago crushed and poisoned rats, vermin so large they rivaled those of Hong Kong. Sparrows by the thousands inhabited the roof joists, chirping deafeningly and drooling tons of guano onto the rotting wooden floors. The tour complete, J.W. duly impressed, they settled onto the deserted loading dock. J.W. envied the man for having built an empire out of nothing.

"The Prince of Packaging," Bernie dubbed himself majestically.

"The King!" J.W. decreed

Bernie rolled a joint, started to offer it to J.W., but pulled his hand back unsteadily. They sat and talked for an hour, Bernie smoking a second and a third, until J.W. pulled the keys from Bernie's pocket and drove the BMW back to mid-town. As they turned onto Madison Avenue, Bernie asked J.W. to drop him off, "Just for a second. I need to buy some groceries," but Bernie disappeared into a laundromat, and when J.W. whirled around the block again, Bernie was standing in the gutter weaving. He stumbled into the car and fell back silently.

Bobbie Jo packed the car while Bernie sat in a corner staring out at the gray city and nodding off every few moments. Khai tried to play with him, for he had been gentle with her earlier, but he was now so nearly comatose, J.W. thought he might have had a stroke. When Bernie half-crawled to the bathroom on his own steam, Bobbie Jo took advantage of his semi-upright posture to guide him to the elevator and off to Spain.

Khai used the potty frequently—everywhere they went. After Bobbie Jo and Bernie drove off, however, she spent a protracted period in the bathroom with the door shut tightly. When she emerged at J.W.'s insistence, her hair was dripping wet, and J.W. growled at her for using the shower without permission. But Khai protested, "Water falling from the sky, just like Chicken Lickin', Daddy."

When J.W. warned her about lying, she made no excuse, but took his hand and pointed to a fine spray coming from the antiquated toilet tank riveted into the wall near the ceiling. Bernie had apparently pulled the pipe loose, having used it to steady himself. J.W. tried to tighten the corroded joint from which the water was misting, but that only worsened the leak. He wrapped cloth, saran wrap, rubber bands, radiator clamps, aluminum foil, kid's glue, crazy glue, and Bernie's Coach leather belt around the leak, but each feat of engineering only jarred the eighty-year-old pipes and magnified the flow.

J.W. knocked on neighboring doors, and though he could hear people inside, no one answered. J.W. went out into the street and found an all-night convenience store. He asked the counter-man if he knew the name of a real plumber, but the clerk spoke no English, and J.W. no Amharic. J.W. searched the shelves for plumbing supplies to fit a 1910s toilet, but there were only candy bars, Twinkies, and beer. It was, after all, New Year's Eve.

J.W. crawled into the attic through an access panel in the ceiling outside Bernie's apartment. He sweat profusely as he unfolded in the freezing loft, one that appeared to have been untouched for decades. It was a shambles, stuffed with the flotsam and jetsam of the lives of generations of long forgotten New Yorkers. A peculiar, yeasty smell, like stale beer, mixed with the musty scent of the old timber eaves. The odor followed him as he navigated by the shafts of colored light from the Empire State Building filtering through cracks in the soot-coated skylight. He crawled into a corner and found galvanized pipe and a box of fittings.

While J.W. pawed through the hardware, he sensed the presence of a being. He shivered and gathered the plumbing supplies, dragging them as he crept back toward the hole in the floor. As he passed a heap of neglected rags, he saw the pile quiver then produce a cloud of oily dust. A fissure opened to reveal the outline of a bewhiskered face. The rest of the corpus emerged, its cold blue eyes locked onto J.W.'s. The torso was clothed in a tattered overcoat, the head in a moth-eaten, wool ski cap. Next to the rags were impedimenta sitting on a decayed coffee table: a metal cup, a chipped porcelain plate, and a bent serving spoon. Behind the apparition were torn plastic sacks overflowing with beer cans.

J.W. could not speak, nor could he make his legs crawl. For an eternity, the two stared at each other, until the light from the great tower outside became so bright, J.W. could not avoid the absence of malice in the man's pale, desolate face. It was the mortified stare J.W. had encountered so many times at St. Augustine's. "Old man, what the hell you doing here?"

The derelict's face twisted in resigned defeat as he gathered his things and placed them slowly in a greasy burlap sack. He stuffed a few rags and the smaller items into his pockets, gathered up as many plastic bags as he could, and began to stand.

"No, sir. You stay here," J.W. besieged. "I'll get you some food. It's New Year's Eve, sir. You're welcome to stay. I swear I won't tell anyone you're here."

Krista made a sandwich. J.W. wrapped a twenty around a beer and held it in place with a rubber band. He reached up and placed the alms on the lip just inside the attic and slid the wooden hatch over the hole. In the morning, J.W. poked his head into the loft. The sandwich, with its edges curled, sat where it had been left, and next to the sandwich was the twenty; only the beer can was gone.

CHAPTER TWENTY-FOUR

R otations at the hospital during the fourth, senior year of
medical school, became less threatening as the nascent physicians began to recognize the words and phrases of clinical medicine. Some of the more verbal began to use the new language with
a slender sense of confidence. What amazed J.W. was the common-
ality of all the specialties, the basics of medicine that appeared
over and over, the same language spoken with just a few new nouns
sprinkled about to safeguard that specialty's turf. They enjoyed a
growing ability to start a new rotation and fit in after day two or
three by applying the primitive concepts of human pathology that
had been stuffed into them during year one. Inflammation, infection, stress, cancer, trauma, all of the primary causes of disease
showed themselves over and over, regardless over which body part
that specialty claimed dominion. Even the interns and residents
who interrogated them on rounds used the same, worn, didactic
techniques. They grilled students day in and day out, refusing to
let them be until the apprentice spit back, maybe not the correct
diagnosis, but the relevant, tired medical cliché.

Differences became apparent in the cast of characters, though. Real doctors were grouped into categories—the mechanics, cold technicians of clinical practice; and those who tempered their science with the art of medicine. The latter physicians did not flutter eyes and twist mouths in contempt, classic resident demeanor, when a student presented a patient evaluation. They often nodded in agreement and mumbled a word or two of praise; some even instituted the student's recommended therapy.

On rounds, when the intern flubbed his lines, medical students were invited to step forward to address the attending physician, to defend the use of so and so antibiotic by quoting scholarly papers from the *Annals of Internal Medicine* or the *New England Journal of Medicine.* From the periphery, it seemed certain students were brighter than the interns, but in fact, while interns had been kept awake all the previous night trying to draw blood from collapsed veins, and running through the halls to see their next admission, or running through the halls to pronounce the next deceased patient, students had been sent home. They were supposed to read about the various diseases for morning rounds, but by third year, most just slept and returned in the morning showered and fed.

Seltzer chortled, after coming up with an obscure fact regarding the nephrotoxicity of certain antibiotics, "We're winning the war with the house staff."

But one of the interns overheard him, shoved his shoulder, and whispered angrily, "Your time'll come, numb nuts."

War or not, the life of a medical student superimposed upon that of a combatant in Viet Nam did not leave a smudge, and J.W. remained excited and content while in the hospital. At home, however, the two Purple Hearts still sat above his desk, gazing down like sphinxes, watching, uttering nothing, but roaring silently in his ears. J.W. knew his war was far from over.

Internal medicine was billed as the black hole of the four years of interminable study. It was long hours, a mountain of mental masturbation, the snottiest of residents, and the very sickest of patients. Most medical students put it off as long as they could. J.W. was assigned to the cardiology service first, near the tail end of students, interns, residents, fellows, and attendings slogging the cardiac care unit. Though a senior medical student, J.W. was still buried deeply enough on the totem to be almost invisible. Fortune had placed him on the service with another medical student, a former NFL center for the Jets, who suffered from an inability to stop eating once he had retired from professional sports. As the man's midsection expanded on a daily basis, it became easier for J.W. to hide behind him at the bedside. J.W. wasn't alone in his ruse, as medical students became so adept at blending into the pea green walls, they were sometimes docked points for missing rounds on which they had actually participated, at least in body.

At night, however, they were the chief scut puppies for the intern. J.W. was assigned to look after a ponderously expansive, though elfinly short, woman with suffocating, crushing, chest pain. It had begun that morning while she was working in the Mahdi Family Pita Bakery in Southey. Still dressed in her black gowns, head covered and face partially veiled, she was brought to the hospital by her extended Palestinian family. She clutched her chest as she was lifted off the gurney onto the bed in the cardiac intensive care unit, crying out softly to Allah in Arabic, begging for mercy.

An army of technicians descended upon her, each armed with a tube or a wire. She was an elderly woman from the Dead Sea, brought up in the turn-of-the-century desert without electricity, running water, or anything more over her head than the bare material of a nomad's tent. Yet, there she lay, transformed within minutes into a technological curiosity that outshone

John Glenn's space capsule. As the pack of hospital technicians stepped back in satisfaction, a switch was thrown, and monitors in her room and at the nurses' station blipped to life, reading heart activity, respirations, and blood pressure, chirping and blinking to the beat of her seventy-five-year-old body.

The family discussed the meaning of the impulses as if they were on the cardiac transplant team themselves, every skipped beat sending the women rushing to the bedside wailing. At 8 P.M., they were ushered out of her cubicle into the waiting room, where the family set up shop. An interpreter was appointed, and only he was allowed in the unit, and only if needed. There was no argument. They seemed grateful to leave Mrs. Mahdi in such professional hands.

J.W. introduced himself to the patient honestly, never using the word "doctor," but she spoke no English. "*Doctori*," she whispered in Arabic then pointed to her chest and grimaced in pain. J.W. flushed her IV line with saline, added a few milligrams of morphine, and in seconds, a gentle smile came upon her. She relaxed and finally slept. So did J.W, but at 2 A.M., while trying to rest on a table in a darkened corner of the deserted dining hall, he was paged stat to the cardiac unit.

Mrs. Mahdi had metabolized the minute amount of morphine with which J.W. had fearfully spiked her IV, and she was groaning in pain. She had waited until J.W. arrived to clutch her chest and point desperately to the IV tubing. J.W. began to flush the line with a drop of saline, though before he had finished with the saltwater, her eyes were swimming in ecstasy. She held his hand. "*Shukron, Doctori, shukron katir.*"

At 4 A.M., and again at five, they twirled through the same dance. She motioned to a half-dozen pictures of young children her family had arrayed by their matriarch's bedside. When she pointed at him, J.W. showed her Khai's picture. She remarked in Arabic about the blond hair while tugging at his thinning, dark locks. She laughed until the pain in her chest reemerged, pointing again to the IV tubing.

At dawn, J.W. left her side for the on-call room and a shower. During his absence, the Mahdi family swept into the unit with a platter of feta cheese, olives, pita, a hard-boiled egg, a brick of halvah, and jabana—thick, syrupy, strong, middle eastern coffee, which she sipped. Before swallowing, though, or so the family swore to Allah, Mrs. Mahdi grabbed her chest and pointed to the IV tubing. The alarms shrieked, and though a nurse flew into the room, Mrs. Mahdi was gone.

When J.W. reached the unit, the family was washing her body with plain water and chanting "*Allah kareem, Allah kareem,*" Allah provides. J.W. stole away from the room to steel himself for the onslaught of recriminations. At 9 A.M., a note was delivered by one of Mrs. Mahdi's grandchildren, a surly, unshaven man in his early twenties. Although J.W. assumed it was a threat of impending legal action, it was actually an invitation to the bakery for the funeral.

J.W. knew in his heart he had had nothing to do with Mrs. Mahdi's death, yet he worried he'd be skewered on rounds that afternoon, for turbulence ran downhill in medicine, gathering speed as it approached those least likely to understand what had gone wrong. But at rounds, as they passed the room in which Mrs. Mahdi had expired, the attending cardiologist just nodded to J.W. and very subtly shrugged his shoulders as they went on to the next bed. And with that, J.W. assumed he had experienced a rite of passage, an initiation into physicianhood, the ritual loss of a patient, a baptism that was to be done quietly. An hour after rounds, J.W. was in the unit working up the next heart attack, wondering if he'd find a few minutes to get dinner.

At the funeral, through the wailing and rejoicing, J.W. barely heard one of the sons assure him he had been a good doctor for having helped his mother with her final pain. J.W. was thrown back, for an instant, to the rare times in his life he had sensed the family of man. For a twinkling, he was proud to be a doctor. Mrs. Mahdi's passing was, nevertheless, an inauspicious beginning to his internal medicine course. Everyone had patients die, but it wasn't good form to lose your very first on so vital a rotation. Internal medicine was the course that had the most extreme effect on finding a good residency, and residency was far more important in finding a job than medical school.

✦ ✦

Two days later, a care package of Middle Eastern goodies was delivered to J.W. at the hospital. One of the secretaries found him eating pita and feta cheese in a dusty, forgotten corner of the micro lab. She snarled, "The dean wants you in his office at noon."

So, he was to be the first doctor in history to be sued for malpractice before he became a doctor, and he stewed over that proposition for the balance of the morning. Over a slice of halvah, though, he thought back to his last act in Viet Nam, to the moment he decided he wasn't going to be the scapegoat again. He'd told a colonel from another unit to close his mouth and just listen to what had really transpired during the calamity du jour. It'd worked, worked so well, when the commanding officer realized Captain Weathersby had spoken the truth, J.W. was made an honorary member the infantry battalion.

And he remembered Dr. Gerstein's musing, "Only if we had fought back," and by noon he was loaded for bear, building a level of anger that surprised him. He sat and planned for half-an-hour, sitting in the micro lab, stuffing pieces of half-chewed pita down his throat. He would start the war hitting the dean with the old Purple Heart, combat veteran ruse, and, if that didn't work,

241

he'd bluster and posture for fifteen minutes and simply wear the man down.

As noon approached, J.W. went to the intern to get permission to leave the floor, but he categorically refused, threatening J.W. with duty for the next three nights if he left before his work was completed. But getting all the scut done, all that had been assigned by the intern, would have made J.W. three weeks late to see the dean, so he left anyway. Sitting in the dean's office were several well-dressed attorneys—for the plaintiff, for the hospital, and for the accused.

"Have a seat, Mr. Weathersby," the dean directed with a dour face.

"I'll stand," J.W. puffed.

"Fine, stand. I would like you to meet some people interested in medical education."

Before the dean could say another word, J.W. added, "Or lack thereof."

The attorneys stared up at him. The dean did as well.

"May I continue?" the dean asked. "These folks are from KKMA in Los Angeles. They're doing a network TV special on medical education. They're impressed with your background and want to interview you for a part."

"I thought I was here for what happened to Mrs. Mahdi. You're not lawyers?"

The dean cocked his head—the others gazed up at him slackjawed. How could one so impressive on paper be such a disappointment in the flesh?

"Mrs. Mahdi was a very ill patient. The attending said you actually did quite well. Have a seat."

The malpractice weight off his chest, J.W.'s mood brightened. At that point in his life, though, he had not an inkling of the number of times he would come to experience that identical feeling of professional dread, the apprehension that he had harmed a patient by his inattention or ignorance, and the realization that he was surely to be sued, that both his professional and personal life were about to be exposed and demeaned. How many times over the next three decades would the torment be relieved when he discovered his medical transgression had not been what he'd imagined? Though the relief was incomparable, it was temporary, lasting only until the next crisis.

The producer interrupted the dean and peppered J.W. with questions about Mrs. Mahdi, turning to one of the lesser suits, grumbling, "Take notes."

J.W. offered to go to his locker and get some of the pita and cheese, but the dean suggested there probably wasn't enough time to fully appreciate the exotic offering. The audience remained poker-faced as J.W. responded to questions. When the producer yawned, signaling the termination of the interview, the dean stood, the producer stood, and the assistants offered don't-call-us-we'll-call-you, wet-fish handshakes.

Two weeks passed before the next pre-sunrise phone call. J.W. lifted the ringing phone and mumbled to Krista, "Hemorrhoids."

It was the dean. "Well, good morning," he bubbled cheerily. "How are ya?"

"Great. Am I getting sports medicine? I'll be there in an hour," J.W. blurted, thanking him with his tone.

"Sports medicine? I don't know. Did you request it? Look, sorry to bother you, but the reason I'm calling is about the TV special. They're really interested in you. They thought the feta cheese was a nice touch. Can you meet with them today?"

"But what about sports medicine?"

"We should talk about that at a better time, don't you think? Let's just be there at noon."

⊷⊱ ⊰⊶

Filming started. Deans, sub-deans, attendings, administrators, secretaries, and alumni flooded the halls and patient rooms, prompting one of the cleaning ladies to mutter, "They is moh attention done bein' paid to da ill dan in da las sixteen years!"

The camera and sound technicians followed J.W. into patient rooms, exam rooms, bathrooms, and hiding rooms. One segment was shot with an attending physician offering him a lecture on heart murmurs while they stood at their respective urinals, though there was so much laughing in the background, the piece wound up on the cutting room floor.

⟩⟨

A few months later, Krista, Khai, and J.W. lay in bed and watched their lives unfold on national TV. "Did you have to talk about my salary and our sex life?" she asked during the first commercial.

"All I said was that it was hard to get home before my wife went to sleep anymore. It's the truth. You haven't been up past ten in the last four years."

"So, I'm supposed to wait for the great one until midnight, with legs spread? That's if you bother coming home at all. No way. Them days is over, buddy boy, oh magnificent one." She jumped out of bed and left the house before the commercial was over.

As the special ended, the phone rang. J.W. wanted it to be Krista, but the first call was from a woman in Georgia whose father was dying of cancer. She asked how to transfer the man to Boston to be placed under J.W.'s care. He explained he wasn't a doctor, yet, and that even if he were, things just didn't work that way in the medical world.

The next call was from a woman who introduced herself as a medical intern at an inner city hospital in New York. She started off gently, with a smile in her voice. "Are you the one who said he loved medical school so much that you wish your life could be freeze-framed as a senior medical student?"

"It's been a good time," J.W. agreed. "Yeah, better than a lot of times I've had."

"Well, you are one grand asshole, my friend. You haven't seen shit. You made us all look like Pollyanna fools. I've got patients asking to leave here and go to see you. I ought to send 'em up. You love medicine so much? Wait till you get into it. Give it a year as an intern. Then let me know."

The phone slammed down so hard, Khai heard it across the room. J.W. wrestled with himself over leaving the phone off the hook to avoid any more calls, but he wanted to hear from Krista. When it rang again, eight seconds later, J.W. answered with a, "What?" It was his mother.

Krista came home an hour later. "I tried to call, but the line was busy. You leave it off the hook so I couldn't get through?"

"What's on your mind, Kris?" J.W. asked gently.

"You just don't understand, do you? I have a life, too. It's all for you, never for me. Hong Kong, pre-med, and now the great one is star of the medical school class. And all I do is take care of your house and your kids."

"Kids? You mean a kid. As far as I remember, we have only one child." J.W. stared at her as hard as she did at him.

"I'm pregnant," she wept.

"How long have you known?"

She wouldn't answer. "How long have you known, goddamnit?"

"Two months."

J.W. tried to touch her, but she pulled away, tears flowing like a river, her sobs bitter. She locked herself in the bathroom, and J.W. soon gave up and went to his office to start filling out the application forms for the residency programs that were to begin in a few months. He tried to start with the first form on the thick pile, but could not concentrate, his eyes fixed on his opium, the

Purple Hearts. While they gazed down, they remained without expression, their indifference not having thawed a trace in the years he'd been gazing up at them, seeking guidance.

J.W. felt small, selfish, and thoughtless for having walked away from his pregnant wife. He sought wisdom from the Hearts, waiting for the gold-plated *alto relievo* images of George Washington to say something, to curse J.W. for having been such a self-centered ass, but the first president's eyes remained unblinking, never answering.

J.W. asked Krista to talk with him about where they should go to interview for residency. "I don't care where we go," she said softly. "Wherever you think will be the least unpleasant. It's not me becoming an intern."

J.W. stared into Krista's eyes. "Got to tell you what happened today. Dean called me in. I was scared he was going to tell me I was going to have a tough time matching with a good residency program. He pointed to a chair. I said, 'Shit, here it comes.' He laughed. 'J.W., I'm not supposed to do this, and I hope you will keep my confidence, but it's important. We want you to stay here for your residency. You have done exceedingly well. You know all the players, the doctors and nurses, even the orderlies. They all know you. You've helped most of them in one way or the other, fixing light switches, tuning carburetors. Took a couple of years, but everyone respects you. You take the crap well for an older student. Lots of practice I guess.'

"I told him that was the problem. That I was tired of the crap. I needed a rest. Engineering, army, a war, graduate school, killed myself to get into medical school, and now all the local programs had you on call every second and third night. I told him I was burned out. I was going for the easy programs.

"He said, 'Well, I understand, but if you leave here, you have to start all over getting to know people. A residency isn't about the hours; well, yes, it is, but it's more about who you're working with. It always is in life, isn't it? It's the people. And I will put our people up against any residency in the country. That's why we're rated at the top. It's up to you. Your Dean's Letter will reflect that you finished sixth in your class. You'll go anywhere you want. But you need to think about it very hard.'"

Rumor had it Cedar Springs was the gentlest residency training program for Emergency Medicine, and the most selective. Every fourth night on call was doable. There would be time to get to know Krista and Khai again. They would explore the Rockies, the most beautiful, gentlest fragment of the country. They had been happy there when J.W. returned from Viet Nam, stationed at Fort Carson. His co-pilot, Lieutenant White, who had died in combat a few weeks after saving J.W.'s life, had been from near there, a place called Black Granite. Maybe someday, J.W. thought, he would keep his promise and visit the man's family.

J.W. told Krista, "My preference is Cedar Springs. Every fourth night on call. I don't want to be medical director at NIH. God forgive me for saying it, but all I want is to sit in an office and see coughs and colds and tell patients they don't have cancer. No need for the most prestigious residency in the world. And you liked it there, didn't you? But if you want to stay here, that's fine. You want to stay?"

"Not particularly. Cedar Springs's okay."

CHAPTER TWENTY-FIVE

K rista and J.W. joined the class for "Match Day," the moment senior medical students are informed where they would do their residency, where the next three to seven years of their lives would pass, and most often, where they would spend the rest of their lives. As they left the house, the brake line on the Buick split again, and they flew through a stop sign into the neighbor's garden. J.W. pumped up the tires on their bikes, and the cycled to Union.

Every graduating senior medical student in the U.S. opened the destiny letter at the same moment. The envelopes were handed out at high noon on the East Coast, on the West Coast at 9 A.M. Those who did not match scrambled to the phones to scratch for the few lifesaving spots.

The wild cards, shy one, gathered toward the back of the lecture hall. They opened their envelopes at the same moment. Seltzer handed Natalie his envelope. She fought with it, unable to get her fingers under the flap, and by the time she got it open, the letter inside had been torn in several places. Seltzer glared, but relaxed when he pieced the shreds together to see they would be staying in Boston to do radiology. "It's the only specialty where you can wear jeans to work, make big bucks, *and* sit and eat while practicing medicine," he laughed grimly.

Jimmy Ray also got his first choice—pediatrics in Stanton. He wanted to go home to the Rockies and practice in a rural clinic someday.

J.W. handed Krista his envelope. Cedar Springs, Emergency Medicine. The best residency in the country, the one with the humane schedule, every fourth night on call, not every other night, like so many of those they had interviewed. Penny Brucker, a fellow graduating senior, due the same day as Krista, came over. As she and Krista hugged, Penny abruptly pushed away and screamed, "Oh, my God!"

Both Krista and Penny looked down to see blood pooling at their feet.

But it was not Penny who had reason to cry. It was Krista's legs covered in the blood. Seltzer muttered that she was aborting, and Krista stood frozen, afraid to move, waiting for the auditorium of physicians to save her, but only a dreadful silence hung over the hall. As several of the women students hurried over to guide her to the emergency room, Seltzer gently placed his suit jacket over her shoulders.

Krista said little over the next few weeks as they packed. She put her bicycle up for sale, cursing it as the source of her loss. As graduation approached, there were still no buyers for their house, and the realtor shrugged and advised they board it up. Promising to forward the proceeds when it sold, the woman asked for an address. "We'll send one when we get one," J.W. offered as Krista left the room.

Graduation was a gathering of the same faces, though the baby fat was gone, as was the sparkle of discovery. The exhaustion was palpable. The speaker's remarks about the art and science of medicine completed, they edged closer to the moment about which J.W. had spent years dreaming. Finally, the dean stood to tell them of the guiding words around which he had built a thirty-year career.

"*Primum non noceri.* First, do no harm. There will be times, many times in your career, when the desire to help a patient will be overwhelming. You will feel a need to know that the years of endless labor, and I might add just plain drudge, that went into getting where you are, weren't for naught. You will be tempted to do a procedure or try a medicine that might hurt your patient.

"It is better, my colleagues, when you are tortured with doubt, to do nothing, and suffer along with your patient, to learn to live with your doubts and failures, than to harm your charge."

It was strangely quiet in the hall when he offered those sentiments, and the Class of '81 repeated the Hippocratic Oath.

"I swear by Apollo the physician and Aesculapius and health and all-heal and all the gods and goddesses that according to his ability and judgment I will keep this oath and this stipulation—to reckon him who taught me as my parents, to share my substance with him.

"I will follow that system of regimen I consider for the benefit of my patients. I will give no deadly medicine. While I continue to keep this oath unviolated, may it be granted to me to enjoy life and the practice of the art, respected by all men, in all times, but should I trespass and violate this oath, may the reverse be my lot."

And it was done. J.W.'s mother approached from behind. "Dr. Weathersby, congratulations."

PART III

CHAPTER TWENTY-SIX

Three days before they left Boston, Krista developed a uterine infection that required a D&C, so she flew to Cedar Springs alone. Khai and J.W. followed in a rental van, dragging the Buick more than two thousand miles.

On the flight to Stanton, Krista's chills worsened, a marker of the persistent infection that lingered in her womb, and of the loss that would trouble her heart for the rest of her life. She searched for an apartment but spent most of her time sweating in a motel bed.

Khai and J.W. arrived six days later. It would have been five, but for yet another Mao the Cat, a stray, moth-eaten calico this time, who befriended Khai the morning before they set out for Cedar Springs. J.W. discovered fleas in Khai's hair the instant they pulled out of their street, and banished Mao to ride in the Buick, towed behind their rented Jartran van. Six-year-old Khai adjusted her side view mirror to keep an eye on Mao as he spent the long days asleep, wedged between the windshield and the steering wheel. As J.W. turned the van, the steering wheel of the Buick rotated, flinging Mao off the dashboard. Each time the cat disappeared, Khai insisted they stop to check on his orthopedic status.

The journey was slow and uneventful until Council Bluffs, Iowa. The night in the cheapest motel on the highway was restless, Mao pacing and scratching until J.W. threatened to exile him to the car. The price of calming Khai was allowing Mao to sleep in her bed, but that also cost more fleas in her thick, blond hair, and another treatment of the powder. When J.W. left the next morning to buy snacks at the adjoining 7-11, he warned Khai, "Sweetheart, don't open the door for anyone, anyone. Okay?"

Mao, however, began scratching at the door to go potty. Khai opened it a crack, ordering, "Mao, don't go anywhere, anywhere. Okay?" She left the door ajar and re-engrossed herself in an argument between Big Bird and Oscar the Grouch.

When J.W. returned minutes later, he walked into the room dumbfounded. "I told you not to open the door!"

She jumped up and ran past him into the parking lot, calling, "Here, Kitty, Kitty, here Kitty, Kitty."

The maid in the next room joined the hunt, and soon, so did the owner.

"He's gone, Daddy," Khai choked with tears.

"Nah, he's just in the bushes chasing bugs. And why did you let him out?"

She wailed harder.

By late afternoon, the local TV station was covering the story of the aged, but brand-new doctor, his six-year-old daughter, and the missing cat, the three of whom were on their way cross country to start a new life. On camera, the reporter asked a tearful Khai why they had named him Mao. "All animals are named Mao," she sobbed.

The mayor of Council Bluffs, saddled with an upcoming election, paid a visit to his wayfaring guests. With cameras rolling, he proclaimed he would personally have Mao the Cat, when located, shipped to Cedar Springs. It was, however, too late to leave that day, and he suggested they remain overnight as guests of the city. Khai left a plate of tuna salad outside their door.

At midnight, Khai woke with a start and shook J.W. "Daddy, I can hear Mao. He's under the bed. Listen, he's scratching."

The base of the lumpy bed was entirely enclosed in wood, nailed and screwed to the floor. He assured her, "Sweetie Pie, there ain't no way a cat, or even a mouse, could squeeze in there. Must be a roach or something."

"Daddy, no, Mao's under the bed! He's calling me. He needs help."

"If I show you he's not there, will you go to bed?"

J.W. squatted down and heaved sighs of sufficient vocal register to convince Khai the maximum effort was being exerted on her behalf. He grabbed the bottom edge of the box spring and ripped it from the floor. Mao was cowering in the corner. He caught sight of Khai, sprang forward, took a swipe at J.W., hissed as J.W. swiped back, and wedged himself behind the nailed-down bedside table.

J.W. left thirty dollars on the bed, but waited until they crossed the river into Omaha before calling the TV station with the rest of the story. He pictured the follow-up, human-interest report featuring the mayor asking for contributions to repair the ripped-out bed frame and stand. The announcer would, no doubt, end the piece noting sadly, "And, once again, we learn that no good deed goes unpunished.

The radio news on the early June afternoon they limped into Cedar Springs advised it was colder in town than it had been on Christmas Day. As they neared Krista's downtown motel, the front bumper and tow bar on the Buick broke away. The car rolled through a rotting fence, across a vacant lot, and came to rest against a garbage container. The dumpster was barely dented, but the fence was shredded. J.W. left his name and hospital address at a nearby house.

Mao's hackles were standing on end when they opened the car door. He flew over J.W.'s shoulder, crossed the street at a gallop, and tore up a Doug fir. J.W. begged Khai to let him stay in the tree, but she cried so hard, the firemen promised to charge J.W. only half the standard pet rescue fee.

⟫⟪

Their rented house was seven miles from the hospital, just vacated by the last of a string of Brookline Union students doing residencies in Cedar Springs. The neighbors advised against commuting on a bicycle, but J.W. wagged his tongue and pumped up El Buraq's tires and zoomed off on a trial run.

An hour later, J.W. faced a gang of early-teen delinquents blocking the hospital entrance, their eyes locked on El Buraq. One snipped, "Hey, lemme drive that thing around the block." J.W. growled like a maddened bear. They scattered, and he rolled past the bike rack, through the century-old, tooled wooden doors, into the stairwell outside the residency director's office. He chained the bike to a banister and went off to find his new boss. The man was gone for the day, so J.W. returned to the stairwell. A gaggle of security police had surrounded the bicycle, arms folded across bloated chests, grunting approval as one of their number hacked at the chain with bolt cutter.

"Hey, gentlemen! What the hell's going on here? That's my bicycle! I'm Dr. Weathersby."

A wheelbarrow of a woman with cropped hair stepped through the crowd and nodded to the saw-wielding guard before turning her attention to J.W. "Doctor, we can't have bicycles within the confines of the physical plant. This isn't the army. You aren't the captain anymore. We won't have this again, will we?"

J.W. attempted to recapitulate his history of bicycle imbroglios, of just what El Buraq had survived, but she glowered and hissed, "Will we, Doctor?"

⊨⊣ ⊢⊨

Sunday morning was the first of the pre-internship get-togethers. Krista, Khai, and J.W. were invited to the chief resident's home. Her husband was a distant man, a pathologist, who grumbled that he hadn't seen his wife in weeks.

"But there's not that much night duty in this program," J.W. corrected. "That's the beauty of it, every fourth night on call. I just can't imagine how good that's going to be. What if it was one of those every-other-night programs? That's why we moved all the way out here. To escape that crap."

"Fourth night, my ass. Where'd you hear that?" He called to his wife, "June, come here for a minute."

She dragged herself over, an emaciated, pale woman with braces. Finishing her three-month stint as chief resident, she had been in control of thirty-six very unhappy, very tired, very exhausted young people. It was hers to produce the call schedule and listen to the grousing of the residents whose lives she'd been tasked to oversee. "What's this about not wanting to do every other night on call? You're not going to start bitching already, are you?" Her eyes reddened as she continued. "Some of the rotations are every fourth night in your second and third years, not this year."

"That's not what we were told!" J.W. protested in a near shriek.

Her eyes moistened. "Don't you raise your voice to me. You're the one who gave Ms. Pote a ration of shit about your bicycle, aren't you?"

"I didn't give her any shit. She hassled me."

"They wanted me to talk with you about that, but I'm not going to waste my time. You keep your bicycle out of the hospital." She spun around and loped to the table to pour herself a tall glass of red wine. The clock was yet to strike eleven.

⚒

J.W. gathered Krista and Khai and left, a resident in hot water before he was a resident, the big guns already aimed. He was suddenly aware that their lives were not to be as predicted, as had been implied, as he had been assured by the residency director during the interview a year before. Leaving Boston, the loss of the baby, Krista's illness—for what? For what?

J.W. was amazed at how fast he had slipped back into the deep black cavern of sadness and doubt that had clouded the earlier years, when medicine had been an unapproachable dream, when he had fought to become a doctor, believing that the profession would allow them to live happily ever after.

J.W. called Seltzer to ask if he knew of openings in residency programs in Boston, offering to set out that night. Seltzer simply blurted, "No," but told J.W. he had some bad news. Natalie had been diagnosed with Parkinson's. Seltzer cried. "I was such an asshole, J.W. How could I have missed it?"

Krista was listening from the kitchen. When J.W. told her, she left for the bedroom. J.W. followed and sat on the end of the bed. "It would not hurt me one little bit to pack up and leave here tonight, and see what happens back in Boston. What do you think?"

Krista was silent for several minutes, but J.W. could see she was seething. "Why did you have to open your mouth? I don't want to move again. I've had it." She began to cry in a voice J.W. had not heard since their great fight years before at the Paris

Inn, waiting to leave for Viet Nam. "Why did you do this to me again?"

"I wish I could take it back, Krista, the whole damn thing. A lot of things."

"Just stay out of her way at the hospital. Can you do that?" she demanded, her eyes pouring tears.

CHAPTER TWENTY-SEVEN

Residency began the next morning at zero six hundred. The eleven interns with whom J.W. was to share the years had been carefully chosen from thirty-six-hundred applicants. His colleagues ranged in age from twenty-five to twenty-six. J.W. was closer to forty. They were kids—J.W. had a kid. The only other male was Sam, a tall, thin soul with the sweet face of an innocent Midwesterner. They were, to an intern, as pale as if they had lived under Alaskan skies for the past ten years. The team of young residents knew and accepted that this was to be their ordeal; J.W. still nursed the scars from the skirmishes into which he had dropped himself over the past decade-and-a-half.

Housekeeping was first on the agenda. The residency director, Dr. Jacoby, introduced the hospital's Chief Executive Officer. "Some of you have met Miss Pote, I understand."

Still stout, still without make up, she marched with a fine tremor to the podium. She wore a wrinkled, puffy, black skirt. J.W. noted that her white cotton blouse was stained yellow under the arms. She had, at one time, frosted her hair, though missed the back. Her black tie was dusted with a patina of gray from frequent washings, matching the salt and pepper behind her head. J.W. wondered how long it would be before he looked like that. She peered down at him, snubbing his apologetic smile.

She addressed them seriously. "You will wonder many times over the next years, as have those who have gone before you, why you chose medicine as a career. The challenges will be profound at times, but in the end, the rewards worth the sacrifice. There will be long and thankless hours, days with meals consisting of a slice of dry toast flavored with packets of ketchup and relish, and a cup of coffee. Interns call it 'bread and water.'"

She paused for a laugh, but there were only edgy stares in return. Her mouth hardened as she went on. "The medical and administrative staff is here to help you. You are essential to the operation of the hospital I administer. No one has ever left this program in the middle. Everyone has finished. That is a feature of the caring we do for you."

J.W. had not heard such a heartwarming welcoming sermon since 1968, on the first day of commando training at The United States Army Ranger School. The cadre had pledged the same punishments and rewards in the wretched swamps of the deep South. There was a difference, though. In Ranger School, Master Sergeant Cowsen warned, "Gentlemen, in a week, y'all gonna be so hungry, you'uns'll trade a piece of ass for half a peanut butter and jelly sandwich. Gentlemen, let it never be said we did not give you choices."

Ms. Pote, having apparently experienced but one of Sergeant Cowsen's two possibilities, did not know the power of leaving alternatives in her wake, of allowing a smidgen of control in the lives she dictated. "For some, this is a baptism of fire," she finished, bobbing her head, then keeled around and marched to her seat, a plastic smile aimed at her clutch of novices.

Dr. Jacoby ran slender fingers through waves of silver hair as he retook the podium. "There's nothing wrong with a little stress," he commenced solemnly, "and there is plenty of support in the program. I reiterate what Ms. Pote said about never having lost a resident. Why, we've never even had a marriage break up. Cedar Springs is a wonderful place to do your residency. J.W., I hope you get to see some of our glorious summer. Enjoy the sun. Let's take a break."

Karla, one of the interns, sighed in a whisper, "It's been years since I've had a free hour to sit in the sun. Looks like a lot more to go." She had started her comment with a smile, though it disappeared as she considered the next three years. "I need to stay out of the sun anyway. My freckles light up bright orange, and my hair turns white if I go out for more than fifteen minutes."

Sam laughed sarcastically, "I haven't had even fifteen minutes outside this building in the past four years." Sam glanced at J.W. out of the corner of his eye.

J.W. asked, "Did you all go to med school here?"

"Most of us did. Right here in this building. They don't like foreigners so much in the program. I think you're the only one. But they told us you were in Viet Nam, so you know what it's like to be, like, different."

"Nah, medical school's medical school—med students in Afghanistan are probably just as pale as us. Anyway, I've had too much sun in my life."

"When you were in the war, huh?"

"Yeah, lots of sun. A real tropical paradise."

"What was that like? I was in fifth grade," Sam chuckled uneasily.

Dr. Jacoby's eyes squinted, waiting for the outcome of this first examination of his decision to have tossed a wild card into the cauldron. Even Ms. Pote paused expectantly for the reply. Though J.W. had not intended to make Viet Nam an issue, or even mention it, it had come around on its own, and far sooner than he had expected. He hadn't planned on what to say, so he looked away, out the window, at the planes approaching Cedar Springs Airport. He thought of his eleven fellow residents, all waiting to hear the answer, and he tried to think back to the day he realized he was an adult and being tested for a first time. He wondered if they were as scared and unsure as he had been fifteen years before. When he turned back to peer at them, he was not sure what they were thinking. Certainly, the women had absorbed through their pores disdain for any older man schooled in the days before liberation, when medical school classes were ninety-five percent male, and any female in white was, at best, a nurse.

His new colleagues' faces, though, were neither wary nor dubious, and when he smiled gently back at Sam, everyone relaxed several quanta. He knew suddenly that there was no need to boast that he had, long before, been through far worse. He understood at that moment he would either befriend them as equals or fail to survive. As his face lightened, so did the tension in their hands. He did not need to regale them with war stories of wounds, silent Purple Hearts, or even his fury over what he had learned at the welcoming party. It was a new day, and nothing in life was as bad as people said it was—except for some things.

Their expectant eyes had not left him. He tapped the side of Sam's shoulder with his fingers, smiling kindly. "Viet Nam? Nah, not as bad as medical school, man."

He glanced at Ms. Pote; her tight plastic grin had degenerated into a miffed scowl. J.W. had not snapped back at the kids, as she'd hoped. He wasn't a violent misfit, the loose cannon she'd presaged during the countless meetings as the administration shuffled through the thousands of applicants. Another early chance to rid the program of Jacoby's Folly vanished before her eyes.

J.W. turned back to the window, glaring, rehearsing a diatribe designed to set the ground rules for Ms. Pote, to notify her to steer clear. "Lady," he would growl, you're dealing with a combat vet. I've been to commando school. If I chain my goddamn bicycle to a friggin' pipe in *my* hospital, you come and ask me politely to move it. Do you understand that?" J.W. took a deep breath, slapped a solemn mien on his face, and turned toward Ms. Pote.

The kids were watching him, their fists tightening again. "It was hot, that was the worst of it," J.W. mumbled, managing a drained smile.

Ms. Pote ordered them back to their seats and presented them with sheaves of benefit forms. The medical insurance contract was stamped in red, "RESIDENT COVERAGE ONLY."

"Excuse me, Ma'am," J.W. interrupted. "Does that mean I have to pay for my family? How much extra for my wife and daughter?"

"A nominal amount," she barked.

"Ms. Pote, excuse me, but my wife is quite ill. She has an infection from when we lost our baby."

"Yes, we are aware of that, but it is a *preexisting* condition. Unfortunately, it won't be covered, even if you purchase the insurance for her." She made a note and went on.

"Sam," J.W. whispered, "what's nominal mean? Do you know? Usually winds up costing me a lot."

"It isn't that much at all, Doctor," Ms. Pote interjected.

"At least The Blob's not suffering from presbycousis," J.W. whispered very softly as a parting fusillade. Though he smiled inwardly at the brief victory, he could not help but smell the stench of battle roiling from the podium.

⋯

Next on the program were physical exams for the new interns. J.W. was examined by June, the senior resident, who was silent as she dropped the ice-cold stethoscope onto J.W.'s chest. He waited with relish for the order to drop his drawers to check front and back, but she ignored the rules that the exam be complete, and made only a written comment on his chart describing the patch-work of scars on his legs. She never inquired about their cause.

The interns were sent to a meeting at which June, back from her medical duties, handed each of them a sheet of paper in-scribed with the tally of a year of neatly planned, one-month blocks of "opportunity", she smirked. J.W. was assigned to sur-gery. "We're throwing you to the dogs first," she laughed. "We figured after your big Viet Nam, it'd be a breeze. Surgery has to come sometime, and better sooner, while you're still in one piece. It's a gift in disguise. Report to Dr. Holderman's service at eight tomorrow morning."

There were hoots from his new friends.

"You mean 'm-o-u-r-n-i-n-g,'" consoled Karla. "I was on his service in medical school. Two times, thank you! You're really going to enjoy him."

"Guy a flamer?" J.W. rolled his eyes in Seltzerian fashion, ask-ing around the room.

There were nods, and Karla added, "Been a pleasure know-ing ya. See ya in about three years." She was about to go on with more about Dr. Holderman, but June cleared her throat, and Karla's face shifted to the doorway where Ms. Pote was listening.

"Just checking on the progress of your orientation," she mut-tered as J.W. turned and looked at her. "Dr. Jacoby would like a word with you at your earliest convenience, Doctor Weathersby."

At first, J.W. thought Jacoby was going to congratulate him for coming through the physical with flying colors, despite his advanced age and receding hairline. Perhaps it was another TV special.

"Sit down, Doctor," he ordered, eyes peering at an open ma-nila folder on his desk. He looked up past his half-focals and stared at J.W. for a second. "Great first day as a doctor. I understand you aren't thrilled with the on call schedule, the insurance plan, bicycle parking facilities, your first rotation, or our hospital administrator. She worked her way up from the typing pool. She knows all about medical terminology, like, ah, presbycousis. Did you think she didn't know that meant old-age hearing loss, Doctor?"

"She deserved it."

"May be, but she wasn't amused, and she's the boss. Anyway, she's younger than you," he reminded. "So, she's not old, she isn't deaf, but she is definitely pissed off." He paused and stared out the window. "I want you to slow down a bit, Doctor. Give the other dogs a chance to sniff you. Sometimes East Coast doesn't fit in around here so good. I don't want to hear anything else about you, not for a long time." He turned back to his desk and closed the folder then a selected a chart from a pile and dictated, "The next patient is a pleasant thirty-eight-year-old female complaining of dyspareunia. She..."

That night, Krista evaluated her husband's initial scrapes with the administration. "You just can't stay out of hot water, can you? But, on the other hand, your Ms. Pote sounds like a real asshole. What's her problem?"

J.W. was shocked, but pleased, by the sliver of Krista's outward support. At least they were in agreement that Ms. Pote had to shoulder a smidgen of the responsibility for the way their lives had soured. It was the first time in a long time J.W. didn't feel completely alone.

CHAPTER TWENTY-EIGHT

I t began in the morning. J.W. found the lead surgeon in the break room drinking coffee. "Dr. Holderman, I'm J.W. Weathersby. I'm on your service, sir." Those words had become a knee jerk, and J.W. smiled to himself at how admirably Union had prepared him for the challenge of internship. J.W. felt at home in the hospital, in a surgical scrub suit. He knew where to get coffee without ever having been in that hospital. He knew where the cream and sugar were stored—in the cabinet above the sink—and where to find the bread and butter. It was in the little fridge under the counter, where staples were stored in every surgical break room in the free world. J.W. made tea and popped Wonder Bread into the toaster then opened drawers and found the condiments for ketchup and relish sandwiches. He asked Dr. Holderman, "Sir, would you like one?"

"We've already done a gall bladder and a breast biopsy, Doctor," his new course director reminded over the rim of his coffee mug. "We start at six, not eight."

J.W. started to tell him that Ms. Pote herself had set the reporting hour, but the military lived deep within him, and so did Dr. Van Noy. J.W. responded without hesitation, "Yes, sir. Won't happen again, sir." That had always worked in the army, and even with Van Noy, for what else was there to say? Okay, I screwed up and I know it; and I don't like screwing up any more than you like seeing me do it. I'm prepared to eat humble pie, admit I was wrong, and assure you it won't happen again. So, from one professional to another, accept my assurances.

"Where were you?" Dr. Holderman asked quietly, but continued before J.W. could answer. "We need you here on time."

Dr. Holderman bristled out of the break room, and the anesthesiologist, sitting in the corner, crooked his finger for J.W. to follow. J.W. crooked his to the medical student. As the procession entered the operating room, a nurse was placing a sterile plastic drape over the tubes of a microscope suspended over the operating table. The drape allowed the surgeon to touch it without contaminating his sterile gloves. Excited at this first opportunity to observe microsurgery, J.W. waited impatiently by the swinging doors. He was placed in a sterile green robe by the scrub nurse, handed sterile gloves by another OR tech, and motioned forward to the sterile operating table by yet another of the myriad nurses who had caught the scent of fresh intern meat.

As J.W. approached the table, the nurse applying the plastic microscope shield put her very ample posterior in reverse, backed into him, turned angrily, and gloated, "He's contaminated!"

J.W. jumped back in surprise, knocked into a portable lamp, and sent it teetering toward Dr. Holderman's head. J.W. grabbed and stopped its pendulum arc, but it was so hot, it slipped out of his hand, brushed the surgeon's gown, and clanged loudly onto the tile floor. The halogen bulb burst into chunks of steaming crystal. Holderman swung around just as J.W. lifted the lamp from the floor.

"That didn't take long," he hissed disgustedly.

Dr. Holderman and J.W. went through the entire scrubbing-and-gowning followed by the covering-the-microscope-with-plastic sequence a second time. It took fifteen minutes before they were back by the peacefully snoring patient's side. "Can we start the operation now? Can it be done without contaminating the surgical field this time?"

"Yes, sir." J.W.'s heart slipped from his throat to a level as low as Dr. Holderman's white nylon socks. He waited breathlessly for the procedure to end. Holderman grunted a few commands, and J.W. watched the surgeon's hands closely, but Dr. Holderman did not share the panorama revealed by the scope.

At lunch came a call from Dr. Jacoby. "What happened in surgery this morning?" he asked resignedly.

"Nothing. I contaminated my gloves."

"And your gown? And his gown? And the sterile wrap? Dr. Holderman thinks your attitude and your surgical technique could use an adjustment."

"Yes, sir!" J.W. added sarcastically and hung up; his decision was made. He did not report back to surgery that afternoon. He called Krista and told her it was over. They would not stay. Her silence was the warmest love she had afforded him in years. At 5 P.M., J.W. strolled, head high, into Dr. Jacoby's outer office. The residency director's secretary nodded superciliously at what had become J.W.'s chair. "I know why you're here," she added matter-of-factly. "Have a seat. He's on the phone. It's an important call."

J.W. could not help hearing through the open door. "Mom, did they tell you where you can live? Are they going to help you?" He was silent for a moment and spoke soothingly, "Mom, I love you. And tell Dad I love him. Everything's going to be okay. I'll fly out this weekend. We'll get things straightened out. I'll be with you. Don't worry."

Jacoby called J.W. into the office. His eyes had lost their sparkle. His lips were tightly closed, and he was silent for a long time.

"Have a seat, J W. Your folks alive?"

"Yes, sir."

"I'm glad for you, but life never stops stabbing people. My mom called to tell me that a gasoline tanker crashed in front of their house, and the fuel spilled down the hill into the living room and kitchen, flooded the whole bottom floor. Police came and ordered them out of the place. My dad's in a wheelchair. They didn't help my mother push him into the driveway. This is going to kill him. He built that house with his own hands thirty years ago. He wanted to die in his bed there."

He shuffled charts on his desk from left to right and asked, "How'd it go this afternoon? I'm glad you took some time off. I hope you talked with Krista. It's important to keep her involved."

"Better," J.W. mumbled, gathering courage to tell him to take his residency program and shove it where the sun didn't shine.

"J.W. I don't like to see people suffer. Not my folks, not you."

J.W. opened his mouth to begin the tirade, to crush the man who held the helm of a ship gone awry. J.W. could bury him with wrath, leave the program, and head back across the States. Jacoby would learn a lesson, and perhaps teach an asshole surgeon and an asshole administrator a modicum of humility.

But J.W. had seen despondency before, and the sadness in Dr. Jacoby's eyes brought him back to, of all things, the man in Hong Kong who had stolen the purse from the rich lady. J.W. remembered how the little thief had been kicked and spat upon, the swollen face, the blows, a man down, the more he hurt, the harder he was pounded. J.W. cringed recalling the Hong Kong judicial authorities threatening to keep him from sitting for the MCAT, for he was a material witness in a felony, and then the news that the wretched bandit had done away with himself. It all seemed so far away, and yet so close. And in the end, all of that had passed. He reminded himself everything does.

"I just came by to tell you how happy I am to be in the program, Dr. Jacoby. Sorry to hear about your family, and about the last couple of days. Things'll straighten out. You'll be happy I came here."

"We already are, Doctor. Thanks for stopping by. I needed that."

CHAPTER TWENTY-NINE

The ride to the hospital next morning began long before the sun reflected off the Rockies. El Buraq rolled to a stop two miles from their house just as the red lights and wooden arms of a railroad crossing came to life. In the distance, he made out the lights of an approaching freighter. The ones he had already seen in Cedar Springs were so long, they took fifteen minutes to pass. Already late, J.W. steered his bike around the barrier and sprinted to the start of a two-mile hill, so steep in places he had to stand on the pedals to get El Buraq going fast enough to remain vertical. Halfway up, a Cedar Springs Police Department cruiser pulled alongside, the lone cop waving in the bare light of early dawn. Nonchalantly, J.W. waved back. When the officer blasted his siren in J.W.'s ear, he pulled over and handed the officer a brand new driver's license explaining, "Hey, sir, I got to get to surgery. I'm a doctor."

"Yeah, right, tell it to the judge." He lit a cigarette and leaned back to wait for the night shift computer operator to run J.W.'s name for wants. J.W. sat on the curb for twenty minutes. The officer finally crushed his third cigarette on the ground, handed J.W. a thirty-eight-dollar ticket for ignoring a railroad crossing, and drove off.

Too late for a shower, and perhaps too late to even show up, J.W. rushed into the surgery suite reeking of exhaust fumes from the engine the cop had not shut off. Dr. Holderman was silent. They spent another surgical session, a master and his manservant, no useful information passing the preceptor's tight lips. The saving grace of the day was that J.W. was on call that night, and the only commute the next morning would be from the on-call room to surgery, two floors below. It felt good to know he couldn't be late.

The interns and residents not on call were out of the hospital by six or seven that evening. J.W. met with them over stale coffee in the dining room—the changing of the guard. Each exhausted intern presented J.W. with a barely legible, penciled list of the ill who would fall under the aegis of J.W. Weathersby, M.D., embarking upon his first nocturnal venture as a licensed health professional. Next to each name was a diagnosis and lists of medications; beside the names of a few players, a star was scratched to warn of impending calamity. As the last intern signed out, a gnawing in J.W.'s gut gave him pause. At first, he believed it was the overwhelming responsibility placed in his hands, but the growling in his stomach reminded him he had not eaten that day. He had been too late to order breakfast, too busy for lunch when Mr. Barmash's Whipple's procedure went beyond the five hours Dr. Holderman had allowed, and now too late for dinner, as the lady in the hairnet behind the tired food display enlightened him. J.W. response was his palm smacking the serving line. When the food manager flew from the kitchen, he called over his shoulder to call security. J.W. retreated to the on-call room to wait for the arrest.

After five minutes, with no detention, he went searching for a vendo-heaven, to stock up for an evening of candy bars and coffee. Dropping a quarter for a Clark Bar, the only remaining selection, his beeper sounded. He was to report to the emergency room, STAT, for the first hit of his career. He was about to enter the fraternity he had driven so hard and long to penetrate, and he sprinted joyously through the halls.

The ER doctor, who was tying the last restraint to the arms of J.W.'s inaugural patient, barked at the new intern to write orders for immediate transfer of the screaming man to an isolation room. The doctor finished his command with the diagnosis, "SAEW. Get 'im going."

J.W. mumbled, "Excuse me, sir, but what is that?"

"Severe acute ethanol withdrawal."

"But, I'm the surgical intern."

"Who knows, you might need to go in and tie off bleeders."

"What do you suggest?"

The emergency room doctor's eyes closed, and he heaved a sigh. "The DTs. The DTs! I might as well treat the dirtball myself. I suggest you fix his DTs, and please do it somewhere else besides my emergency department."

"Well, excuse me," J.W. whispered, hoping the doctor shared Ms. Pote's affliction of exceptional auditory acuity. The doctor turned to stare back at J.W., but Weathersby had gone to his patient's side to stroke his arm and quiet him. The vibrating drunk's face relaxed, and he stopped tugging at the restraints. J.W. glanced superciliously over his shoulder at the ER doctor, for he had just demonstrated his aptitude in the art of medicine— the skill to sooth the violent beast. It was a talent polished by years of acquaintance with real-world tragedy.

From behind, Nurse Princeton called to the ER doctor, "Good, that shot of Librium's kickin' in."

J.W. turned to leave for the hospital library to investigate the treatment of "Acute Ethanol Withdrawal," to assume responsibility for the life of his first patient.

"Hey, where you goin'? Let's get him outta here."

J.W. hesitated. At Union, in patrician, gentile Boston, even physicians-in-training didn't wheel patients to the floor—that's why there were orderlies. "Come on, let's get him tucked in."

As J.W. struggled to move the gurney toward the elevator, Nurse Princeton huffed and walked over and touched the wheel with the toe of her white sneakers. "There, the brakes are off. Think you can handle it from here?" J.W. pushed the gurney to the elevator, but before he could push the button, his beeper detonated. He was to return twenty paces back into the ER for the next hit.

Instead, J.W. got the drunk to a room, removed the restraints from his patient's hands, and wrote orders for admission and medications, verbatim, from the little cookbook, the spiral medical guide every intern carried in his short white coat. J.W. drew blood to check the man's serum alcohol level then trotted the stairs back to the basement ER.

Patient Number Two was an unfortunate older gentleman suffering from Acute Ethanol Withdrawal. "Goodness, Doctor, is this the first time you've seen the DTs? Let's get 'im outta here! Get the place cleaned out before the evening rush."

J.W.'s beeper rang again in the elevator. J.W. ran to the first phone he came to. It was the lab. "Ethanol level on your patient—167."

"Which one?"

"Your drunk patient."

But even J.W. knew that made no sense. One-sixty-seven was far too high for withdrawal, and far too low for a chronic drunk to act so drunk. At that level, even Ms. Pote would not have been all that much fun at a party. J.W. wheeled Number Two into a room three floors above, and a building-and-a-half away from his first admission, just as the floor nurse called him to come back and reevaluate Number One, who was exhausting his slug of ER Librium. J.W. could hear the man screaming in the background, "My ears are buzzing. Stop the buzzing."

When J.W. got there, he asked, "Are you hearing voices, sir?"

"Voices, goddamn buzzing voices. Buzzing, buzzing voices," he bellowed on and on.

The diagnosis was finally clear. This wasn't the DTs; it was a schizophrenic break, like the dozens J.W. had witnessed at St. Auggie's, back when life was good, and there were honors for those who tried hard. Had J.W. been able to spell "haloperidol," that is exactly what this patient would have gotten from him, the staple medication of the psychotic population of America. It was providence that J.W. was a poor speller.

The patient leaned forward, gripped his stomach in pain, and puked up some dinner tainted with what appeared to be coffee grounds, the curdled blood from the torn veins in his gut, paper-thin vessels from years of alcoholic excess. J.W. ordered more tests, x-rays, electrical studies, and more x-rays, to appear assiduous while he waited for the senior resident he'd paged breathlessly.

A new stream of phone calls and pages began to arrive from the nurses on the floor where J.W. had parked Number Two. There were requests for admission orders, treatment orders, and medication orders, intermingled with pleas to issue orders to place him in restraints before he made good on his threat to beat the nursing staff to death if they didn't find him a bottle of Thunderbird. "We need orders, Doctor, and we need you here stat."

The senior resident did not answer, having retired to his on-call room to sleep, husbanding the scarce moments of quiet he could eke out of the first few months of the medical year. June to September, the phase of the cycle that witnessed new interns descending like a black cloud upon the teaching hospitals of America, was a challenge at every level of the medical establishment. Senior residents slept early in the evening, for how much trouble could even an intern foster in the first two hours on call? Their years of residential duty had made the seniors past masters in the art of safeguarding precious moments of sleep before the babysitting commenced. It was a nocturnal watch over apprentices that would not totally wind down until a full year later when the next class of neophytes arrived, and the seniors were elevated to practicing physicians.

J.W. ran from his patient to the sixth floor, to the penthouse on-call room, pushing through the locked door with his shoulder.

"Hey, Doctor Tizzuto..." but he was cut off.

"Whatever it is," he grumbled, "handle it!"

J.W. ran back to the floor in time to witness a second round of black retching. He filled a paper cup with the sepia sauce and carried the sloshing vomit back up the five flights to the senior resident's cubicle. Tizzuto sat up, gagged, and paged the chief surgical resident.

J.W. ran back down to the floor, cup in hand. The eight-month-pregnant chief surgical resident wobbled behind J.W. She examined the coffee cup of puke, retched, and paged the attending surgeon. Dr. Holderman stomped in belligerently an hour later, having just removed what was left of the leg of a helmetless, insuranceless, inebriated motorcyclist who had kissed the ass-end of a stationary, 1950s Buick at forty-miles-per-hour. According to the police report, the patient, driving a '54 Indian, had spied a slinky prostitute exposing one of her ample breasts. Dr. Holderman's chief resident asked how he knew all of this if the guy hadn't been wearing a helmet. "Wasn't he gorked?" she laughed.

"Asshole was gorked before the accident. He talked a lot, but mostly bitched about not seein' her other boob."

J.W. piped up, "Hey, I got one of those."

"Dr. Holderman grunted, "What, a boob?"

"No, sir, a '58 Dynaflow Buick."

"Huh. Good for you."

Their present victim, with ear cocked as if listening to Dr. Holderman's narrative, suddenly bent forward and urped up more coffee ground sludge, now tinted with a streak of bright red blood. J.W. blushed, realizing the ER doctor had been right. This was a surgical case. But Holderman took a better look at the vomitus. It was floating with chunks of dinner and a hundred little white dots. To J.W. they looked like undigested pills. Dr. Holderman groaned, "A goddamn suicide. Betcha a quarter he ain't got no means."

The nurse pushed her way into the medical conference for her hourly check of vital signs. "His breathing is rapid and shallow, doctors," she advised as she snapped the thermometer in her fingers.

The chief medical resident was summoned. He was an anxious little man with a generous nose and thick lips that trembled. He had the look of a scared rat. He folded his arms in intellectual contempt at the gathering of surgical hacks before pronouncing the patient a victim of an obvious aspirin overdose.

"Who's the surgical intern?"

J.W. raised his hand.

"Your boy's one blood test away from a good stomach pumping, Doctor," he snarled.

Dr. Holderman held up both palms to the medical resident. "We don't do stomach pumpings on surgery service anymore. Your attendings wanted to expand their repertoire? Make a few extra bucks, do procedures. Board approved it. So, he's all yours. I recommend you drop a tube and treat his acidosis. If he doesn't stop bleeding, *then* you may page my service for a consult."

With just those few words from Dr. Holderman, the patient was transferred off the surgery service to medicine, and that meant one less patient for J.W. to take a history on, to do a physical on, or to present on morning rounds, and have his butt chewed for the predictable gaps in care. It was one less patient on whom he'd have to gather lab results, and, best of all, the surgery senior resident clucked, "Next time the drunk comes in, if you had been the last intern to see him, he'd be yours, even if you weren't up for the hit. But now he's medicines', and that's a good thing. Now, I am going to try to get some rest before the serious drinkers show up."

J.W. nodded and smiled. He didn't bemoan the two hours he'd squandered on the man. In fact, he was elated to turf him to another service. The rub was that, as a house staff virgin, Dr. Weathersby was unaware that purging the man from his personal venue automatically added the next to hit to his inventory, now swelling with another ailing creature lying supine on a gurney in the overflowing ER. And there was still the alcoholic on the floor two buildings over for whom J.W. had not yet written orders.

But certainly things would change. J.W. felt it in his bones. This was going to be a lucky night, one on which Cedar Springs's ill and maimed reported to the hospital early, one on which the intern's supplication bore fruit, the prayer that it would be over soon, that the spasm of admissions would burn itself out by midnight. In just eight minutes, though, the distant alarm of an incoming ambulance heralded the approach of yet another desperate life.

In his past life, J.W. had paid no heed to a blaring siren, other than to pull off the road and shake his head that some poor fool's life was about to be changed, probably forever. In J.W.'s new world, the siren became a gut-knotting misfortune of his own as the ambulance drivers rid themselves of their nuisance, dumping the cargo onto J.W.'s life.

⊨⊣ ⊢⊨

There soon came nights, nights so dark and rainy, so lonely, so hungry, J.W. resorted to pinching congealed, curled slices of ham and wilted strawberry shortcake off the dinner plates of comatose patients. He had become a master at ordering special meals of his personal taste for inmates who clearly would not be sufficiently alive by six to eat. But that did not always work, and when the menu became "liquid diet," or the patient had expired and the meal was taken away before the family arrived, he had to divert time from healing to hunt for cans of Ensure. Then he'd hide in darkened corners of the admissions waiting lounge on worn chairs to sip Strawberry Ensure and melt specks of chocolate from stale Mars Bars on his tongue. Though he'd nod off between swallows, the longest respites were not even ephemeral, for the beeper detonated every two minutes, driving him back to the ER. And each iteration was the same bump in the night—an ambulance crew off-loading another miserable creature for J.W. to torture through the last hours of life.

"Did you hear us coming or what? Love that new siren," a semi-toothed driver grinned.

The latest player, a Mr. Abraham Cohen, was assigned to J.W., because J.W. was the next up. Hoping for justice, though, J.W. sidled up to the ER doctor, reminding that he had just taken an extra hit because he'd been the one to sign the discharge orders two weeks before, and that he had a player on the floor for whom he had not yet written orders, and a star suffering from acute ethanol withdrawal in the ER whom he had not yet welcomed.

"Weathersby," the ER doctor hissed, "Here is a dime. I want you to call the fire department and tell them your story."

"Fire department?"

"Yeah, they're paid to care. Abraham Cohen's yours. Enjoy him."

Mr. Cohen's gurney shook in a seismic rumble. "Guess who's seizing?" the ER doctor questioned sarcastically. "The usual, Nurse Princeton."

She rolled up with the stainless steel cart, a cornucopia of IV's, Valium, and fishing-tackle boxes of medications J.W. had never before seen or heard of. Working as a team, J.W. held Mr. Cohen down until Nurse Princeton emptied the contents of the syringe somewhere into the man's wasted buttock. The shaking ceased, and J.W. smiled, but Nurse Princeton did not, for she knew, even without a program, the next act with Mr. Levy. And when it came, she shook her head as Mr. Cohen's pants filled with urine. It flowed off the rubber-coated gurney, onto the shiny linoleum floor, to pool next to J.W.'s sneakers. As he jumped back, there was a loud grinding and an awful stench.

"Weathersby," the ER. doctor uttered professorially with fluttering eyes, "this man has demonstrated incontinence of both urine and stool. He is yours. Be a doctor. Treat him."

"But I was just told surgery doesn't treat drunks."

"Take it up with Mrs. Pote. Just get him moving."

Mr. Cohen's room on 3-South was semi-private. The nurse told the other occupant, an elderly rabbi who had just had his prostate carved out because he hadn't been able to pee more than two drops a minute for the past fifteen years, that a Mr. Abraham Cohen was to be his new roommate. The rabbi was ecstatic. "Tanks Got," he moaned. "He vas in my congregation. Vatta you talkink? I know Abraham Cohen. Tanks Got."

But the rabbi's euphoria was fleeting "*Oy vey! Oy vey is mir!*" he wailed as they wheeled Mr. Cohen in. "Oy Got, vat did zey do to you, Abey?"

The religious leader's new roommate had not been a member of his congregation, or any other congregation for that matter.

Mr. Cohen was black. The rabbi continued grumbling in Yiddish, becoming louder and louder as more of the rank air from his new companion collected in the tiny hospital room. The floor nurse, responding to the commotion, stuck her head in. Watching Mr. Cohen commence round two of incontinence, she turned to run but stopped, shook her head in resignation, and pleaded to J.W., "Could you give me a hand cleaning him up? It just isn't right to leave him like this."

It was the only moment of residency so far that had a trace of meaning, the first time J.W. had been invited to be on a team, to work with a professional, not as a slave for a professional. As they stripped off his clothes and sealed them hermetically in plastic, she handed him a surgical mask to ease the stench. Next, they bathed him in strongly antiseptic soap. Mr. Cohen opened his eyes and peered into the two covered, hovering faces. He shouted in panic, "I dead! I done gone to hell!"

The rabbi shouted, "*Oy vey is mir!*"

A lady in the next room screeched in Vietnamese, "*Trời đất ơi!* Oh, my God!"

The nurse calmed Mr. Cohen, who sank back into his postictal stupor, while J.W. calmed Mrs. Tran in the adjoining cubicle. In minutes, they had a sterilized, sleeping Mr. Cohen. This was a gift. One cannot take a history from a snoring, post-seizure patient, and how much of a physical exam could a young doctor be expected to perform on a comatose alcoholic? Make sure he's breathing, look for bleeding, for broken bones poking through the skin, abscesses, and maybe comment on a bloated belly to confirm advanced liver disease. But J.W. could take blood, aliquots of it, for tests and more tests, and without even having to say, "I'm sorry for having to poke you, sir."

There was also time to go back and finally see Hit Number Four and write admission orders. While Mr. Cohen slept, there would also be time to see Player Number Three, wherever he had been stowed, and there was a full thirty seconds to spend standing by the window, to stare out at the normal people walking the streets at 4 A.M., humans left alone to do as they wished. J.W. tried to ignore the sound of sirens closing on the hospital.

⇥⇤

By the time J.W. finished washing his hands, he was paged again to the ER, to enter the life of his next victim, one Bertha Petersdorf, an elderly soul who had fallen in her apartment three days before and could not get to a phone. Her daughter received no answer when she made her daily phone call from up the block, and though surprised, as her mom was a shut-in, thought her mother was simply too busy to answer the phone—for three days. When the daughter finally became suspicious, twenty minutes ago, she ran up the street in her robe to find her mother on the floor, dehydrated and delirious.

The ambulance driver was direct when he radioed the ER to warn the doctor that while Mrs. Petersdorf's vitals were stable, she had not been in control of either bowel or bladder over the past seventy-two hours. The driver wheeled her into ER wearing a surgical mask. The daughter was furious with the driver for the fifteen minutes she'd had to wait for the ambulance. She warned that she was watching closely, and that she intended her mother be admitted and kept in the hospital until able to care for herself, "…and I mean completely. My husband's a lawyer," she snarled with a sufficient volume to wake Abraham Cohen five floors away.

"Yeah, and I'm Clara Barton," Nurse Princeton mumbled.

J.W. introduced himself. The daughter glared at the nurse. "What the hell did you say?"

Nurse Princeton walked away, leaving J.W. standing by the gurney. The daughter eyed him suspiciously, her stare focused on the J.W.'s scrub shirt and the chocolate stains. "Thank God they didn't stick us with some baby-faced intern," she screamed into her semi-conscious mother's ear.

As J.W. pushed the gurney into the elevator to set sail for a room on 5-North, a wheel on her rolling bed caught in the aged carpet, and the doors rolled shut on her. While struggling to pry them apart, his beeper went off. He pulled Mrs. Petersdorf out of the elevator and made for the nursing station phone. Mr. Cohen was seizing again. J.W. could hear the rabbi in the background groaning that this was the wrong Mr. Cohen, and Mrs. Tran in the next room shouting in Vietnamese that she had to go into fields to shuck rice, to get away from all the craziness in her hut. J.W. slammed the phone down, shoved Mrs. Petersdorf back into the ER, then sprinted through the empty corridors, encountering dead ends, surgical suites, and the psychiatry ward. He exited through a fire door into the darkened business office and past the hospital administrator's door.

Ms. Pote was at her desk and looked up as J.W. flew by. This section of the hospital emptied into the area around the dining room. The scent of bacon and eggs and toast drifted into the corridor as J.W. dragged himself up onto 3-North.

Mr. Cohen had stopped seizing and lay in his bed snoring, fresh urine soaking fresh sheets. J.W. helped the nurse rediaper Mr. Cohen, ordered a few more milligrams of Librium, and ran back to the hallway outside the ER for Mrs. Petersdorf. Her daughter was asleep on a wooden chair. J.W.'s beeper sounded, startling them awake. It was the nurse on 4-South. A patient for whom J.W. was responsible, an ancient man on another intern's service, had just expired. A doctor was needed to pronounce him. J.W. felt a wave of guilt and fear wash over him, as if it were his doing, or lack thereof, that cost a human life. It would eventually come down to being his fault for not having attended his colleague's patients. Worse than that, the deceased wasn't even on his special program of critically-ill players, the ones with stars scribbled next to their names. J.W. checked the other list, the one noting the healthy patients scheduled for early morning discharge. The man was on that list—at the top.

How could he have known? "It's the other intern's fault," he spit, but that did not quell the wave of dread descending over him as it had on the morning Mrs. Madhi had died under his care. It had happened again—J.W.'d killed a perfectly normal being.

The departed patient's wristwatch slipped down to his elbow as J.W. lifted the man's arm to search for a pulse. It reminded him of a wounded, hospitalized friend in Viet Nam, the loss of substance so marked by the ravages of illness. At least for this man, the insults were done. The watch read 5:37 A.M. J.W. recorded the time and gazed down at a time-worn, but serene, face. The tubes and IV's had been removed. The family sat quietly in the visitor's lounge. The deceased's son, a man of many years himself, thanked J.W. for the kindness the staff had afforded his father in his last days.

"He's very peaceful now," J.W. assured them.

"Thank you, Doctor," they offered, as each of three generations took his hand.

"You're very welcome. I'm sorry we couldn't have done more."

⊱⊰

Mrs. Petersdorf was awake. She complained she was thirsty, and J.W. tugged at the skin on her forearm. It tented up and stayed there. She was critically dehydrated, and he ordered a stat IV. In the moments J.W. waited, she started to cry that her knee hurt. J.W. pulled up her gown. The knee was normal, but there was a mass of swollen black-and-blue in her groin. He ordered an x-ray of the hip. He couldn't leave, but he had to, so he walked to the nursing station to call surgery and let Holderman know he'd be late. No one answered. He was down to thirteen minutes.

When J.W. got back to his patient, a siren was approaching, and J.W. froze, eyes cast down. As he looked up, he saw the daughter holding a glass of water to her mother's mouth. "No, ma'am," he snapped, "She's NPO. She can't have anything by mouth. She's got a broken hip. She needs to go right to surgery."

He started the IV in a huff, and when he was sure the fluid was flowing, ordered pain medication and took off at a sprint for surgery, his beeper bleating like Mao the Sheep.

CHAPTER THIRTY

J.W. flew into the OR at six-oh-seven. "Late again," Holderman grumbled. J.W. had not managed to make it to the dining room for breakfast, nor to the shower. When Dr. Jacoby called J.W. at 8 A.M., J.W. noted with a distant laugh that he had never gone this long without bathing, not even in commando school.

"I didn't call to check on your personal hygiene, J.W., just to ask why you were galloping through the administrative offices so early this morning."

"Yeah, I remember, or I think I do. I got disoriented when they paged me stat to 3-North."

"And?"

"And I had to cross a lot of buildings."

"But administration's two buildings over. Look, J.W., it's probably best not to hang around administration after dark; lots of papers and things over there. Let me get one of the senior residents to give you a tour of the escape routes."

On rounds with Dr. Holderman, J.W. tried to present the four pa-tients he'd admitted, willing to trade ass chewings for teaching. Dr. Holderman, though, had little to say. Mostly, he just grunted as they went from room to room, shaking his head at the state of flux left in Dr. Weathersby's wake, particularly when they arrived at Mr. Cohen's room, for the man's ethanol withdrawal had not gone well at all.

J.W.'s relationship with the rabbi had deteriorated when Mr. Cohen spent much of the night howling, in between sedative dos-es, that he had, indeed, been a member of the rabbi's church. He threatened to report the matter to the hospital director, who really *had* been a member of the rabbi's congregation, so Dr. Holderman had the man transferred to the internal medicine service, "Where you should have made sure he was admitted at the beginning. And this room stinks of stale urine. Make sure it gets cleaned up."

J.W. had not met the last hit of the night. The patient had been admitted, though, and when they got to his room, Dr. Holderman introduced J.W. to the man. "Dr. Weathersby," Holderman grum-bled, "it's supposed to be the other way round. You're supposed to tell me about the patient, not vice versa."

"Yes, sir."

Mr. Allen Bray, a gargantuan man, had presented with ex-cruciating pain in his stomach, the one that served his three-hundred-and-ninety-pound frame. The problem had begun at two, worsening insidiously until right about the time J.W. was called to pronounce the unstarred old man. When Mr. Bray couldn't take the pain anymore, his wife called the aid car.

Actually, Mr. Bray was a very pleasant gentleman who had no history of abdominal problems, but was now a corpus of undu-lating pain, and even Dr. Holderman was moved. There could be no pictures of the inside of the patient's abdomen, for the x-ray table weight limit was three-hundred-and-fifty pounds. Dr. Holderman retreated quietly to the corner of the room to ponder his options on this poor surgical candidate. He could undertake a risky exploratory operation, or watch him suffer and maybe die.

"Roll up your sleeves, Doctor," Holderman suddenly called brusquely, as if they were going to go dig a ditch. "We've got some heavy work to do."

In surgery, J.W. was briefed momentarily in the art and science of suspending a panniculus, the mass of abdominal fat, out of the path of Dr. Holderman's scalpel. "You hold the Richardsons until I tell you not to hold them. Questions?"

"No, sir."

Dr. Holderman stepped to the table and waited patiently for the anesthesiologist as she poked the endotracheal breathing tube into Mr. Bray's mouth, sweating with effort to snake it through his twenty-five-inch neck, past his vocal cords, and into his trachea. She probed over and over, pushing and twisting the tube, coating it each time with ever more massive dollops of KY Jelly. Had she been a summo wrestler, it would have been a task, but as the patient's throat swelled from the trauma of the increasing number of attempts to intubate him, it became nearly impossible for a hundred-pound Chinese woman to drop the tube, and she began stammering in something other than English.

"*Gei wo kan kan. Ke yi ma?*" J.W. asked in Mandarin Chinese.

The endotracheal tube dropped out of her hand to the floor. "You can try if you want," she answered, slack-jawed, and unwrapped a new tube and handed it to him. Her mouth remained limp as J.W. growled in Chinese for effect, using every ounce of strength and finesse he could muster to slide the tube into place. For a moment, there was a bit of background gabbling, though the room burst into absolute silence as J.W. entered the trachea on the first stab.

J.W. held the panniculus with retractors until his arms became numb, each hand supporting fifty pounds of adipose tissue. J.W.

was determined not to let the rolls of fat slip a single centimeter until Dr. Holderman discovered the source of the man's agony. Finally, J.W. was really part of the surgical team, useful, like when he and the nurse had bathed Mr. Cohen. The numbness in his hands was reassuring.

Dr. Holderman searched Mr. Bray's abdomen for the needle in the haystack. An hour slipped by. J.W. did not let go of what he held.

"There it is. Got it!" Dr. Holderman laughed toward the end of the second hour at the table. A small, but very swollen, red, hot, pus-filled pocket lay halfway down the duodenum. Dr. Holderman excised the dead tissue, and amid the stench of rotting fish, discovered a white sliver, a needle-like foreign body. He placed it in a specimen jar and had it transported, via the pneumatic system, to the path lab for analysis.

They asked Mrs. Bray what it could have been.

"Maybe it's a fish bone," she suggested. "He eats so damn fast, you never know what you gonna find in the man's stomach. Y'all ought to tell him to slow down."

In the surgeons' lounge, Dr. Holderman spoke to J.W.

"I'll take a piece of toast if you don't mind. You speak Vietnamese."

"Yes, sir, I do, but that was Chinese."

"No, I mean you spoke with Mrs. Tran last night on the floor. Do you know why she's here?"

"No, sir."

"She has a brain tumor. They say it's from Agent Orange. When she came to the U.S., my church sponsored her family. Lousy deal. Get some lunch and a shower, please. And good work dropping that tube."

⊷⊶

There were calls from the floor, calls from the ER, and a call from Dr. Jacoby. Mrs. Petersdorf had been transferred to the orthopedic service for the fractured hip, though her surgery was going to be delayed until late that night because the intern had allowed her to eat, according to the floor nurse. "Now, doctor, I know you know that we don't allow people to eat for eight hours before surgery so the stomach is empty, and the patient doesn't vomit on the operating table and suffocate. Let's make sure that doesn't happen again."

And there was a call from Krista. Mao the Cat had captured a bird, eaten it, then vomited bones and feathers. Should she take him to vet for a stomach pumping?

J.W. thought of the man with the aspirin overdose and remembered he had promised to call the family with results of his cholesterol count. They were apprehensive about that, for one of the man's brothers had high lipids. Though the patient smoked a carton of cigarettes every three of four days, and downed a six-pack or two after dinner most nights, and was suicidal, the family was obsessed with controlling his cholesterol. By the time J.W. found the lab results on Aspirin Man, there was another admission to process. There was a handwritten note on her chart: "Personal friend of Dr. Holderman."

Mrs. Koppenberg was a sixtyish, red-headed woman with a penchant for greasy food and cigarettes. While taking her history, J.W. noted her hands shaking ever so daintily, and, also, the thick odor of stale alcohol steaming from her pores.

"Do you drink, ma'am?"

"It is Listerine, Doctor!"

J.W. called a nurse to chaperone his physical exam, and a teenager appeared in the private room still wearing a yellow gown, surgical gloves, and a mask, having just assisted another intern on a fecal impaction case. Without a word, the nurse sat in the corner and closed her eyes to rest.

"Don't trust me, Doctor?" Mrs. Koppenberg asked sarcastically.

It was not until five P.M. that her labs were drawn and all forms and releases completed, and six when the EKG tech called back to say she would be on the floor to do Mrs. Koppenberg in a jiffy, right after she answered a stat call from the ER. J.W.'s mouth watered. All that was left to his day, night, and day on call was a screening EKG. J.W. conjured visions of hopping on El Buraq and pedaling home, standing under a hot shower for half-an-hour, inhaling a roast chicken, and most of all, sleeping. It was just minutes away. J.W. calmed himself and smiled.

When J.W. called the EKG tech back at six-thirty, she was still in the emergency room, "But it won't be long, I promise. We're gonna get you home." She was waiting for a man who had called the ER complaining of crushing chest pain, shortness of breath, and nausea. Nurse Princeton had urged him to call 911, but had forgotten to take the victim's name and address. That was at five, and the troops were still standing by, waiting to converge and preserve a life.

J.W. went to the basement to watch. As he passed through the automatic doors, the man called again, complaining that his pain was worse, but he had forgotten the number Nurse Princeton had told him to call. The ER doctor snatched the phone from Nurse Princeton, demanded the man's address, and called 911 for him. When the medics got there, the patient was unconscious. Though they revived him, he denied chest pain and asked the medic to call the ER doctor on the radio and get a prescription of Antabuse, a drug to keep people from drinking. The medic refused, proposing the man come to the ER for a full evaluation. Instead, the patient vomited and demanded, "Hey, Doc, get on the radio and get me some pain meds. This is gonna be a hell of a hangover."

On the floor, Mrs. Koppenberg had become progressively more jittery over the planned surgery and couldn't get to sleep.

The nurse paged J.W. and asked for a sleeper, but it was only 8 P.M., too early to give her a pill that would only last for six hours. When J.W. got back to the floor, the EKG tech was on break. Mrs. Koppenberg had fallen asleep, dreaming eagerly, no doubt, of surviving her medical difficulties and returning home to sip Daiquiris for many years to come.

The EKG tech was also happy, for at nine, when she wheeled her cart up to Mrs. Koppenberg's bed, she was able to remove the woman's bra without waking her, hoping to finish her work before Mrs. Koppenberg ever knew they had tapped the secrets of her heart. The bra came off without a hitch, but every time the tech placed one of the suction cup electrodes on her chest, Mrs. Koppenberg called out in terror and violently ripped the electrode from her skin. J.W. held her arms down, but she continued to wriggle, and the tracing on the EKG looked as though it was a map of the Himalayas.

Around eleven, J.W. signed out to the on-call intern and headed down the hall of 3-North toward the backstairs, where he had hidden El Buraq for the past forty hours. He heard the rabbi grunting painfully and stuck his head in to see how he was. The old man mumbled, "You're da vun who svitcht da name of mine frent, Abey Cohen." He turned away in disgust, took a bedpan brimming with foamy, bright red liquid from under his covers, and placed it on the bed stand, next to his untouched dinner.

The graveyard shift of nurses and aides was returning to duty. They had been home twice and back to work twice since J.W.'s arrival at the hospital the day before.

⚊⚊ ⚊⚊

J.W. mounted El Buraq and rode numbly through the wet streets of the North End, rolling into his driveway after midnight. Krista was asleep. Khai was reading in bed.

CHAPTER THIRTY-ONE

The ride back to the hospital at 4:30 A.M., five hours later, was cold, but only at first. J.W. passed over the railroad tracks and spied his police friend lurking in the shadows of an all-night convenience store parking lot, head back against the seat. A burning cigarette hung from his lips, but his eyes were shut tight. J.W. started up the hill, though the grade and his weariness soon overcame him, and despite standing on the pedals, the bicycle hardly moved. Very little air passed over his him, and he fell deeper and deeper into a stupor until the pain disappeared. He surmised he had ridden into a sauna, and was enjoying the heat and moisture. There was no more pain in his legs from the struggle up the hill—he had reached an exquisite steady state with nature, as if a blast of endorphins was now carrying him on the climb toward the hospital.

That feeling lasted until his head slammed against the concrete. For a moment, there was no pain, no time, just gray-black. But his nose began to hurt, and J.W. opened his eyes to blood dripping to the ground. He took a tee-shirt out of his pannier and put pressure on his nose. By the time he was shaving in the men's surgical dressing room, the area around his left eye was swollen with a hint of deep blue. J.W. flew into the surgical suite at five-thirty, just steps behind Dr. Holderman. "You got blood coming out of your nose," he observed cryptically. "Have that taken care of before we start."

The ER doctor fluttered his eyelids in disrelish as he cauterized the bleeder and sent J.W. back to surgery.

Dr. Holderman made the opening incision for the hernia repair in a fluid swipe of his scalpel. He picked at a ligament.

"You know what this is?"

"Ah, well, let's see. Let me get a bit closer, okay?"

"Don't you move, Weathersby. It's the inguinal ligament. Ever heard of it?

"Yes, sir. I think so."

A few more swipes of the scalpel, a line of sutures here and there, and Holderman snorted, "I'm going to close now."

Another surgical session passed in which J.W. stood in neutral while the master performed. He shook his head and started for the door, but Dr. Holderman called out, "What happened last night with Mrs. Koppenberg? You ruffled her feathers. Why'd you have to wake her up so many times? Patients are nervous the night before surgery. You were lucky she had fallen asleep. Why'd you do that?"

"To get an EKG."

"You could've gotten an EKG any time during the afternoon. You need to plan your day more efficiently, Doctor. You can't be annoying my patients like that." He popped a few more staples in the incision, keeled around, and walked from the operating room to the lounge to wait for the next patient to be wheeled down. It was Mrs. Koppenberg.

She was still jabbering when Dr. Holderman lifted her tiny frame onto the operating table. He nodded officiously to the anesthesiologist, who drew up a syringe of golden fluid and injected it into the IV tubing, sending Mrs. Koppenberg drifting off into a realm of endless Daiquiris. As surgery began, J.W.'s arms were still numb from the day before, but Dr. Holderman handed him the retractors, and J.W. accepted them without comment. At the gall bladder, the surgeon discovered a round mass of green-stained tissue the size of a small olive. His tongue clucked as he picked carefully at the gooey surface, and sent a bit of it off for biopsy.

He clucked again when the frozen section report came back from the pathology lab. "Cancer. I'm not surprised." He tugged at the tiny tumor, removed what he could of it, and directed J.W. to close. "Do the skin sutures, Weathersby. I'll talk to the family."

Moments later, as the nurse and J.W. moved Mrs. Koppenberg to recovery, J.W. spied Dr. Holderman sneaking out of the hospital in his suit and tie. J.W. was by Mrs. Koppenberg's side when she woke up. "It's you!" she cried as her eyes trembled open.

"No, no, actually, it's my twin brother you're thinking of," J.W. reassured her. "We're both residents here, identical twins, really. I heard what he did to you. He's been like that all his life. Imagine our poor mother."

Mollified, she asked for water, but everyone in medicine knew that patients, both young and old, took nothing by mouth for long periods after abdominal surgery. J.W. wet her lips, but she didn't like the taste of the moist paper towel and demanded to see Dr. Holderman.

The Koppenberg family stood outside the recovery room cubicle, listening. Her husband walked into the room and took J.W. by the arm, leading him into the hallway. "I apologize for my wife, Doctor. She's changed since her gall bladder's gone haywire. She was a great lady. Why did this have to happen? She was really something. You would have loved her. Everyone did."

Dr. Holderman arrived quietly, met with the family again late that afternoon, and apologized for his intern. J.W. peeked into the room. Holderman clasped Mrs. Koppenberg's hand for a moment before placing a moistened paper towel on her lips. She asked, "Could you do that again?"

By 5 P.M., there was peace on the surgical service for the first time since J.W. had arrived in Cedar Springs. His work was done: lab results were recorded on charts, medications for comfort and sleep ordered, and lists turned over to the intern on call. J.W.'s patients were stable. It was time to head home to see his family for the first time in days, grab a quick dinner, and escape into sleep before his on-call day and night began again in a few hours.

As J.W. strutted out the main hospital doors, his beeper went off. He laughed. He was history; whatever the problem, it was no longer his. J.W. had signed out to the intern. The beeper rang again. J.W. laughed again as he unchained El Buraq to the tone of the beeper squawking a third time. Through his addled consciousness, he imagined an emergency had surfaced. Why else would he have been paged three times after he had signed out? Perhaps it was his family. Maybe Khai had seized; worse, maybe Khai had stuck a bottle cap up her nose.

J.W. could do the smart thing and turn off the pager, as he should have when he walked out of the hospital; or, he could answer it, like he knew he would, like he would answer a ringing phone, even if he knew it was a wrong number. J.W. went back, found a phone outside Ms. Pote's office, and responded to the page.

"How am I supposed to know who's on call and who's home?" the page operator snapped. "I'm not a mind reader, Dr. Weathersby. Are you on call or not? If you are, contact Mrs. Koppenberg's nurse."

"Why didn't you call the intern?" J.W. growled at the nurse.

"You never told us you signed out, Dr. Weathersby. Mrs. Koppenberg's spiked a fever. She's hallucinating. Her family wants Dr. Holderman to do something."

"They want The Man? Call The Man. I'm just a lowly intern, sweetheart."

"We're not supposed to call him. We're supposed to call you. You're the intern."

"But I'm not on call!"

"Well, why did you answer your page?"

"Look, Holderman makes twenty times what I do and ten times what you do. Call him, not me." J.W. tossed the receiver onto the phone.

"Just turn around and walk out," J.W. screamed at himself, and he actually spun for the exit and took a few steps toward the door, but his next memory was of trudging up the backstairs to 3-South, driven by a force outside his person. He had visions of Ms. Pote's frown at the podium that first day, visions of her call to Dr. Jacoby, and of his grimace. J.W. imagined Jacoby's desk piled with medical charts, and one folder standing open—his. J.W. could see the dejected frowns on his parents' faces when he told them he had been kicked out of the residency for ignoring a call from his dying patient because he was tired and hungry.

Mrs. Koppenberg was sweating, her head flopping from side to side. She was no longer the formidable enemy she'd been just a few hours before. J.W. sat on the edge of the bed and took her hand, as had Dr. Holderman. She calmed almost immediately, looked at him, and whispered, "Robbie?"

Her family interjected from behind, "She seems so confused. Please help her."

She wouldn't let go of his hand. J.W. felt the fading of her spirit as he tried to pull away, so he sat there until she fell asleep.

Primum non nocere, first do no harm. It rang in his ears, over and over, an echo of the oath he had sworn at graduation, only days before leaving their only worldly asset, the house, in the hands of a real estate agent. His adventure crossing the country with Khai emerged from the torpor, their time together, hearts brimming with hope. And then his mind swam back to the day his greatest fear had unfolded—the upheaval in their lives growing out of a two-second puff of air that J.W. had heard as "every forth night," but everyone else as "every other night." Three lives were torn asunder by a single word. He'd have to abandon his family to fulfill the machinations of aging, stressed, overworked, angry doctors who had been forced to undergo the same ordeal a generation before. He would lose his family one way or the other—all he had promised Krista, and himself, was a lie.

"Do no harm," he heard himself whisper. "Do not leave her. This, too, shall pass. Get the job done. You'll get home." In his near-stupor, what J.W. saw most vividly was Mrs. Koppenberg's matted red hair, roots dull white. She appeared years beyond her age, and the senselessness of his enmity toward her struck him like a bolt of lightning. They were not enemies, just victims, she fearing the ebbing of life, of the now-demarcated approaching end; he of his fear of endless years of on-call nights awake, away from home, of more of the loneliness he had already suffered, of constant judgment, of never rising above the status of wild card. Out of the clear blue he mumbled to Mrs. Koppenberg, "It's only been eight weeks."

Mr. Koppenberg leaned forward and asked, "Did you say something, Doctor?"

J.W. examined the surgical wound, ordered more blood tests, and walked them down to the lab himself. The night lab tech had but one real eye. Perhaps that had soured her on the world, for she moved with such lack of purpose and dispatch, J.W. observed under his breath, "About as useless as tits on a boar hog."

"What did you say? Did you call me a dog?" she sneered, and it took an hour-and-a-half for the numbers to come back. They weren't good numbers. Mrs. Koppenberg was sick. Her white blood count had doubled since admission. An infection was eating at her, one that had to be treated before morning, but the senior resident was busy in the intensive care unit; the second-year resident did not answer her page; and the on-call intern was lost in space, probably devouring pilfered tins of chocolate Ensure before heading off for his next hit.

J.W. considered leaving a message with the medical student to ask the intern to look in on Mrs. Koppenberg, so he could leave the hospital with a clear conscience. But medical students disappeared at night. The decision was his alone. J.W. could do a more thorough physical exam and more tests. He had the power to order everything under the sun to try and find an answer to Mrs. Koppenberg's problem. His only limitation was to ensure that she not wake up, even if it meant she died before dawn. Or, J.W. could call it a night, let the nurse hit the intern with a barrage of pages, and force his involvement.

J.W. told the family they would let her sleep until the intern came by, or until morning, when Dr. Holderman was back on the job. The way J.W. said it, in soothing tones with an air of certainty, the family relaxed, and J.W. escaped in just minutes. He switched his beeper off and informed the operator, twice. El Buraq sailed down the great hill in a minute, but as the cold, wet Cedar Springs evening washed over his face, pangs of conscience bubbled. By the time he got the bike stopped at the railroad tracks, J.W. was boiling with guilt. "Son of a bitch!" he screamed aloud to the stare of a man sitting on the tracks, a bottle tipped to his lips. J.W. turned El Buraq to start back up the monster, but first rolled up to the drunk, hopped off the bike, and with another blast of profanity, dragged the man twenty feet away to a bench. J.W. forged the hill without sensing the pain in his legs until the chain popped off the sprocket. It caught in the spokes and toppled him to the ground. He smacked his already mauve right eye and reopened the bleeder in his nose.

At the hospital, J.W. ran to the surgical dressing room and changed back into a scrub suit before charging furiously through the halls to Mrs. Koppenberg's room. As he ran, he concocted every manner of justification to save face and undo the last excuses he had made to the Koppenberg family, the nurse, and the page operator. J.W. settled on a story that the lab had called him at home and told him there was a small question about one of the results, and they needed to do further testing. The family was still there. "Don't you ever go home?" they laughed nervously.

"I'm not comfortable waiting 'till morning. I'm going to call Dr. Holderman and discuss Mrs. Koppenberg's situation with him right now." They said nothing, but the distressed faces softened.

"What is it?"

"Sir, Mrs. Koppenberg has a temperature."

"I should certainly hope she has a temperature. Mammals are warm-blooded. Do you mean she has a fever?"

"Yes, sir. Sir, could you come in and take a look at her?"

"Let me talk to the senior resident."

"Sir, he's in surgery. I already tried to call him. He wouldn't come either."

"What's her white count?"

"Twenty-two thousand."

"Start her on some IV diclox. Can you do that? I'll see her in the morning."

"Yes, sir," and the phone went dead.

By the time J.W. figured out diclox was dicloxicillin, a powerful anti- staphylococcal antibiotic, and how to administer it, it was midnight. He phoned Krista. She growled, "Why didn't you call earlier? Khai was worried sick. She fell asleep on the

couch waiting for you. You have a mistress, don't you?" she accused angrily.

"I do not, goddamnit."

"Yes, you do. It's that damn hospital. Where the hell is your
head, J.W.?"

"Bitch!" J.W. screamed into the line that had slammed down
on the other end. She had no idea what was going on behind
these walls. Nobody did. People puked and cried and bled, and
a hell of a lot of them died—it was a lunatic asylum. People's
lives were entrusted to those who didn't trust themselves. Worse,
people's lives were entrusted to those who trusted themselves
far too much, shamans whose conceit obscured the demons that
lurked deep in their hearts and minds. The place stank of pain,
fear, and death, and Krista didn't care. She hadn't even tried to
understand.

Mrs. Koppenberg's white count had risen to thirty thousand by
morning. J.W. stayed all night and drew blood again at 5 A.M.
The beeper had been silent while he spent the hours in an empty
bed two cubicles away.

Dr. Holderman brushed into her room quickly minutes before
surgery. He glanced at the lab results then at Mrs. Koppenberg
tossing and sweating. He called the surgical suite. "I need to
get an emergency case on *right now*," he spat. They wheeled
Mrs. Koppenberg back to the OR and opened her fresh scar. A
pocket of yellow pus squirted from the wound as Dr. Holderman
drained the abscess. They inserted a drain, and J.W. pushed Mrs.
Koppenberg's gurney back to the recovery room. Dr. Holderman
disappeared to dictate his operative note, and J.W. talked to her
family. "They found the problem. She'll beat the infection, but
the cancer is a different matter."

"Cancer?" Mr. Koppenberg gasped, surprised, his face sour-
ing into a frightened hue of red.

"Yes, sir. I thought Dr. Holderman told you. The tumor they found by her gall bladder. It's going to be a difficult road for her."

Mr. Koppenberg faced the family, jaw slack, his beaten shoulders drooping even further forward. It was if he had just been told she had already passed. Robbie took his father's arm and walked him gently out of the room. They retired to the lounge at the end of the hall. J.W. stayed with his patient.

CHAPTER THIRTY-TWO

B y late that afternoon, it dawned on J.W. that his night on call had rolled around again. He figured it out because a column of residents and interns were grinding about the hospital looking for him. No one listened to his objections that he had been home for only a few hours in the past week. "That's why they call you residents," the old lady in the hairnet behind the serving line laughed.

As J.W. babbled protests, his colleagues shook their heads in sad realization that J.W. had gone 'round the bend, and so soon. There were still two years and ten months to go. Didi asked, "Wasn't combat worse than this?"

J.W. began to answer, for she seemed concerned, but she added without waiting, "Hey, my sign out's quick and dirty. No sick players. Now, you're gonna get a call from Mr. Crutcher's nurse in 345. He's my star. The guy's gorked. Starts yelling that he's in pain, screaming that an elephant's sitting on his chest. Don't get excited, don't get an EKG, and for God's sake, don't call McMurtrie, his attending. Go by the room, say hello, and forget it. I'm tellin' ya. This has been going on for a month. Have fun!" And she, too, was OTD—out the door.

It was comforting to know that one professional had communicated with another, and J.W. was relieved of the tension and concern he might have otherwise wasted on a squirrel of a patient. The pleasant emotion vaporized abruptly, though, as the buzz of sleep deprivation grew louder and louder in his ears, and night had not yet fallen.

J.W. had lived with the buzzing for months in Ranger School and for a year in Viet Nam. He had grown, not used to and comfortable with it, but in dread of the noxious humming, for it was the harbinger of pain, the misery of endless days and nights trudging fields, paddies, forests, jungles, and elephant grass. It was a portent of starvation, the loss of forty pounds in forty days, of bodies and bodies, some his pals, some his enemy, all of it so confusing that after a time, J.W. couldn't tell who was who. The expressions on the faces of the dead in those ghastly days were not terribly dissimilar to those on the souls he was pronouncing twice a night at the hospital.

That's what the buzzing culled from his heart, a reminder of his fractious past, the one he had worked so hard to escape, the one in which he found himself again mired. There was nothing but bleakness, not a sliver of light in the tunnel that stretched for years and years. Worse yet was the knowledge that at least in the war, everyone was affected. There weren't cohorts of the privileged, bands insulated from the insanity. In warfare, before long, life became an eccentric act of God, every life painfully and relentlessly intertwined with the madness. It was what you did and saw every day. Here, only interns and patients suffered.

J.W. left the cafeteria for the on-call room, determined to sleep, to rid himself of the buzzing, to function normally again, to serve the beings incarcerated in the little cubicles of his hospital. Just a little catnap, and he'd be back on track. He'd done it a thousand times before. But with the first strike of the beep-er, J.W. cursed aloud that he was the prisoner, that the patients were the lucky ones—all they had to do was lay there and take it. There would be no escape for him. The fatigue would grind him down again, depress him as it had in the past. It was no way to live, fearing the future during every moment of the present.

Patients and their families walked past quietly, smiling, nod-ding respectfully, though J.W. could not imagine why. Those in wheelchairs, the fragile and the ancient, even those nearing the end, smiled to him. One sallow-complexioned waif, the tiniest of little old ladies, rode the halls in her wheelchair, tied to life only by the tubes bristling from her neck, her nose, and her hands. She reached out weakly for his arm. "I love the marble in these hallways, don't you, doctor? You're so lucky to be a healer in such a distinguished hospital. Did you know I was born in this hospi-tal on the third floor?"

The beeper rang again. J.W. shuddered but smiled, "Ma'am, I wasn't aware someone so lovely was brought into the world on this very spot."

She smiled back graciously. "Doctor, if you have time, come by my room. I have pictures of the hospital eighty years ago. You can have one."

The gentleness of the woman's hand and her offer was broken by the second call of his beeper. Mr. Crutcher was complaining of pressure in his precordium, as Didi had prophesied. "I'll be up to see him in a few minutes," J.W. promised the floor nurse as he headed for the ER to welcome his next hit. But when the page came a third time, J.W. detoured to 5-South to calm the nurse.

CHAPTER THIRTY-THREE

Now on his eighteenth admission, or some such number, Mr. Crutcher was widely regarded as a crock, with little need for a seasoned professional to tend to his medical needs. A second-year nursing student was waiting outside his room with wide eyes and a trembling lip. "Mr. Crutcher's acting funny," she whispered breathlessly. "He says he's having chest pain."

J.W. laughed at himself for having allowed a student nurse drag him away from his next hit, snickering at the neophyte for how deeply she had fallen into the man's web of secondary gain. Had he really been ill, the nursing supervisor would have taken over his care and called the senior resident, the attending physician, the janitor, someone, anyone but the intern.

"Mr. Crutcher, how are you, sir?" J.W. asked, peering around the corner into his room.

Mr. Crutcher was supine on the floor, having rolled out of bed past the rails that had been left down when the student nurse ran from his room. She had retreated from her patient to escape his rantings that it felt like an elephant was sitting on his chest.

J.W. thought about his next patient, the one waiting in the emergency room. That man was also screaming about elephants, though they weren't sitting; they were flying and they were pink, and they were dancing circles about his gurney. J.W. knew all this because had heard the patient over the phone when Nurse Princeton paged demanding J.W. transfer the man from their venue to his. J.W. felt more a zookeeper than a doctor, and wondered why he hadn't been offered a single course in veterinary medicine during his four years at Union.

Elephants! J.W. knew little of elephants. His pre-med biology professors taught that pachyderms had been designed without knees, an important observation for an orthopedic veterinary surgeon, but of no help in caring for patients on cold, wet, Cedar Springs autumn evenings, on which J.W. sought to survive the next eight hours, a night during which his only fantasy was not a secret rendezvous with one of the nurses in the on-call room, or even a night with only five hits. All J.W. dreamed of for those hours was the dim possibility of a few crumbs of breakfast at the far end.

J.W. lifted a writhing Mr. Crutcher onto the bed. Not to be fooled by the theatrics, J.W. searched out of the corner of his eye for the TV control, hoping to catch the last few minutes of *Hill Street Blues*. J.W. patted his patient on the shoulder, reassuring him, "You're gonna do fine, sir," remarking to himself that Crutcher really was well versed at the game.

That was it! This wasn't heart disease; this was J.W.'s first von Münchausen's Syndrome. Here was a pathological, but brilliant, liar who had fooled the best of physicians. J.W. marveled that the man had even perfected labored breathing. Crutcher must have pawed through a dozen medical texts and studied the symptoms of heart disease for years in order to mount such a performance.

Mr. Crutcher gurgled and stopped moving. The line on his heart rhythm monitor decayed from sharp, regular spikes into a curious pattern of pretty waves then, abruptly, into a flat line, only occasionally disturbed by rough patches of chaotic electrical vibration. The emergency horn at the nurses' station came to life as Mr. Crutcher's spirit drained away. J.W.'s heart choked into his throat, for it was the same whine as the twenty-minute fuel warning on the helicopters whose gas tanks often ran dry in Viet Nam. But in those days, J.W. knew how far he could push the HUEY with nearly empty tanks. J.W. could feel it in the touch of the cyclic, the way the ship vibrated just a little differently with no fuel aboard. Pilots got that way after months and months of living in the helicopter.

Through the haze of his fatigue, it dawned on him that someday he would have the medical hours under his belt to look at the Mr. Crutchers of the world and feel the warning siren before it sounded. But that night, he was not yet sufficiently astute, and when the alarm rang throughout the hospital to draw teams of resuscitation specialists, all J.W. could do was stand by dumbfounded.

The nursing student jumped to Mr. Crutcher's side and thumped him in the chest with her fist. The heart monitor on the wall vibrated with the shock of the punch, but the line on the screen barely wavered. She socked him again. The monitor rocked, and there was the most subtle twitch of Mr. Crutcher's eyelids. The thin green line on the screen began a reversal of the decay seen seconds before. Neat, even, organized prickles rose out of the flutter to move at a snail's pace across the screen. In seconds the barbs grew into spikes, towering waveforms that accelerated into a reasonably normal cardiac rhythm. With that, the whine of the bedside alarm became still. J.W. wondered if the monitor and the horn were aware of what they had just witnessed.

As hordes of resuscitators raced toward the dying man, the tiny, hard-rubber wheels of their carts hummed like a dozen crazed contestants in a supermarket shopping spree. They pushed into the tiny room, shoving compatriots, fighting to attach *their* personal array of monitors, tubes, and needles, the cumbersome tools of the basic bodily functions they were trained to restore.

J.W. stood in a corner and marveled at how a house fly survived on its own.

The agonized expressions of determination on the technicians' faces degenerated into annoyed boredom when Mr. Crutcher's eyes quivered open. J.W. nodded his head in confident reassurance and thanked them for their grand efforts as they rolled their carts away to dens in far-flung corners of the old hospital, to nooks J.W. was never to visit in the nearly five thousand hours he would serve that year of internship.

The room hushed, and the student nurse fixed Mr. Crutcher's pillows. "Good work. Very professional," J.W. called to her. "Give his attending a call and let him know what's happened."

Mr. Crutcher had been revived on J.W.'s watch. One of the resuscitation techs would remember his presence and word would surely spread that the new intern had been instrumental in saving a patient's life. The hospital would be abuzz with the tale of his heroics, and while J.W. fully planned to afford the nursing student her due, he was desperate for the recognition, for something positive, and he nurtured the thought of a complimentary word until, in just seconds, his beeper sounded.

Mrs. Koppenberg was gagging up green-stained mucus from a stomach that had not been challenged by food or drink in days. J.W. rubbed her forearms after she informed him her acupuncturist massaged those points to quell nausea. Her queasiness passed, and she smiled. It was the first time J.W. had seen her happy, or any of his patients happy, or his colleagues happy, or the attending physicians happy. "I'll call Dr. Holderman. Maybe he'll want you to have something."

"What is it?" he demanded.

"Well, sir, Mrs. Koppenberg's been vomiting. Would you like me to treat her with Compazine or something?"

"Or something? Jesus Christ! Cut her toenails," and he hung up.

His observation was astute. Her nails had grown long and thick, and had putrefied into a deep, malodorous, repulsive yellow. She was pleased when J.W. offered to trim them, but the clippers on the surgical tray were in the minor leagues compared to the hardened, neglected claws on her feet. So, J.W. snuck into to the basement, to the darkened maintenance department, and borrowed a pair of shiny, new, tin shears.

"Would you also do the calluses? Oh, God, there's such pain when you grow old. You should never have to know."

As J.W. carved with a scalpel at the years-thickened mat of tissue on the bottom of her feet, she reached back and fixed her pillows, as if settling in comfortably for a long movie. "Do you know my first days in America? Nobody knows I came from the old country. You won't say a word, will you?"

"No, ma'am."

"You can't tell, but I came from Poland. My father, Nathan, Nathan Levy, a *mensch*, that man. He came ahead of us. Do you think it was easy to make a living in those days? Selling underwear and socks door to door? You think that was easy?"

"No, ma'am."

"It wasn't. I'll tell ya. You know how hard that man worked? A *mensch*. He got good, too, at his trade, Nathan Levy. No one helped him. He did it on his own. Then he went into umbrellas. Door to door. With each sale, he put half into a sock, and then he put that sock into a little metal tin. He kept it under the floor of the loft he rented on the Lower East Side. You couldn't trust a bank in those days, could you?"

"No, ma'am."

"He saved passage for us to America. And he saved for us to go on the train across the country. And every day, he sat back at the end and smoked a stogie. I know you shouldn't smoke. Don't remind me, but he loved it so. *Luzzem alain*, leave him alone. After dinner, he sat in an easy chair. The blue smoke from his cigar was all around. Clouds and clouds, and he drank his small glass of schnapps. Not a lot. He wasn't a drinker, my father. Just a *bissel.*

"I sat by his feet every night. I wish I was there now. He promised someday we would live across America, in the mountains. No filth, no *dreck*, none of it.

"The persecution we had to suffer in Poland. In America, my father could take us anywhere we wanted. I never saw evergreen forests or wild rivers until I got here.

"His *zaydeh* promised my father the same thing. He smoked a cigar, too. They lived in Mesritch. Oy, I could write a book."

J.W. handed her a tissue to dry the tears then gave a final tug at the callus, just to neaten his work. But the piercing cry of his beeper startled him, and the blade, that had grown dull quickly from the thick, cornified skin, dug into her foot.

Mr. Crutcher had crashed again. The hordes redescended. This time they had an excuse to execute their trade. He was shocked with electrical paddles repeatedly, the increasing injections of current bringing him further off the bed into arched spasms. After each salvo, the nursing student knelt by his side, pushing gently on his chest, sobbing as the cardiac monitor maintained its flat hum.

J.W. elbowed toward his patient, telling the nursing student he would take over the CPR, but with his first compression of Mr. Crutcher's chest, there was a series of cracks, one that brought an end to the chatter in the room.

"Good job. You just busted his ribs," the senior resident yelled above the warning siren. J.W. stopped CPR. The senior resident shook his head in disgust and through gritted teeth hissed, "Might as well keep goin', Samson."

In the reflection from the window, J.W. witnessed the flat green line on Mr. Crutcher's heart monitor grow thinner, until even the tiny fibrillations faded away. The paddles were applied one last time. They delivered great voltage in a final bid, though did not convert the line into life. The senior resident mumbled, "Stop CPR. Call the code."

The resuscitators relaxed, and there were sighs. But J.W. snapped back, "Bullshit," and resumed pumping, easily compressing the organs beneath his victim's flail chest. He pushed harder and more fiercely, for there was nothing to lose at this point but his patient's life. His beeper went off. "Kiss my ass!" J.W. grunted, but no one laughed. He was in the throes of a drama he had waited nearly forty years to savor. No matter that the line on the monitor line had flattened into a perfectly horizontal trace, J.W. pumped with the fervor of a crusader, sweat dripping from his face, until his arms became painfully heavy and so tired, he asked breathlessly, "Hey, man, we could use some help here."

"Like I said, call the code," the senior resident spit, and J.W. checked the cardiac monitor. All electrical activity had ceased. Mr. Crutcher, the great thespian, was gone.

The troops repacked their carts, policing up some of the spent syringes, catheters, and adrenaline bottles, piles of debris that had accumulated nearly ankle-deep on the puddled floor. As they rolled away, there was nervous, very quiet laughter about the miscues and blunders that accompanied so absurd a pursuit as resurrecting life. A woman from the records room appeared brandishing forms, and J.W. snuck off to answer his page.

The nursing student opened the curtains around Mr. Crutcher's roommate and sat on his bed holding, his wrinkled hand while the elderly man gazed at the teams of youngsters who had worked so frantically. It was the first time his dulled eyes had seen them, and he cowered against the corner of the bed rails asking, "Why did they laugh?"

CHAPTER THIRTY-FOUR

When his beeper rang at 5:55, J.W. feared, through his stupor, it was a fourth post-midnight hit that just couldn't have waited five more minutes, until the watch changed and the next intern was on the hook. It was, though, the senior resident searching for him. "M & M conference. Seven on the dot. You're doing Cruzer. Questions?"

"Yeah. What's M&M?"

"Where did you say you went to medical school? Morbidity and Mortality Conference. You will present the saga of his final hours. Meet me in the cafeteria a few minutes before seven. I'll tell you what not to say."

For fifty-five minutes, J.W. ran from patient room to patient room, drawing blood and delivering it to the lab, running results back to the floor, and recording numbers in charts before the attendings arrived for morning rounds. Back and forth, back and forth, like a hamster, redrawing blood on patients whose lab tests had been lost, redrawing blood on players for whom the wrong tests had been ordered, attending the bevy of meetings with residents and returning interns, and reporting on the status of the patients who had survived the night under his care.

At three minutes to seven, the senior resident sat over a steaming cup of hospital coffee into which he slowly, deliberately, sprinkled precious grains of brown sugar scooped off the top of his piping hot, butter-covered oatmeal. In the concha of the senior resident's ears were traces of shaving cream. J.W. enjoyed the clean, pleasant scent of the man's fresh scrub suit.

"You need to get organized, Weathersby. Are you prepared to defend Cruzer's bungled resuscitation?"

"That's Crutcher."

"Whatever. You knew he had serious coronary disease," he accused around a mouthful of oatmeal, "and when the floor called, you were off cutting your toenails. What kind of shit is that? His attending's pissed. So's Jacoby. Them boys don't like early morning surprises."

The buzzing in J.W.'s ears had risen to an almost deafening roar. He had not felt the weight of such weariness and hopelessness since the night his helicopter crashed into the bomb crater. He thought back to Lieutenant White, who had stayed with him that night, and the next day, and into the next night. He heard himself hiss through gritted teeth, "That kid's gone, and I'm alive, and I'm all hot and bothered about my problems? I'm lettin' this little piece of shit scare me? This ain't stress; it ain't even work." He chuckled again sourly at his weakness, at how he had let his eye drift from the target. But he also felt a sense of relief for simply having defined the problem. Just having a diagnosis made him feel better.

That was the moment J.W. heard the crash. The senior resident's sweetened coffee spilled, and the bowl of oatmeal lifted off the plastic-coated table. Ms. Pote, who had been moving along the serving line with a tray of napkin-wrapped donuts, stopped and looked over. By the intensity of her eyes, J.W. realized it was his own fist that had hit the table.

The fatigue whined louder and louder in his head, reaching an almost deafening clatter as he fought to stay awake in M&M Conference. He barely heard the other attendees blather themselves into a tizzy over Mr. Crutcher's demise. "Here was a patient with known coronary disease who was left in the hands of a student nurse and, of all things, an intern!" complained Dr. Jacoby.

J.W. was shaken out of his reverie by that remark. He was being presented to his colleagues, and more importantly, to his superiors, as a dull, incompetent cretin, the professional equivalent of a nursing student. On the other hand, there was a bit of relief, for Jacoby had implied it wasn't his fault. He was simply at the wrong place at the wrong time. He relaxed, dreaming of lunch. M&M conference adjourned, Dr. Jacoby grasped him by the arm, and led him back to the office. Jacoby pointed to the chair at the business end of his desk. J.W. refused and stood. "Relax, J.W. This isn't the South Bronx," he offered in a reassuring tone. "Take a load off. Let's talk."

J.W. continued standing at attention.

"Place your butt in that chair. Now! People die in the hospital, Doctor. That's why they come here. Where you went wrong was going it alone on Crutcher. What you should've done was call the senior resident the first time there was trouble."

"I told the nurse to call his attending!"

"Did you ever check to see if she did? She didn't. He just found out this morning."

"Then the nurse should have her ass chewed."

"Get serious. You raise your voice to a nurse and the next stop is federal court. And stay out of the maintenance area. Don't, ah, get involved with hospital property."

"I was getting a pair of shears to cut the toenails on one of my patients."

"Right. Read any philosophy, J.W.?"

"Yeah, sometimes during my copious off hours. What do you mean?"

"J.W. there's no such thing as luck. No event in life just happens. You wish upon yourself all that turns up, my friend. Good and bad. You want to trace the road between the first day you entered this hospital with your bicycle and what's going on now? Go ahead. It's a simple path. You're a bright guy. What's happening here is a self-fulfilling prophecy; the more you expect trouble, I mean in your gut, the more you want it, the more you'll find it. You're in a daily waiting game for the call from me or Holderman, aren't you?"

"No."

"Yes, you are. Everybody in the hospital knows about you. It's a hot topic, Doctor. The nurses on 3-South wager how long you can go without getting your ass chewed. They bet cans of pop on when I'm going to call you."

"So, I'm not paranoid! It is real. Every time I fight back, every word of derision about the absurd hours, every comment about wishing I was home with my kid, crazy shit like that, all of it gets back to you, doesn't it?"

"Does that surprise you?"

J.W. sprang to his feet. He hissed, "You folks really believe you're doing the right thing here, don't you? Carrying out the will of God, huh? Your little patches of turf are so important, you just can't see how far your heads are up..." He spun about and marched from Jacoby's office before the man could answer.

At home, J.W. related the story to Krista, the stranger who shared his bed. "My life's a joke. I'll never survive what's happening."

"There's nothing at the end of our rainbow, is there, J.W.? We took one step forward and fell back two. You were the only anchor I've ever had in this life."

"Were?"

"I went along with your dream. Remember? We were going to be happy. 'Just hold on a little longer.' And a little longer and a little longer. I want a future, but there is no such thing with you, is there?"

J.W. closed his eyes and tried to bolster himself, recalling the Viet Cong troops who had refused to submit, no matter who dumped their dreams into tiger cages and mass graves. But as his eyes relaxed; all he could imagine was the never-ending procession of sick, needy patients flowing in over the wearisome days and longer nights. He asked himself if he was simply a psychological pansy. "Am I being tortured? Is it being done to me, or is Jacoby right? Am I doing it to myself? How much of a hand have I had in what's happened?"

His colleagues had more staying power than did he. Why? They took the crap with a smile, never breathing the word "quit." Why? They spoke of opportunities to learn new procedures, to see another patient with a rare disease. "What is wrong with me?" he asked himself aloud once again, if the pedestal on which he had placed doctors was indeed real. What if it was drive, just hard work, not quality of character and intelligence that had delivered him to this residency program?

⊶ ⊷

With each on-call night, his vision narrowed, funneled into a black cavern through which J.W. regarded the world. He had been lost in that tunnel before, in high school, when he was taking heat from teachers and football coaches, and in the army, when every move he made, every command he delivered, was thrown back in his face, and he was held up as Darwin's theory in reverse, an incompetent monkey. It was back, the darkness. He was finally a doctor, and he had no idea what that meant, other than it brought a ration of pain no different than all the other pursuits of his life. He hurt like hell, and he didn't know where to dump the blame.

CHAPTER THIRTY-FIVE

It was in mid-November, while J.W. was on the obstetrical and gynecology service, mostly the latter, that the walls closed in nearly all the way. Sometimes, if the attending liked interns, they were allowed to deliver the occasional baby. Usually, however, interns just nursed patients in labor until the attending physician whisked in at the last second to complete the process, and share in the minutes the family would treasure and relate to their friends. Yet, even watching was good. J.W. still revered the first moment of life and remained smitten with each birth, just as he had in medical school and when Khai had come into the world. He missed her so.

After deliveries, he often sat on a radiator in the hall looking out at the desolate streets, in awe of the wonder he had just witnessed, of the new being that had been protected for nine months from the storm. That was all to change. The new life would start fending for itself, each year taking on more, until it paid for crazy decisions like his.

On a rainy night, he watched the orange light of the hospital reflect on the puddles, the beating of the wind distorting their surfaces. No matter how J.W. tried to see his reflection in the water, nothing was clear. A homeless man trudged by. J.W. was jealous of his freedom.

＝＋＋＝

There was little rest on that two-month rotation, and by early December, J.W. didn't expect any. He had become adept at sleeping on his feet during rounds, meetings, and classes, especially x-ray conferences, where the lights were turned off as the first film was popped onto the view box. Didi was somewhat more sophisticated, keeping her eyes open for the first glance at the image, so when she was called upon to proffer a diagnosis, at least she knew the body part under consideration. She'd guess at an answer with just enough certainty in her voice to stave off total humiliation. She had confided in J.W. one very early morning on call, an hour or two before dawn. "J.W., you know, I've begun to accept worthlessness as the norm. How do you do it? You're the one who has it all together. This is nothing for you. I wish I had your experience."

＝＋＋＝

Cicely Sanchez was beautiful. She was fifteen when she presented to the emergency room, sweating, vomiting, bleeding vaginally, and crying for help. She had had no prenatal care, for neither she nor her twenty-nine-year-old mother knew she was pregnant. Cicely was assigned to Dr. Pickworth, on whose service J.W. was taking hits that night. She was going to be a freebie, and he knew it. So did the hospital.

J.W. pushed her on a gurney from the ER toward the elevator. "What are you going to do to me?" she whimpered through building tears. Her voice was so weak, J.W. had to lean forward to hear her.

He looked down at Cicely and smiled. "Just going up to your room. We'll give you some medicine, and you're going to feel a million percent better."

"What does that mean, a million per…?"

"Little one, we're going to take good care of you. You'll see. I promise you'll be happy." He paused and took her hand. "You know what, you remind me of someone I knew once. A very long time ago."

But as the doors opened on the OB floor, she screamed in terror and grabbed her belly. Blood trickled through her knit pants onto the gurney. The OB nurses pushed J.W. aside and moved Cicely to a labor room, started an IV, and draped her in a blue hospital gown. A more matronly nurse snapped, "*Hable, no grete!*" then turned to J.W. and added arrogantly, "Spanish for 'Talk, don't scream.'"

Instead of shrieking, Cicely began to shake uncontrollably. J.W. took her hand. "Pumpkin child, don't be scared. You're okay now. We've got you covered." But her hands were burning. When the lab called with the results of her blood tests, J.W. was more scared than she was. Her white count was triple normal, like Krista's when she had become sick from the infection in her womb.

"Is your baby old enough to be born?" the nurse questioned roughly.

Cicely wept, "What do you mean?"

"Well, when did you get pregnant?"

"What do you mean? I don't know what you mean!" Cicely cried.

The nurse drew pictures of a penis and a vagina, and Cicely sort of recognized the parts, but not the names. "When did the man put his dick in your cunt?" the nurse demanded.

Cicely turned her face away from the nurse and now cried quietly. She didn't know. She told them her mother had talked to her of sin, of not letting that boy touch her down there, but just where in the process all this trouble began, Cicely simply did not know.

The fetal monitor on her only slightly distended belly displayed a baby's heart rhythm that slowed repeatedly, every time she tightened in contraction. With each of Cicely's screams, the baby's heart rate took longer to return to normal. If the infant was not born soon, vaginally, she would have to have a cesarean section, and Cicely, burning from a deep infection, was a lousy operative candidate.

J.W. tried to explain. She asked for her cigarettes.

"Sweet Pea," J.W. laughed, taking her hand again, "we don't smoke in the hospital. They'll shoot the both of us if you light up. Picture it. We're in jail. Once a week they let you out of the cell for your appointment with the felon doctor over at the prison clinic." She smiled weakly, but another contraction wracked her, and she began to scream.

"You heard the nurse, '*no grete*,'" but J.W. also promised, "Okay, okay, okay, after the baby's born, I'll sneak you out to the patio where the staff smokes."

With each more closely-spaced contraction, the beep of the fetal monitor slowed and more blood spit onto the sheets. J.W. called the attending physician at home. Half-an-hour later, when he called again, Mrs. Pickworth assured J.W. her husband had just walked out the door. J.W. saved the chucks, the blue, plastic, cotton-lined pads placed under wet things, and J.W. weighed one dry then weighed all of the soaked chucks. She had lost two units of blood, just since they began saving the pads. He called Pickworth's home again. His wife informed J.W., "The doctor walked out the door one minute ago."

"That's what you told me a half-hour ago," J.W. blared as he jammed the phone down.

The nurse looked up from her desk and wagged a finger. "*No grete*, Dr. Weathersby."

The baby was born at midnight, minutes after Dr. Pickworth rolled into the delivery room. He was out of the hospital at 12:30 A.M., and Cicely started bleeding again at one. J.W. called Pickworth at quarter-to-two, who suggested, "Get some cryopre-cipitate from the blood bank to stimulate coagulation. And don't you ever snap at my wife again. Am I understood?" He slammed his phone down before J.W. could smash his.

The blood bank had cryoprecipitate in stock, gallons of it. The technician on call invited J.W. down to pick it up. "Yeah, I'll dash right over. Look, lady, I can't even leave here to take a leak. I'm an intern. Do you know what that means?" There was a dreadful silence. He wondered if she was cowed by the fact that a doctor was yelling at her, or perhaps her silence was out of pity.

"I'll send it over by taxi," she offered, "but you have to pay the cabby."

J.W. borrowed the eight bucks from the nurse who spoke Spanish, but when J.W. asked the cabby for a receipt, he laughed, "A what?"

Cicely went through the two units quickly. She kept bleeding. J.W. ordered four more units. Eight more dollars. The bleeding slowed, and for a time it looked as though the years of study and work had finally borne fruit, though the chucks became soaked again at four, and the taxi driver wouldn't accept his Visa Card. "Come with me," J.W. ordered, and the driver followed reluctant-ly up to Labor and Delivery. "This is Cicely. She's the one getting the blood you've brought. She wanted to thank you for saving her life."

He glanced up at the spent bags of cryo, touched Cicely's arm, left the room, and hand-carried the four bags to the floor, as well as the next delivery at four-thirty. By five, Cicely's bleeding had stopped. By seven, she was sitting up in bed consuming the bacon and eggs on the morning menu. J.W. wondered if he had ever been that strong.

"Can I see my baby? I promise I won't try to keep him, honest."

But the infant had been transferred to another section of the hospital during the long night. The adoptive parents had been notified, and neither Cicely nor J.W. were allowed to meet with them. "Those are the rules, Sweet Pea. I'm sorry."

"Who do I remind you of?" she asked.

"A little one, like you."

"Who?" she demanded gently.

"A woman I knew in medical school. She was fifteen, too, when she had her baby. Then she finished high school, graduated from college, and went to medical school. Now she's a doctor. A good doctor."

"Honest? Did they take her baby away?"

"Yep," he lied.

Dr. Pickworth blew into Cicely's room, consulted her chart, and asked how she felt. Without giving her a chance to answer, he asked J.W. to step out into the hall. Fightin' words, J.W. assumed, and he took a position in the hallway as far away as he could from the obstetrician. But the doctor looked down, avoiding eye contact with J.W., and J.W. thought it a ploy, a ruse. Pickworth would draw him in and coldcock him.

"Thanks for the help last night," Pickworth muttered.

"Cocksucker." J.W. whispered under his breath, but Pickworth continued.

"Look, I'll be up front with you. My wife and I are splitting, and it's tearing both of us apart. I owe you one."

━┿ ┿━

J.W.'s beeper sounded, heralding a request for his presence at the front desk to meet with the Koppenbergs, to be served with papers, J.W. imagined. They were, however, waiting with smiles. Mr. Koppenberg held a large, brown cardboard box under his arm. He shook J.W.'s hand. Mrs. Koppenberg remarked, "You look so thin. Have you lost a lot of weight? You need to eat, you know."

"Yes, ma'am."

Mr. Koppenberg stepped forward and handed J.W. the package, a telescope. "It's for your son," Mrs. Koppenberg offered, barely able to raise the sallow corners of her mouth. "Our company makes them. Your son needs to get used to sleeping outdoors and reading the sky if he's going to go into the army."

"It's a girl, Bubbie, the doctor has a beautiful daughter," Mr. Koppenberg added gently. They stood awkwardly for a moment after J.W. thanked them. As they left the hospital, J.W. allowed it had been a good day and night and day; perhaps not great, though at that frozen moment in time, maybe worth what had cascaded under the bridge. He passed Ms. Pote in the hall and smiled. She stared, and J.W. laughed and pulled out his beeper, to turn it off, to block the call sure to come from Jacoby.

━┿ ┿━

Cicely was propped in a recliner, picking at dinner. Her fever had remitted, the infection succumbing to the expensive new antibiotics dripping into her IV. J.W. wondered if Dr. Flowers was using them yet in Hong Kong.

"What was her name? The one who looks like me?" Cicely asked.

"Sharra. Dr. Sharra. I wish I could have her talk to you.

That night, J.W. pulled from his wallet the scrap of notepaper Sharra had left for him two years before. He focused on the letters 'Aysa' written in tiny script at the bottom. He stole into the Medical Director's office and dialed the phone in the pitch blackness. An operator answered. "Beth Israel Hospital." J.W. froze and began to shake. He dropped the receiver, tiptoed out into the area outside the cafeteria, had coffee, dragged himself to an on-call room, locked the door, and lay on the bed in the dark, ruminating. There was no choice. He would call again and just ask for her.

The operator put him on hold. After two minutes, he heard the door to Administration open, so he hung up again and waited silently. As he looked at the number a third time, it struck him like a tank crushing his chest—the letters, Aysa. "Ma'am, is Doctor Aysa there?"

"I'm sorry, I don't see a Doctor Aysa on the staff. Who are you, again?"

"Oh, I'm sorry, I'm Dr. Weathersby. We were medical students together in Texas. I'm organizing our reunion. I think she got married. Her last name used to be…" J.W. stopped in midsentence. "Ah, here it is, her name used to be El Buraq. Hope I'm pronouncing that properly."

"Ah, let's see. Well there's an Aysa Nur. A resident in medicine."

"Of course, that's her. Foreign names are so hard, aren't they? And then they get married…It's impossible. Could you put me through?"

"Give me a minute, Doctor."

"Of course."

An exhausted voice answered, "Medicine. Dr. Nur."

"Aysa? Is that you?"

Her end of the line was instantly and deathly silent. J.W. was not sure how long it took for a weak, "J.W?"

"Yeah. Aysa, I'm sorry to bother you. I know I shouldn't have—only. Hey, are you okay?" When Sharra did not answer, J.W. blurted, "Hey, look, I have this patient. I want her to talk to you. She's fifteen. Just had a baby. She thinks her life is over."

"J.W., I...Oh, the note, the letter."

"Like I said, Aysa, I know you won't talk to me, but will you tell this little girl everything's gonna be okay? Everything always is."

"Will it be, J.W.?"

"I don't know. Time might tell."

"Of course, I'll talk to her. Is she there?"

"Can I call you back in five minutes?"

"Cecily, you remember that doctor I told you about? You want to talk to her? I'll give her a call. You can speak to her in Spanish. She's real nice."

"Honest?"

"Honest."

Cicely started to cry as J.W. asked for an outside line. "Hey, Doctor, I got a great kid here. Her name's Cicely. She's fifteen. On my OB service. Tell her how hard you worked. She speaks Spanish even better than me."

After "*Buenos tardes*," J.W. did not understand until Cicely covered the receiver with her hand and asked, "How is your wife? She wants to know."

CHAPTER THIRTY-SIX

J.W. thought of telling Krista about Cicely, but what he really wanted her to know, and never know, was about Sharra, to get it over with, to apologize and swear he would never, ever, think of Sharra again. Krista knew he was restless, but he didn't want to lose what he had. He would start over, make amends, and never cheat in his heart again. But as soon as he started pedaling home in the driving rain, Sharra was all he could think about. He was still drenched when he looked in on Khai, asleep with *Charlotte's Web* on her chest. She moaned as J.W. kissed her and took the book away.

"Separation anxiety," Krista whispered from the door. "Just like when you kissed her good night after taking a break from Mao, the cat cadaver. Remember? It's hard to believe, but in the greater scheme of things, those were better days, weren't they? The journey was better than the inn. Anyway, the basement's flooding, Plumber Man. You need to do something down there."

Water trickled across the cellar floor, and J.W. followed the trail back to the corner wall, where it puddled around the mountain of moving cartons they had not yet unpacked. As J.W. lifted the soaked cardboard boxes out of the water, several collapsed, their memories spilling into the silt-thickened water that flowed through cracks in the foundation. A thin, black book caught his eye, his flight logbook from the army, and he sat on the floor, dreaming back to the initial entry in 1965, his first lesson in the air.

J.W. had worked hard to be accepted into flight school, losing nearly eighteen pounds in one weekend, transforming his Sterling College linebacker weight to U.S. Army flight weight in less than three days. He recollected the master diet he had commenced upon a Friday noon, on the eve of a big game, after he'd run to the gym and weighed in twenty-one pounds over the army's maximum for pilot training.

J.W. raced back to the fraternity house, pinched a roommate's rubber rain suit, and returned the two miles to the gym. He worked out in the boiler room until that evening, when his new friend, the custodian, had to turn down the boilers because Ray Charles was performing on the main floor and had bitched about the heat.

J.W. ran back to the fraternity house at midnight, took a fistful of Ex-Lax, turned up the heat on the furnace, and did pushups until the floor was soaked with the sweat that seeped from the steaming rubber suit. The Ex-Lax acted mightily, but not until 5 A.M., and again at 5:03, 5:09, and every few minutes until game time. His pants were up and down so often, he was afraid to tie the belt of his uniform. Two-and-a-half-hours of chasing receivers over Ridgeway Stadium bought him another eight pounds and a series of ass-chewings from his coach. "Weathersby, you're running like you got a load in your pants. What the hell's wrong with you?"

At the Saturday night fraternity party, J.W. was so thirsty, he snatched the orange slice out of Krista's wine punch and chewed it into a puree, but expectorated the bulk of his indulgence as he ran for the toilet.

Sunday was not a day of rest. The hours saw trips to the scales and the men's room at the gym, the men's room at the fraternity, and every men's room in-between. The final journey to the scales was at midnight. The custodian kept the building open until everyone else had gone, so J.W. could strip nude for the final weigh-in.

By 6 A.M. Monday morning, the hour of departure for the air base two-hundred miles from campus, J.W. was so shaky from starvation, thirst, and his rapid heart rate, he had to be helped up the stairs of the bus. He told Captain James, the local ROTC commander, that he had been hurt during the football game.

Captain James laughed, "Don't worry, we'll be stopping along the road for sausages, pancakes, home fries, and eggs. An army travels on its stomach, and this army's picking up the tab. That ought to make you feel better, Weathersby." As the other flight cadets inhaled their meals, J.W. dreamed of a glass of water.

The flight physical at the military hospital was divided into twenty stations, most of which involved needle pokes, some drawing vital fluids, others adding. J.W. started a record of the net balance of liquid transfer on the back of his physical exam form, hoping more had been extracted than received. A sergeant saw him writing on his own records. "Hey, that's government property you're defacing, Cadet." He snatched the record out of J.W.'s hand.

"Hey, Sarge, when do we get weighed?" J.W. asked.

"Oh, we got us a wiseass cadet. You get laid when you earn it, college boy."

The scale loomed at the far end of a long hall, still hours and a dozen stations away. It was the very last stop, for body weight was not an important medical statistic. At the urinalysis station, J.W. was unable to produce even three drops. The sergeant commanding that station ordered him to drink four gigantic glasses of water and try again. "Hey, Sarge, I'm not even breathing deep. See, I'm trying to lose this weight, because I had to gain weight to play football, and..."

"Sounds like a personal problem, Cadet. I need a bottle of piss from you. Any other questions?"

J.W. cornered one of the other flight cadets by the urinal, who shared his wealth, but J.W. was so tremulous from low blood sugar and dehydration, most of the ill-begotten urine spilled on the sergeant as J.W. handed him the little paper cup.

The psychoanalysis station, next to last, was manned by a fully uniformed woman military psychiatrist, across from whom J.W. sat in his shorts.

"Cadet Weathersby, how do you feel about your mother?"

"I don't know, ma'am. We had our good times. Yeah, we got along pretty good."

"What do you mean by that?"

"Well, ya know, good times, bad times, ma'am. Sometimes she yelled at me. There was the time she got angry when she came back from seeing the president, because I wrote some curse words."

"The president. I see. How did you feel about that? And why do you keep covering yourself up?" She looked down at his exam form and asked, "What's this scribble on the back? 'One-ounce in. Half an ounce out.' Okay, report to the final station."

"Well, did I pass, ma'am?"

"Just move on to the next station, Cadet."

J.W. mounted the scale as if stepping onto shards of razor sharp, poison-coated glass. The sergeant ordered, "Come on, move your ass, Cadet." He threw the sliding weight to the right in a brutish toss, far beyond the one-hundred-eighty-two-and-one-half pounds allowed for J.W.'s height. J.W. exhaled and the bar teetered at one eighty one! He danced off the scale and hugged the sergeant, who tore off to report the incident to the psychiatrist.

Flight school commenced on his twentieth birthday. How he had loved to fly, screaming during his first solo, lying in bed at four in the morning in flight school, waiting for sunrise so he could soar again. He was the last in his class to start, and the first to earn his wings, graduating a month after turning twenty-one.

＊＊＊

Next to the entry in his logbook for 2 May 1969, summarizing the crash of his HUEY into the B-52 bomb crater, was scribbled, "1st. Lt. Robert White, Black Granite, Deep in the Rockies," and beside that his co-pilot's lyrical words celebrating the jagged mountains, white-water rivers, and the warm forests of his home. It was all that was left of his poetic friend. J.W. looked on a local map and saw that Black Granite was only forty miles from where he sat on the soaking floor. It was a discovery that stripped his last excuse for avoiding Lieutenant White's parents. Just the same, J.W. tossed the logbook back into the carton, wondering if there was any reason to reopen their wounds, or his. The logbook was a relic, and J.W. wouldn't need it, for he knew he would never fly again, and he would never visit his dead co-pilot's' home.

＊＊＊

Krista called into the basement. "Long distance, Dust Man."

There was an uneasy quality about Bernie's voice. "Just want to let you know. Not using any more. Bobbie Jo's not, either. Hey, we're coming out to Cedar Springs. Would you like to see us? It's okay if you say no. I know how Krista feels about me and my habits."

"Come on, we'd love to see you. Got a big bathroom. The two of you can sleep in the tub together this time."

J.W. mentioned that Bernie and Bobbie Jo were on their way and watched Krista's eyes. She nodded in acceptance, yawned, and went to bed. J.W. sat alone in the living room, ruminating about the day's ups and downs, a peculiar day, as full of pain and happiness as any he remembered. For one second, it had been marvelous, her voice, the thinnest slice of her presence, and in the next breath, he had tasted the loneliness of her absence. For a last time, he relived the benchmarks of his short career as an aviator. It made him happy, but just for the instant before he realized he'd be pedaling back to the hospital in a few hours.

J.W. awoke on the couch at dawn, hours after his team had finished morning rounds. He rode to the hospital without shaving, and when Dr. Pickworth saw him, he must have assumed J.W. had been on call again, for he walked away quickly, his eyes cast down as usual. J.W. imagined divorce was awful.

As J.W. came onto the OB floor, a well-dressed man carrying bright flowers walked jauntily past him into Cicely's room. J.W. wondered if it was her minister, but in Cicely's bed sat a pretty Caucasian woman nursing a newborn. The man bent over and kissed her. The room was lined with flowers and cards. "I'm sorry. I must have the wrong room." J.W. smiled. "I must've been on call too long. I can't remember. Hey, congratulations anyway."

J.W. left the room and stared at the number. It was indeed Cicely's. He felt a soft hand on his shoulder. "I'm sorry. It happened so fast."

It was the bilingual nurse. J.W. stared wordlessly then ran to the nursing station. As he snatched Cicely's chart from the rack, Ms. Pote walked to his side. "May I have that chart, Doctor?"

J.W. pulled it away from her arrow-straight, outstretched hand. The final entry read, "Patient deceased 3:54 A.M., secondary to septic shock. Willis Beardshear, M.D., Intern."

J.W. dropped the chart at Ms. Pote's feet and charged off to find Beardshear, fuming aloud, "That son-of-a-bitch. He wouldn't even call a cab to save a patient."

Beardshear was clipping toenails on 5-North for the old lady who had been born in the hospital eighty years before. "Beardshear, I want to see you out here in the hallway. Now!"

"Dr. Weathersby," the old lady looked up. "I thought you had the day off. I'm so glad you stopped by. I want you to have this picture."

"I couldn't take that from you, ma'am."

"Oh, I won't be needing it any longer." She offered a framed, sepia-tinted photograph of the hospital at the turn of the century. The bricks and mortar had a crisp, new cut about them.

Dr. Beardshear watched the scene dully, as if he had not slept in days. "I want to see you outside," J.W. reiterated heavily.

Beardshear stared at J.W. for many seconds, though his eyes soon closed and his head slumped. J.W. shook his shoulder until the man looked up. He followed J.W. into the hall. "What's your problem?" he snarled.

"Cicely Sanchez, that's what."

"Who?"

"The fifteen-year-old on OB. I want to know what in the hell happened to her. She was my patient. You were on call. Why didn't you tell me?"

"You're not the attending. I called Picksteen, or whatever the hell his name is. Go talk to him."

J.W. crossed the street to the Medical Arts Building and marched blindly to Pickworth's private office. Though he was with a patient, J.W. pushed past the nurse and knocked on the door, seething, until Pickworth answered, "Yes?"

"May I see you out here?" There was long silence, and J.W. heard him excuse himself.

"What is it, Dr. Weathersby?"

"Why didn't you call me? Did you bother to go in?" J.W. demanded.

"I don't need to justify myself to you, Doctor. And, in case you haven't noticed, I'm seeing patients at the moment. I'll talk to you later. I am sure you have duties on your service, Doctor."

J.W. walked toward the hospital's main doors and glanced at El Buraq, chained to the railing, dusted again with snow, as it had been during so many of the phases through which J.W. had dragged it over the years. Dr. Jacoby was standing inside the doors waiting for him. "J.W., we haven't talked in a while."

"I got nothing to say."

"Good, then listen for a change."

"Pickworth and your intern friend were with Miss Sanchez all night. Along with an infectious disease internist, an intensivist, and half the hospital. Put yourself in his shoes for a moment. He was pretty shaken up when she died. All of them were, not just you.

"Take the day off. Let me handle Ms. Pote. And Pickworth. And Beardshear. Anybody else?"

J.W. walked in the snow, conjuring images of hospital board members convening in extraordinary session to decide his fate. He wondered what incentive they might offer him to leave quietly. It was a proposition that made J.W. scared and hopeful all at once. But no call came that day, or the next. By the end of the week, J.W. had forgotten the incident and chalked Cicely's pain up to ignorance, more on her mother's part than theirs. Everything was forgotten in four days.

Sick patients continued flooding the hospital, as they had for generations. There had been mistakes, and J.W. felt sorry for those who had suffered the imperfect abilities of the medical staff, and for those who had committed the errors. Time, however, was irreversible, that much J.W. remembered from thermodynamics, and each painful day passed with its unhappinesses and fights and tiny euphorias, all piled upon the eruptions of the day before. The entire morass continued to build like a glacier, each Earth-shattering event crushed and soon buried under the next snow storm, until, even after just a few hours, the most recent tragedy was just a remote shadow.

By month's end, on the final night of OB, J.W. sat with another Hispanic patient. Her eyes, too, were as dark as Sharra's, her smile as unsullied. J.W. felt even more alone. Sharra was out of the hospital. The operator said she was off for a while, but wouldn't say where or for how long, and wouldn't give J.W. her home number. J.W. started to leave a message about Cicely but became scared, fearful of further rejection, and hung up.

CHAPTER THIRTY-SEVEN

The next rotation was a two-month marathon, internal medicine, the black hole of internship. There were few sensational cures, and seldom a happy ending on that service. Decisions were slow, deliberate, and stewed in endless reference to the latest medical journals. Treatment was usually instituted only after the dance of man-pimping-man, one doctor perpetrating the utter humiliation, the public castration, of his colleague at the bedside of a dying patient.

Six and seven admissions were processed each night, many of them patients suffering acute heart attacks, some J.W.'s age. Crying men, still in their jogging suits, clutched their chests as they were off-loaded from helicopters that had carried them from miles south of Stanton, and from deep in the mountains. At the helipad, J.W. stole glances at the pilots, asking who had flown in Viet Nam—most had never been in the military, just local boys who had paid for flying lessons. They were unimpressed by his tales of countless, frightful hours at the cyclic, and ignored his feeble attempt to validate what he had once been.

The helicopters made J.W. want to fly again, to fly something, and during rounds, J.W. gazed out the windows, deaf to the pontifications of attendings and senior residents, as he stared at the jets approaching Cedar Springs Airport. Instead of his dreams of flying again, J.W. faced only the next call night; six hits if the God of Ethanol Abuse had had a pleasant day, maybe nine or ten if she was pissed. Even the prospect of Bernie and Bobbie Jo was empty.

Jacoby saw J.W. in the halls at the end of the fifth week of medicine. "Haven't heard a word about you for ages," he beamed. "Go ahead and take the day you requested to be with your friend. You can make it up in the spring."

Bernie and Bobbie Jo walked through the jetway and stared for a moment, to be sure it was J.W. Shaking his head, Bernie lit a hand-rolled cigarette and pacified Bobbie Jo, "This doesn't count. It's just a joint." He laughed gruffly through the thick, yellow smoke. "Hey, J.W., you look great. Lost a lot of weight, huh? Almost didn't recognize you."

"Krista's at home. She made your favorite."

But Bernie only picked at the red, paprika-coated roast chicken. "Looks like you've taken off a lot of weight," he quipped again lightheartedly, though there was more worry in his face than admiration. Bobbie Jo added quietly, "You've already said that. Why don't you cut back on the wine a little, sweet child?"

"And why don't you mind your own glass?"

Bernie turned away from Bobbie Jo and gushed, "I really enjoyed that evening in the anatomy lab. I miss that medical stuff. Who gets a chance to see behind the scenes like that? God, you're lucky!"

They drove to the hospital in the morning. Bernie hovered outside rooms, waiting for J.W. to ask patients for permission to bring in a visiting physician. Bernie stood silently at the bedside of J.W.'s players, watching open-mouthed as J.W. performed his tricks. Bernie gaped when J.W. added a few drops of morphine to the IV of an elderly patient with crushing chest pain, then applauded when the man's face relaxed into a vacuous smile. He blurted, "Wow!"

The old man tried to speak around his breathing tube, but there was barely a guttural bark. Bernie patted the patient's shoulder. The old man took his hand and held it tightly. Outside the room, Bernie whispered, "You're privy to some powerful mysteries. You don't understand that, J.W., do you?"

"There aren't any secrets, my friend. It's not what you think."

Over coffee, Bernie described his new gig: the sale of reclining hospital beds designed for the aged, shut-ins, and the maimed. "You must've seen the spot on TV. The company hits a region of the country hard, you know, a target area, a state or something. We fly out and set up in a hotel room. They put a no-obligation, 800 telephone number on the screen every half-hour. The customer calls, and we drive over to the house. It's a brilliant business model. That's the way it's done these days. Think about it.

"See, where we beat the competition is that we care for the customer—soup to nuts. They never leave the safety of their own home. All they have to do is pick up the phone and open the front door a day later."

J.W. laughed sparingly, "And the price of the beds is very reasonable, a nominal amount, I bet. Tell me you're giving the product away to aid the elderly."

Bernie watched J.W.'s face. "Hey, look J.W., this is a win-win deal. A lot of those folks can't even sit up in bed. What the hell are they saving their money for, anyway? Look, what we're giving them is a new lease on life. Just like you. See, but you gotta show people what they're missing, what's out there. Otherwise, how are they going to know? Yeah, I feel real good about this one."

"Soup to nuts," J.W. laughed, now sarcastically. "Sounds like you're driving 'em nuts. How much did you say those things cost?"

"You mean the beds?"

"No, the goddamn nuts! Yes, the beds, Mr. Sears Roebuck."

"Well, I think they retail for about twenty-eight hundred."

"What the hell do you mean, 'you think'?"

"Well, there's a small delivery and installation charge, a bit of tax, but that's local, not my fault, and we offer a financing plan. Lot of people take advantage of that. It's a blend of loans and prescriptions from Medicare. Boils down to ninety-days-same-as-cash."

"That certainly clears things up."

"Look, J.W., what the fuck do want me to do? I needed work. Nothing doing in the City. I got a right to live, too. Even if I'm not a doctor."

At attending rounds, J.W. introduced Bernie as a visiting resident from Romania, Dr. Valentin Petre. Bernie spoke in a broken Eastern European accent that everyone, including J.W., found unintelligible. The two were left alone to fly about the hospital and minister to the ill.

When Bernie was introduced to Ms. Pote, he grabbed her in a Russian bear hug and planted a flurry of European kisses over her cheeks. She flushed, almost as deeply as J.W., but bowed and asked if there was anything she could do to make his stay more comfortable. He turned his head in question, and J.W. translated in Chinese without tones. Bernie thanked her in Yiddish and hugged her.

Though they laughed for an hour, J.W. perceived a deeper sadness in Bernie's eyes than he had seen before. "I probably couldn't have made it into medical school, but I sure as hell wished I had given it a shot. I had more in me than folding beds and dust machines. Now, I don't have a damn thing left in me but joints and roast chicken." He laughed, though half-heartedly.

Bernie decided to stay in the hospital for the night. The first call of the evening was the ER. "Sick lady. Asked for you specifically," the ER doctor smirked. "Must be a psych case."

Hill Street Blues had already started. That made thirty-two straight weeks J.W. had missed the beginning. For nearly eight months, he had had to invest his sagging energy into piecing together the plot when he could sneak away and duck into a patient's room to watch for thirty seconds. "That's the worst part of the residency program. They have no respect for your individual cultural needs."

Bernie was quiet as J.W. continued to carp, even when they entered the cubicle of the patient who had requested his services, a gray-haired, sunken-cheeked old woman. She was covered with a blanket up to her face, and the entire bed vibrated with her bony tremor. Bernie peeked in but retreated from the odor that hung thickly around her body. The apparition on the gurney stuck a spindly arm out to touch J.W.

"Thank you for seeing me, Dr. Weathersby," she whispered. It was a familiar, but weakened, voice. J.W. picked the chart off the bed: Gertrude Koppenberg. "Does your son use the microscope?" she asked in a barely audible, high-pitched squeal.

"He loves it."

She became short of breath, and her head fell back onto the pillow after she shook Bernie's hand. "Are you the new doctor?" she mouthed.

"No, ma'am." J.W. answered. "He's a visiting physician from Romania."

Mr. Koppenberg laughed from the shadowed corner of the room, "Bubbie, he looks like a guy I used to know in New York, a momzer that one."

At midnight, Abraham Cohen was brought to the ER by ambulance. He reeked of stale urine and stale alcohol. The front of his tattered coat was stained with black oil from sleeping in the street or under the Bailey Bridge, where the cops had found him shaking and screaming. Mr. Cohen opened his eyes to stare into J.W.'s upside-down face. "Hey, it's my main doc. Man, could you let me hold a few bucks? I need to get sump'n outta da pawnshop. You know what I mean? It's my ring, man, my weddin' ring. I'm gonna patch it up with the old lady."

Bernie glanced surreptitiously around the room, slipped a fifty out of his wallet, and pressed it into Mr. Cohen's palm. "Hey, doc. Lord bless you."

Bernie and J.W. laughed until dawn, until it was time to start morning rounds, and for Bernie and Bobbie Jo to board their plane. J.W. hugged Bernie. It would be the last time he ever saw him.

⚊⧓⧓⚊

A week remained on medicine, three nights on call and a couple of dozen hits. Pediatrics followed, tending ear infections and colds for eight weeks, then five days off. J.W. was scheduled to commence Year Two on a surgical rotation. Dr. Holderman had been promoted to Chief of Surgery, and directed the training of second-year residents.

The first of J.W.'s final three nights on call brought only eight new patients, and he was done with his work by nine the next evening. Mrs. Koppenberg had been transferred to the brand-new hospice, and he checked the computer for her room number, but all that flashed was "DECEASED," in Hong Kong-green florescent, as if advertising the hospital's failure. J.W. found her chart in the record room, halfway down the pile of those to be reviewed by the coroner. The final entry was in Dr. Holderman's hand. He had been called at midnight to pronounce her. The cause of death was listed as pneumonia, a complication of widespread cancer.

J.W. phoned Holderman at home. "Why didn't you tell me Mrs. Koppenberg died? I spent a hell of a lot of time with her. I think you owed me at least that," but Holderman hung up without an answer.

Dr. Jacoby summoned J.W. for a chat the next morning. It was the first time J.W. had heard him raise his voice. "Sit, goddamnit! You stop playing games with us, Doctor," he snarled, waving his finger as J.W. stood to leave. "Go, but remember you're on the streets with three mouths to feed, the past months for naught. We've got you by the short hairs, and we both know it."

"Yes, sir, won't happen again," J.W. spat, heels locked at attention.

"See that it doesn't." Jacoby glanced at the papers on his desk, and J.W. turned to leave. "I'm not done with you. Consider yourself on call tonight. That's pay-back for the vacation I gave you to spend with your friend from Yugoslavia."

"Romania."

"You really are a gem! Outta here."

⊶ ⊷

The sick worsened at night. That was an immutable law, for they were fearful of the long hours of darkness that loomed, as fearful as was the intern. J.W.'s first hit was a man in his thirties who had passed out at home. He'd been feeling out of sorts for months and presented panting rapidly and shallowly, his breath sickeningly sweet, his pants far too large for his frame. It was a diagnosis even an intern could make—diabetic ketoacidosis, new diabetes out of control. His blood sugar came back from the lab over one thousand, and minutes later, he had been injected with subcutaneous insulin, and an IV insulin drip had been started. J.W. loaded him with fluids and called the senior resident to let her know Mr. Hoeprich was on their service.

Hits Number Two, Three, and Four were alcohol-related and comfortable on 3-South by midnight. Number Five was a black male with a harder problem than the diabetic: priapism, an erection that wouldn't go down. The patient also suffered from sickle-cell anemia, and J.W. treated that first. A few hours later, the man was bitching that he wanted out of the hospital to go home and try again with his lady.

Hit Number Six was cooking in the ER at 3:30 A.M., ready for the floor. "Go get yourself a cup of coffee, J.W.; it's just another drunk," Nurse Princeton assured.

It was a black male, only semi-conscious, his scruffy overcoat more familiar to J.W. than his beaten, pulpy face. "Been rolled, I guess," Nurse Princeton tsooked derisively as they moved toward the elevator. J.W. picked the chart off the patient's chest, scribbling orders as fast as his pencil could fly. Seconds saved now were seconds added to his dream—hot breakfast.

"Abraham Cohen," was typed in faded letters on the thick chart. He looked up feebly from the gurney. "Doc? That you?" He raised his hand to show J.W. his wedding ring. It was huge, studded with diamonds. But as J.W. was telling him how good it looked, and that he would let Dr. Petre know, Mr. Cohen became comatose, the first drunk J.W. had seen do that. J.W. called the attending at home.

Dr. Jackson advised, "Make him comfortable. Give him a bolus of morphine."

"Yes, sir."

"He may not wake up from that, you know, but we are going to treat his pain this time. Enough is enough."

"Wait a minute, sir. What are you asking me to do?"

"Just make him comfortable, I said."

"I won't use morphine, sir. It'll put him into respiratory arrest."

The phone clicked down, and an hour later, Dr. Jackson appeared in the doorway of Mr. Cohen's room, consulting with the senior resident while a diminutive Filipina nurse and J.W. changed Mr. Cohen into clean pajamas. Halfway through that task, J.W. was paged to meet with Mr. Cohen's wife, brother, and daughter. Though it was before dawn, J.W. snuck them up the service elevator and through the dimmed halls of 3-South. Dr. Jackson and the senior resident were still standing in the doorway, debating the care of a man J.W. had not dreamed was the patriarch of so handsome a family, of any family.

Mrs. Cohen, an attractive Jamaican woman, sat by the bed; the daughter was a magnificent. Her piercing, turquoise eyes reddened as she watched her mother take Mr. Cohen's hand, touching his gold wedding band. "He just got that back," she mentioned sadly. "Can't imagine where he got the money to get it out of pawn."

J.W. asked how long they had been married. "Twenty-five years. You should have seen him when he was playing for the Lions. He was so good, they called him the Black Rabbi. He was one of the highest paid linemen in the NFL. And then the headaches and the depression and the drinking. Lord above, he tried so hard to stop. He hated it."

J.W. could not speak. He watched the senior doctors in the doorway, arms folded, chins resting in palms, speaking in increasingly hushed tones as they occasionally glanced at Mr. Cohen, who had not stirred. One sophisticated treatment after another was parlayed in the spirit of friendly, professional discussion, snippets of fascinating medical dialogue passing across bare, arrogant smiles. Obviously, Abraham was receiving personal, world-class care. The Filipina nurse weaved past the conference to recheck Mr. Cohen's blood pressure. She bent over the man, twisted her head questioningly, adjusted the cuff, and re-flated it several times. The tremor in her fingers deepened with each try. She walked past J.W. and whispered, "Doctor, may I see you in the hall.?"

"Doctor, I am sorry. Your patient has become deceased."

"What?" J.W. blurted. "Dead?"

"Yes, Doctor."

"What?" J.W. whispered again loudly. J.W. Weathersby had ac-complished the impossible—credit for a hit on which the attend-ing and the senior resident had become entangled, and would have to do some of the paperwork *and* accept a portion of the blame.

"Mr. Cohen is gone," J.W. offered solemnly to both Dr. Jackson and the senior resident, who were still considering treatment op-tions in the doorway.

The family cried. J.W. relaxed. An admission had been ex-punged from his workload, but added to his tally. He tipped his imaginary hat and sailed through the next admission, a young alcoholic who had attempted suicide with Valium.

It wasn't until his third cup of coffee and the last scrap of scrambled eggs, his first leisurely breakfast in many months, that the rejoicing over the passing of a human life began to curdle in his stomach. At first, he thought it was the cafeteria food, but it soon became plain that a soul who had done him no harm, an innocent man who had drunk himself into the grave, had been more of a teacher, a deeper source of learning, and far more decent and peaceful, than the attendings who had profited from his presence. As peculiar a companion as Mr. Cohen had been, he had had more innate value in J.W.'s life than almost anyone whose path J.W. had crossed that year. He had even tapped into Bernie's compassion.

J.W. wondered if Mr. Cohen's mother had held him when he scraped his knee as a baby, and how he had felt the first time he had tasted a woman's kiss. Had he prayed the snow would never stop so he didn't have to go to school? In the morgue, J.W. stared at him. Even in death, Mr. Cohen had more hair than did he. The man's painful death—what did that mean? What had J.W. become? Even Viet Nam had not made him scream for joy when the enemy was destroyed, and Mr. Cohen was the farthest thing from an enemy J.W. had encountered in many years.

⟞⟊ ⟒⟝

J.W. slept in the on-call room for a few moments, until the weak rays of a gray sun passed unevenly through the smudged and dust-caked windows. He dashed into the shower, but as he sought to cleanse away the sins of the past night, the dream he'd just finished recrystallized. He knew it was important and tried very hard not to think too deeply about it and scare it away. Though already late for rounds, J.W. could not force himself from the hot water, and he played snippets of the emerging dream over a dozen times until it began to fit together. He saw he image of a dirty man on the ground in a forgotten alley between two taverns. His beard was caked with filth, his rough clothing threadbare. He sat cross-legged, quietly, his palm outstretched, begging, his eyes and face reflecting sadness and need. As patrons entered and left the taverns, they passed the miserable creature. Some displayed compassion, some guilt. Some gave him money; others ignored him. A few tormented him. One of the drunks screamed, "Get off your lazy ass or I'll take you, you worthless bastard, to the hospital and have them kill you."

At first, J.W. did not appreciate the significance of what was holding him in the shower, but he remembered from psychiatry that in a dream, one was all the actors, good and bad, and that every sentiment came from within the well of the dreamer's heart.

Instead of joining rounds, J.W. shaved, dressed in a fresh scrub suit, ate a full breakfast, and walked with his head a fraction higher than the night before. Dr. Jacoby was at his desk. J.W. knocked and entered before Jacoby had a chance to look up. "Sir, in the interest of no more games, I will drop it on you directly. When I got to Cedar Springs, I knew right from wrong, who I was, and what I stood for. And now, I don't know shit. All I think about, twenty-four hours a day, is avoiding the next hit. I've become a lazy piece of crap. I don't care who lives or dies. I'm not the same guy who rolled in here a year ago."

"And you're blaming us."

"Us? No! I'm blaming myself for getting sucked in. You taught me that. I don't want to be like the rest of you."

"Don't you drag us into what's going on inside your head, Doctor. There's nothing wrong with a little stress."

"A little stress? It's not the stress. It's the doctors who don't give a shit, who would rather belittle than teach. It's a doctor who just ordered me to murder a patient. He did it over the phone without even examining the guy. Sir, I came out here to work in a center-city program. I never dreamed I'd rejoice at the passing of some poor drunk bastard. Look, I need to finish the year, just the internship. Another few weeks, and your headache's gone. It's a win-win."

"I'll put your proposal before the board," Dr. Jacoby paused. "It's a good idea, though. Best idea I've heard all year." He shook his head knowingly. "There won't be any problem."

CHAPTER THIRTY-EIGHT

The next page was from the hospital operator. She blurted, "Long distance." She paused, and her voice softened. "We're not supposed to put personal calls through, but I hear you've had a bad day. We'll just let this one slide."

Though static distorted the voice, J.W.'s bowels gripped as his subconscious enveloped the gentle accent. "J.W., is that you?"

"Sharra?"

"Hi. Just calling to see how that young Hispanic patient's doing. You heard from her?"

"She's fine...I... No, Sharra, she's dead. Okay? She died the night after you spoke with her. Okay? Look, I need to talk to you, but I'm shaking myself apart. I'm frightened. Can I call you back? Tonight?" He realized he had used her name, and waited, knotted in a ball, sick at his mistake.

"I need to talk to you too, J.W. I'll let you go, but please call tonight. Please."

She spoke her number, and J.W. wrote it on his palm so brutally, he tore the skin. And she was gone that fast. Left behind was but the drone of a distant dial tone, a hum that roared in his ears through that endless day. Though his work was done at five, J.W. hid in the on-call room until Jacoby left then stole into his suite. In the darkness, the air seemed purged of the months of angry confrontations, of the loss of spirit they had both suffered. Nonetheless, J.W. couldn't bring himself to sit at Jacoby's desk, so he sat on the floor in a corner and dialed.

"J.W.?" she answered after the first ring. "Thank you for calling back. I had no right to upset you today. I don't want to get you involved. Just let it drop."

"No. Tell me. It's okay. Don't worry about me. I'll do anything for you."

"I think he's found me."

"Who?"

"Hassan, J'Aveed's father."

"Tell me what's going on, please, Sharra."

She was quiet for an eternity before drawing a gloomy breath. "Okay. We moved into a Turkish neighborhood in LA when I started my residency. My mother and sister and I took Turkish names, all different. Your government gave us new identities. They said we could live here because we speak Turkish, but they warned us not to tell anyone where we were going. They even arranged for my residency. You are very lucky to have been born here, J.W. It is a great country.

"My poor mother. Even though we are nowhere near the Persian community, she never leaves the house. Too scared. And my sister just graduated from law school, but she can't pass the tests, whatever they are, to get licensed. They go around and check where you grew up and ask questions, I guess. And she has a different name. It's a mess. It is no way to live."

"Why do you think Hassan is going to find you?"

"Some neighbors mentioned that those dirty Persian Savak holdouts have been snooping around, asking about Iranians living in the community. I don't know if they're looking for me, but they are making lists of all the Persians, of every one of us in the United States, maybe in the whole world. I mean, Hassan would not recognize me. I was fifteen when we left, but they would start looking into who we were. We have accents, and we look different than the Turks. It wouldn't take long. They would sell us out to the fanatics in three seconds. A bribe here, one there. It is how we lived in Persia. It's worse now. Sometimes I am happy my father is gone, away from the threats.

"I'm talking too much."

"Please don't stop. I want to hear your voice for a hundred years. Do you have friends in the residency program?"

"No. I can't. I see my patients and go home when they let me off. I hate it. I don't see J'Aveed, or my mother, and we don't know where my sister is from one day to the next. I don't know what to do.

"J.W., I can't take it anymore. The walls are closing in. I hate it."

"Do you want me to fly down there?"

"You can't. I can't. I just needed to tell someone. You're so all together, J.W. I haven't stopped long enough in the past two years to talk to anyone. I can't sleep unless I take something. I can't stay awake unless I take something. And when I do sleep, every dream is a nightmare. I wish I had never gotten into medicine. I'm leaving the program at the end of the year."

"Oh, my God. So am I. I just quit today."

"Oh, J.W., I'm sorry. Why am I bothering you?"

"Let me come there. I'll be good. I promise. Please."

She was silent again for a moment. "Thank you for listening." After another painful pause, she whispered, "I can't forget you. I never will." There was a click, and the line fell still.

The weight that should have lifted from his chest bored more deeply. J.W. thought of telling Krista that he planned to withdraw their savings, and lie that he was flying back to Boston to find a job. But when he called to tell Sharra he was coming, her phone rang with no answer. The hospital operator said Dr. Nur was on leave.

⊷⊶

Residents who J.W. felt had treated him with disdain for ten months stopped and chatted, sharing their wishes they'd had the guts to halt the process years earlier, before it had drained their spirits so inalterably. Several of them passed J.W. headhunter notes, which covertly offered jobs in emergency rooms and in non-teaching hospitals, where neither intern nor resident meat plied the halls as an endless inventory of slave labor. The salaries written in big numbers on the notes offered seven times the pittance J.W. had accepted during his hazing.

CHAPTER THIRTY-NINE

On the fifteenth of June at 1 A.M., J.W. walked for the last time from the hospital, numbed, saddened, and joyful. Six hours later, he drove forty miles west for his first day at a walk-in clinic. He travelled the interstate, past green flatlands, a crimson sunrise lighting the snowcapped, towering Mount Brickner. He passed Black Granite, looking away from the logging town, forcing from his heart the tug of Lieutenant White's spirit. He refused to let himself believe the man's worldly remains were coffined so nearby. The Buick rolled ten miles further north into the gravel parking lot of an old house whose backyard opened into the Rockies.

By noon that first day, fifteen patients had passed through the little clinic, thirty-six by the close of business. The nurse commented it had been hectic, an awful day; for J.W. it had been the most peaceful day of the last year. The sun had set an hour before J.W. locked the doors, the last to leave. Though it was very dark, there appeared a sliver of light.

PART IV

CHAPTER FORTY

I t wasn't until several trips past Black Granite that J.W. allowed himself to look down from the highway into the town. He could make out the green of parks in which he imagined his co-pilot had played helicopter hero two decades before, and he saw the signs for Royal Field, home of SkyCo Aviation, where the Ellison 3D was manufactured; an aviator's dream—half-helicopter, half-fixed wing. J.W. imagined flying again, and his heart clutched with such passion, he could hardly sit still. It was not long, though, before his spirit sank as he grasped he would never again be a pilot.

For the first weeks of his commute, he ignored the highway exit that would have taken him into Black Granite, but on the last day of his first month as a physician, he left home early and drove the streets of Black Granite until he passed a monument set in a tiny park outside the courthouse. A bouquet of cheap flowers sat at the base, wilting under the names of the forgotten. "BLACK GRANITE WAR MEMORIAL" was chiseled in the top of the ebony stone. The Buick rolled past and back onto the highway toward the clinic.

By his second month at the clinic, J.W. had seen an impressive array of extraordinary diseases: ear infections; fishing hooks embedded in fingers, cheeks, and eyelids; and a puppy with a barbed lure in its tallywacker. He treated muscle tension head-aches and migraine headaches, abdominal pain and back pain, diaper rash, scabies, and VD, all manner of illnesses to which J.W. had never been exposed in the hospital setting, and about which his mother knew more than did he.

His last patient on Sunday night was so sick, J.W. heard her wheezing through the clinic door after the nurse slid the bolt shut. They saw Mrs. Pineda anyway, and he sat with her as she sucked the curing vapors from a nebulizer. As her color returned, she asked for a prescription of theophylline, for she had left her pills at home in the Philippines. She was sure it was six hundred milligrams, three or four times per day—she was absolutely sure.

As the nurse was leaving, she asked what J.W. had given Mrs. Pineda to make her comfortable for the night.

"Theophylline, 600, tid to qid."

"Whew! That'll get her attention."

"What do you mean?"

"Sounds like a lot of theophylline to me. That stuff makes me throw up. Two hundred milligrams do. What the hell, you're the doctor," she laughed as she walked to her car. J.W. went back inside to consult the *Physicians' Desk Reference*, which also advised that eighteen-hundred milligrams per day was sufficient to burn a hole in a defensive end's gut, to say nothing of the seizures and circulatory collapse theophylline guaranteed at that dosage.

The "local" address on Mrs. Pineda's chart listed an alley in the Tondo District of Manila. Her telephone number had only four digits. J.W. called there to ask where she was staying in Black

Granite, but he had not heard Tagalog since the dean's office in Manila, nearly a decade before, and the old man who answered the phone had apparently not heard English in those years, either. He had not an inkling of what J.W. was asking, and J.W. left the clinic concerned. By 3 A.M., J.W. was pacing the living room.

The next morning, a man in a dark suit sat in the waiting room, a tooled leather briefcase by his foot. "May I speak with you, Dr. Weathersby?"

"About what, sir?"

"A medication, Doctor. I think you may want to hear what I have to say."

The outside line rang. "Dr. Weathersby," Brandi, the receptionist, called out loudly. "It's the pharmacy. He says it's important."

"Dr. Weathersby, do you remember a patient named Pineda? She just walked in with a prescription for theophylline; eighteen hundred milligrams a day? Excuse me, Doctor, but is that what you wanted her to have?"

"How'd that happen? Of course, she shouldn't be taking eighteen hundred milligrams a day. Let's give her two hundred twice a day. Anything else?"

The white-haired man in the suit was by his side before the phone was nestled in the cradle. "Dr. Weathersby, let me introduce myself. I'm Donald Douglass with Tompkins Labs. Is there someplace we can sit and talk?" He pulled a metal, copper-colored, pill-shaped paperweight from his briefcase and handed it to J.W. with great ceremony. J.W. hesitated. "Just a little gift. Go ahead, take it. It represents a new, once-a-day anti-inflammatory medication. Really quite revolutionary, Co-Rouzene, kinda like 'cozy'. That's what all the doctors are calling it. Just once a day. Can you believe that? It's revolutionary!"

He proffered samples along with a hat emblazoned "CO-ROUZENE" and a dozen pens engraved with J.W. Weathersby and the Co-Rouzene logo. When J.W. promised to try the medication on his next dozen patients, the detail man produced pre-printed prescription pads for CO-ROUZENE—all he'd have to do was write in the patient's name and scratch a signature. J.W. mumbled, "Gotta admit, would save a lot of time."

As the man left, he admonished Brandi, "Hey, Sweetheart, make sure he uses Co-Rouzene, you know, cozy." He winked and was gone.

Several patients in need of anti-inflammatories presented before noon. J.W. regaled them with the virtues his groundbreaking medication.

"Side effects?" one of the patients probed warily.

"None that I know of. Hey, this stuff's been through the FDA approval process. Are you kidding? Nothing gets dumped on the market in this country until it's damn near perfect," J.W. reassured. "This isn't like Russia, you know."

It was gratifying to hear his new medication cited on the car radio the next morning. J.W. turned up the volume comfortably on the Buick's AM radio. Co-Rouzene had just yesterday been pulled from the market for devastating side effects, of which the manufacturer had been well aware for a very long time. The detail man had overlooked mentioning that Co-Rouzene had rotted many a pancreas in the Soviet Union, where the drug had been long outlawed. The company's drug information hotline was out of order, as was the drug rep's local office phone. J.W. called the FDA. "Doctor, you had better contact everybody you poisoned."

Several of the doomed had already phoned the office demanding to know why they had been given a medication that, after the first pill, had generated nausea, vomiting, headaches, sweats, yellowing of the skin and eyes, double-vision, loss of vision, loss of balance, priapism, and impotence.

Brandi called the rest of the patients to whom J.W. had dispensed samples and told them to stop the medication, and if they were smart, to toss it in the garbage. One patient, a bearded old man from the woods deep within the mountains, had not listed a telephone number. J.W. ordered Brandi not to open the clinic, and set out for the man's home, driving thirty miles along Route 4 to the tavern outside Bender's RV Park. Five bucks for the morning imbibers bought J.W. slurred directions to a point another three miles up a dirt road that snaked the logging roads above the banks of the Salmon River. The drunks laughed, "You ain't gonna get that tank into the hills."

J.W. pushed the Buick across a wooden, one-lane bridge and up a dirt trail until the pits and the rocks overwhelmed the nearly thirty-year-old car. He climbed the next mile on foot, his loafers saturated as he slogged the deep mud and, soon, the first traces of snow. He came to a decrepit, six-by-eight travel trailer. Quivering light silhouetted a ski-capped head through a filthy, cracked window. Outside the door, dried-food-crusted white linoleum squares, a hundred of them, sat in a loose pile. It looked as if they had served as paper plates and then been tossed aside and forgotten. J.W. knocked, and the figure in the ski cap came to life.

"Huh?"

J.W. slid aside what was left of a sheet metal portal. Mr. Shelton's feet were propped on a rusted half-55-gallon oil drum. Next to his worn, stiffened socks sat, unopened, J.W.'s medicine. Keeping it company were scraps of curled bread and soft, blackened vegetables.

"Mr. Shelton, I'm Doctor Weathersby, sir. You came to see me yesterday about your back. I gave you that medicine. I'm sorry, but just today the government said it isn't good for you. Screws up your pancreas if you take it too long. Can you believe that?" There was not a flicker of the man's eyes.

"But, of course, you didn't take it at all. That's good, sir. Well, just wanted to tell you, sir. Probably best if you throw that shit away."

Mr. Shelton lifted a thick walking stick and pointed it in J.W.'s direction. As his eyes adjusted to the darkness, J.W. realized the walking stick was the barrel of a very old pump action, 12-gauge shotgun. Mr. Shelton swung the barrel horizontally over his makeshift table, sweeping the medicine and food scraps onto the floor.

A breeze puffed through an open space in the wall that had held a window years before. The frosty air rustled the far reaches of Mr. Shelton's flowing beard. His piercing blue eyes turned away from J.W. to fix on the walls of the rotted metal hovel.

"Good day, Mr. Shelton. Why don't you try this stuff instead?" J.W. left a bottle of aspirin. "But only two, twice a day."

Driving out, J.W. stopped to watch the salmon fighting their way upstream. While he had never before seen the creatures, never privy to the spawn, he did not find the inexplicable, mad drive that pushed them into roiling waters that great a mystery.

⊷ ⊶

Each clinic morning began with a promise that he would not fall behind, that patients would not wait more than seven minutes, for that was the standard established by the owners after there had been an incident with the mayor's wife. She had written to the medical director that she'd been kept in the waiting room for fifteen minutes, causing her to miss her plane for Acapulco.

J.W. remembered the episode well. She had blown into the clinic and asked at the front desk for a quick prescription of Valium, declaring a semi-emergency, for she was in a hurry and already late for the airport. She hated flying, she hated doctors, and she didn't need to be seen because she knew exactly what she wanted. Her request refused, she left, raving, "You haven't heard the last from me! I'm the mayor's wife."

The medical director, Chuck Ezron, wrote in reply that Valium was not a drug dispensed at the front desk, especially to patients the doctor had never seen. "If you dropped in on your hairdresser or your mechanic unannounced," he asked in his reply, "would they have taken you ahead of everyone else?"

The mayor's wife did not respond directly to the hypothetical. She filed a complaint with the county medical society which included the clinic owners in California in the correspondence. She alleged the clinic refused appropriate medical care, and had kept her waiting an inordinate amount of time for the sole purpose of forcing her to see a doctor, and thus pay for an office visit. She threatened to sue for malpractice.

Drs. Ezron and Weathersby laughed when the CEO and owner, Charlie Braunwald, appeared at the clinic with the corporate attorneys. But the smiles faded when the meeting began with the presentation of a legal journal, their attention drawn to the brief about the woman in Woodside who had won a substantial malpractice suit, her doctor having been judged guilty of inadequately treating her pain. The patient, a known and admitted drug abuser, had presented to an emergency room very drunk, and with an excruciating headache. She demanded narcotic pain medication and was appropriately denied.

The patient ran out of the ER before the doctor could examine her, went home, and slammed a closet door on her head several times because the pain was so crushing. She showed up in another emergency room when she sobered up three days later, with the same headache, but this time she couldn't move her left leg and had to be carried in by her boyfriend. Nor could she run out when the second doctor refused pain medication and ordered a CAT scan, which demonstrated a lemon-sized tumor in her brain. The court ruled the first doctor had failed to treat his patient's pain, failed to diagnose her tumor, and failed to call her at home to insist she return to the clinic for further work-up. That judgment cost the hospital over a million dollars.

The present attorneys suggested Ezron and J.W. offer repentant letters, cross their fingers, and keep in mind that their patient had three years to file her suit. J.W. laughed again, for by that time he would be thousands of miles away, enjoying his own little practice back in Boston. Braunwald turned to the medical director. "You will write a letter of apology to this patient. You will not piss her off again. You will not piss off any of our patients. The customer is always right. Your job is on the line."

The medical director unbuttoned his white coat and dropped it in front of the board of inquiry, allowed himself a smile, and turned toward the door. Apparently, the CEO had forgotten the man's very direct association with the Ezron motorcycle fortune until Chuck sneered, "This is just a hobby, pal. Fuck you and the horse you rode in on."

Braunwald belched, "Dr. Weathersby, you're interested in the medical directorship, I presume? There is a substantial stipend attached to the position."

"Sir, I'm outta here in about three days. Taking the family back to the East Coast, ya know. That was the deal."

"Do you have a job yet?"

"No, sir."

"Meeting adjourned. Think about it. We could use you. You're an excellent physician. Call me this afternoon."

There wasn't time to consider the future, or even call Krista, for J.W. was pressed into service at the clinic to cover the shift the medical director had just abandoned. As J.W. entered the first exam room in jeans and the medical director's discarded white coat, he tried to ignore the chorus of grumbling protest wafting out of the waiting room. A newcomer had appeared, the mayor's wife, crying about a painful tumor she had just discovered, "Down there."

"It's bleeding. That's a danger sign, isn't it? It's cancer. I just know it is!" she wept as Brandi spirited her into an exam room ahead of the rest of the players, most of whom had been waiting for over an hour.

As J.W. completed the emergency ligation of her hemorrhoid, she allowed that she really hadn't intended to bring suit against the clinic. "I was just very upset about flying. I only wanted a little help. And, will you continue to be my personal physician?"

Apparently, she called the home office with her request, for an hour later, a thousand-dollar bonus check made out to Dr. J.W. Weathersby, Medical Director, was delivered to the clinic, signed in the CEO's hand. A scribbled note invited him to the quarterly corporate meeting at the swank Walser Club in Cedar Springs the following morning.

Brandi was excited. "They like you here. If you leave, the clinic's going to close. Braunwald says you're our last chance."

"Who told you that?"

"He did."

"Do you know him personally?"

"Let's just say I knew him."

Krista loved the two-dozen roses. "You're promising me, right? Only one more month, right? You won't let Khai and me down, will you? I want to go home."

⊷ ⊶

At quarterly meetings, the clinic medical directors were required, before the coffee and donuts were unveiled, to respond to the litany of complaints filed by unhappy patients over the past three months. Next came the inventory of lawsuits and big settlements corporate had defended. The principal case of the latter featured a drunk who had presented to one of the clinics after having fallen and broken his right arm. He was so inebriated, the doctor was able to set the bone without anesthesia and place him in a cast, all without a whimper of protest. J.W.'s eyes rolled toward the ceiling, for everyone knew you didn't cast a broken bone for at least forty-eight hours. A splint was the proper treatment—to allow the swelling someplace to go. But the doctor in the trenches that evening made a tough call, based on his judgment that the patient would never keep a splint in place. He refused to give the patient narcotic pain medication because of his obvious addictive proclivities, and even more so because, if there was painful swelling, the patient would have no choice but to seek medical care and have the cast removed.

A letter virtually demanding the patient return for a follow-up appointment in twelve hours was placed in a clear plastic bag and taped to the cast. But he was a no-show the next morning, the next day, and the day after that. The phone number he had listed was a phony, as was the address.

He turned up drunk at another emergency room three days later, claiming he had had to keep drinking because the first doctor had refused pain pills. The arm was gangrenous, and much of it had to be carved away in surgery later that day. "His right arm, no less," the plaintiff's attorney squawked in court. "A negligent doctor," he screamed, pointing at the physician, "has cost this man his profession. How in God's name is he supposed to hold his carpentry tools with no right arm?"

Clearly, it would have been better if the doctor-defendant had not jumped up and screamed, "You mean, how's he supposed to hold a six-pack?"

The award was in excess of half-a-million dollars. The attorney who related the story allowed there was a silver lining to every cloud—with all that money, the patient had the means to finally pay his medical bills.

J.W. looked around the room at the depressed expressions of the senior physicians who had pushed themselves through college, medical school, internship, and residency, twelve years of study after high school. Most of the doctors in that room had seen in excess of fifty thousand patients. They cared, and they were confident in their abilities to address the suffering of their fellow man, but they were being warned to think of themselves first, to practice the art and science of defensive medicine. They shook their heads in resignation at the punch line of each legal decision, and at the cure recommended by the attorney.

"That's ridiculous. That'll cost three times what it should. Who's gonna pay for it?" J.W. asked. "And then you blame the doctor for driving up health costs."

"That's right. Who said you were put here to understand it, or that it's rational?" answered the attorney. "You must understand that you are responsible for your own tail from now on. Oh, and by the way, also for everyone you talk to or don't talk to. You folks aren't members of that part of the American society entitled to be cared for. No. You chose to put yourself in this position, and now you're responsible—for everything. You are hereby nurse-maid for your patients and your staff, for what they do or don't do. You will mollycoddle, or you will not survive.

"Doctor Weathersby, you're shifting around in your seat again. You're the new guy on the block, but surely, they covered all of this with you in medical school. How long have you been in practice?"

"About two weeks, and I never heard a word about this until I started at the Clinic."

"If that wasn't so funny, I'd cry. Still, you're the one we're here to help. You're on the up part of the learning curve. Your buddies here are getting medically long of tooth. Hard to teach 'em anything. Let me give you a good example.

"How many times have we stood in front of so regal a gathering and warned physicians that receptionists who give medical advice over the phone do so on their doctors' malpractice nickel? *You* should be fielding the calls, not the youngsters at the front desk. And yet we have the case here of the overbearing doctor who won't talk to his front desk staff."

He pulled a sheet from his briefcase. "Try this one on for size. A local patient calls the clinic wondering if it is safe to use her douche bag after her husband has just employed the device to siphon gasoline out of the family station wagon. You can chuckle, but your ass is on the line every time the phone rings, *and* every time it doesn't. The receptionist is afraid to bother the physician. Sound familiar? She recommends the patient rinse it and 'just go ahead and use it.'

"The patient fills the bag with water, turns it over, and pours out the mixture, twice to be sure, but is unaware that gasoline is less dense than water and floats. A few molecules of the gas never flush out. The patient, unbeknownst to her at the time, is pregnant. She develops a raging, painful vaginitis from the gasoline, and a week later miscarries. She brings suit against the clinic, the doctor, and the receptionist. The receptionist has no insurance, and the case against her is dropped as a waste of energy. Even if the nineteen-year-old were convicted, there would be no monetary result for the plaintiff or her attorney.

"Ladies and gentlemen, this case went to trial. The plaintiff would not budge from her belief that the gasoline had caused the miscarriage, despite evidence that twenty-percent of pregnancies end in miscarriage, and that none of the gasoline probably ever traveled past the sealed cervix into the uterus. They won the case for the doctor, but he spent six weeks in a courtroom without pay, and his name is tarnished forever.

"How do you feel about that, Doctor?" the attorney nodded toward J.W.

"I can carry the load."

"You mean you won't die if you're sued?"

"I can carry the load," J.W. said. "Court is bullshit."

"Pretty cocky for two weeks under your belt. Look, a malpractice suit is more than an insurance matter, my friend. It means having your personal life splashed across the newspapers. Ever had a fight with your wife? Ever gotten drunk? Ever taken a leak in public? Yes? Someone else knows about it, and they're going to tell someone, and it's your ass. Maybe your pecker's not worth the court's time, but presumably your intelligence and abilities are, and I can assure you they are going to be impugned. And all the time you sit and tell yourself you can 'carry the load,' some attorney's going to pat you on the back and say, 'It's not personal. It's just the way we make our living.'"

The meeting concluded with tales about doctors who, in their late fifties, were served subpoenas for cases that had begun a decade before. Many of the older practitioners left the profession in despair—a few committed suicide.

CHAPTER FORTY-ONE

The next meeting of the medical directors was scheduled for late January. J.W. drove along the snowy Cedar Springs streets, reeling from the all-night battle he and Krista had joined over their extended absence from the East Coast.

"Sweetheart," J.W. had begged hour after hour," this is the first goddamn time in eight years, really ever, that I've made a living. I'm making twice what the average guy at the mill is. Last year at this time, I was making a third. Folks are beginning to come in droves. Please don't make me start over."

All that came through her sobs was, "You promised us. You swore."

J.W. set out for the quarterly meeting with every intention of attending, looking forward to the catered luncheon the owners from California provided to make up for the trivial salary they provided their physicians. As he neared the exit for The Walser Club, the Buick refused to leave the highway, and it continued west. At the Black Granite war monument, J.W. stopped and found the chiseled inscription, "First Lieutenant R.D. White,

1947—1969, 33rd Mechanized Infantry Brigade, Killed in Action, Lai Khe, Republic of Viet Nam, 28 March 1969."

J.W. rejoined the highway and headed north along the edge of the Salmon River, up the snow-choked roads to the little trailer, wondering if Mr. Shelton had enough left in him to pass the freezing winter. He trudged through the snow to the shanty, greeted a hundred yards away with a thread of smoke spiraling from a hole in the roof. The old man sat with his shotgun by his side, though this time he left the butt on the floor. J.W. dropped off the half dozen donuts from Eason's Bakery, thirteen miles back along the highway. He asked Mr. Shelton about his back, and took from the grunt that he was muddling along. J.W. nodded and left the hovel. Looking back, he thought he saw Mr. Shelton staring out the window toward him, but there was too much dirt and ice caked on the glass to be sure. He walked toward the river.

The Salmon widened into a gentle lake at the point J.W. had abandoned his car in the snow. At a cedar chalet along the shore, J.W. tried the door. It was unlocked and he took a seat on a decades-old, tattered easy chair facing the river. He plugged in a space heater and covered himself with a moldy blanket. The minutes melted into an hour, time he spent recounting his good fortune over and over, seeking to convince himself he was the luckiest man on Earth. The next minute, though, the desolation picked up where it had left off, and the sense of emptiness that had been his minder for so many decades curled about him. At sundown, he abandoned his chair reluctantly and drove back to Cedar Springs, crawling home to an uncertain reception, knowing tomorrow he would again serve as a doc-in-a-box for twelve hours, the cycle churning, whether he cared, or whether he showed up.

Krista had waited up for him. "One of the owners called. Braunwald. He missed you today. He wanted to know if you were okay. Are you?"

"Yeah."

"He said you've turned the clinic around. They're happy you're working there." Krista looked away to stare at the wall. She barely whispered. "I'm sorry. I'm just lonely. Can you understand that?"

"I more than understand, and I'm sorry, but I gotta make a living, Krista. Can you understand *that*? For ten years, we haven't had a life. I'm changing that. Going back to the East Coast to start another residency program, it'll be the same. I'll fail again and again. What is wrong with me? What, I didn't try hard enough? What the fuck is wrong?" He began to weep then pulled at his hair and slapped himself. His sobs deepened as the hopelessness drowned him. "I'm so fucking scared of failing again. At least I'm in neutral now; they haven't found out yet. I'm more scared than when I got back from Viet Nam, and there was *no* future."

"I'm scared, too. Always have been, ever since the day you stepped off that plane. What the hell did they do to you there? Fifteen years. It only gets worse." She filled her tumbler with wine and stared harder at the wall.

⊷┼┼⊶

On Valentine's Day, Brandi called J.W. out of a room to the phone. He recognized the long distance static, but even more critical was the long pause. His heart gripped. "Sharra?"

"Hi, J.W. I'm sorry to bother you."

"Are you okay?"

"Yes. I mean no. I don't know what I mean, I... Why do I keep bothering you?" Her words were slurred.

"You're not a bother. Tell me if you're okay." There was no answer, and J.W. asked with an edge in his voice, "Have you been drinking?"

"You're not going to get on my case, too? Are you? Yeah, I've had a little to drink. Does that surprise you?"

"Sharra, look, that's none of my business. If I can help you, please let me."

"Oh, it's nothing. Just a little wine."

"How much?"

There was no answer. "Do I have to come down there and spank you?"

She started to sob. "I…J'Aveed's gone. His father's got him. I don't care. I can't go on. What does he want from me?"

"Sharra, call the police; take the son-of-a-bitch to court."

"*They* gave him to Hassan."

"Who gave him to Hassan? What the hell is going on, Sharra? Courts don't take kids away from their mothers."

"There were problems with my papers. The right hand doesn't know what the left hand is doing. There is no record of my having gotten political asylum. I, the names are all confused. And anyway, now your government is licking up to the Iranians, so they decided to respect *Sharia*, Muslim law and give him to the father. J'Aveed is in protective custody until the case can be decided by your Immigration Department. I'm not allowed to contact him. They want to deport me and my family. We will be executed if we return. All of us. I worked so hard to get here, and I don't know why. I'm still a pariah. Do you know what that means? I'm trash. An enemy of your government. J'Aveed is gone. There's nothing left. It's all gone."

She cried so hard, all J.W. could make out was, "I want to die. I want to die."

"I'm coming to LA. Please don't argue."

"No. You can't."

"Sharra. You're all I've thought about for years. I'll be there tonight. Tell me where I can find you."

"J.W., it's too dangerous. You're playing with fire. I know you care, but I can't drown you in my troubles. I love you too much, more than any man I've ever loved in my life."

"I'll send you the money to come here. Just say yes."

"Pleeease don't send the money. I can't trust myself," she sobbed. "I won't ruin your life, too." The phone went dead, though J.W. stood there holding the receiver for a minute before he let it drop numbly into the cradle. Brandi looked over at him then quickly away.

After hours, Brandi came by his desk and made him promise again he wouldn't quit. Her eyes reddened as she brooded, "The clinic's all I've got. Please don't let us down."

"I won't, if I survive." J.W. asked if he could tell her a story. She listened for an hour, her eyes becoming even redder.

—⊰ ⊱—

As J.W. lay in bed that night, he felt Sharra really meant she wouldn't see him, but as her choking words played over and over in his head, the emotion in her voice slowly became, "Please don't send the money, because if you do, I will come." J.W. tossed for hours, fighting with himself over whether he would break what was left of his life with Krista and send the money, or take the high road and let his fantasy go.

At noon, J.W. left the clinic unattended and wired five hundred dollars to Sharra. Two nights later, on J.W.'s day off, Brandi called him at home from the clinic, having just spoken with a woman asking for Dr. Weathersby. "She wouldn't leave her name. She had a funny accent, and she sounded real close, like no static on the line. I said, 'Are you Sharra?' but she hung up. I'm sorry. I hope I didn't screw up."

J.W. realized he had relinquished to Sharra, to a voice on a phone, every fiber of control left in him. He could not answer Brandi.

"You be careful," she said sadly. "We can't lose you."

Krista had been standing in the hall outside his little office in the basement when J.W. said good-bye to Brandi. As he opened the door, she pretended to be folding the wash. He forced himself forward to put his arms around her, but her body tightened, and she shivered when he whispered, "Hey, you wanna go upstairs and mess around?"

"Sure," she answered without emotion, "but a little later."

When they crawled into bed at midnight, J.W. held her and kissed her shoulders and drew circles on her tiny nipples with his finger, but they stayed soft, calm, and her breathing slowed. She turned toward him and asked, "Do you think Stanton's going to get into the playoffs?"

J.W. bolted to his side of the bed. "You wanna know why we're unraveling, Kris?" he exploded. "Each time I get near you, it gets uglier. Why the hell do you always have to ruin it? Is that your Catholic upbringing, some kind of shame? I'll find somebody else, and you won't be able to say a damn word, because you earned it."

J.W. turned away, allowing himself the outrage of her insensitivity, savoring the vindication for his transgression. The guilt in his darkened heart softened as he convinced himself he was justified in having sinned by loving Sharra, but a fist in his mind knew well the absolution had been carved by his own hand.

At 5:30 the next morning, as J.W. left for the clinic, Krista sat up partway and took his hand. "I'm sorry. You forgive?"

"Yeah, Kris, no problem. We'll talk tonight."

The past months had been easier, as their sullenness had sharpened the blade that was gutting the nearly twenty years of life they had shared. He glanced down at Krista, telling himself to hug her, to love her again, before it was too late. But as J.W. bent closer, he felt the tow of a driverless locomotive dragging him away. As hard as he told himself to jump from the train, he could not muster the strength to bend forward a few more degrees and kiss her good-bye. What burned in front of him was the memory of Sharra's scent and her cocoa skin. All J.W. could do was wish it were her looking up at him.

⇥⇤

At the close of business, a bit after nine, J.W. sat at his desk in the clinic facing forty incomplete charts, having let them heap, unable to concentrate on either his patients or their paperwork. Brandi walked past on her way out and put a hand on his shoulder but left without a word. Her tired Ford Falcon pinged out of the gravel driveway and faded down Route 4, along with the lonely drone of a passing train. The back door of the clinic opened slightly from the vibration of the train, and J.W. rose to close it in the ritual they went through six and seven times a day. He sensed a cold wind and shivered as he began to pull the door shut, but he stopped breathlessly, aware of another presence nearing the rickety back steps.

As dark as the mountain night had fallen, the first thing J.W. saw were her black eyes then her soaked, ebony hair. Her make-up had been washed away, and J.W. wondered how long she had waited in the rain.

Tears ran down her cheeks as J.W. offered his hand to bring her out of the cold. She began to cry uncontrollably, and J.W. tugged her into the warmth of the clinic. "I'm sorry. I shouldn't have come. I have no right to drag you into my problems."

It was the first time J.W. had seen Sharra Bakhtian truly vulnerable. He was scared, for he had always thought of her as a rock, impenetrable, hardened by the trials through which she'd clawed. He wanted to throw his arms around her and hold her until she stopped crying, as if his body could erase her desperation. But he became frightened she would pull away, compose herself, and leave him standing there, exposed, the fool, again.

"It was the only way I could get away from them. I shouldn't have come. I don't want to hurt you."

They sat, their hands so close, J.W. could feel the warmth of her delicate fingers, so small, so perfect, so powerful, the hands Dr. MacDonald had held up as the ideal years before. J.W. dared not touch her, but it was she who slid her hand forward and brushed his. It was the first time they had ever touched. His stomach churned. He did not know if he was about to die or be reborn. It was he, the football player, Army Ranger, combat pilot, who was helpless, vulnerable. Sharra was in command, and J.W. could not tell if he was savoring those few moments, or dreading that they continue. She leaned forward and touched his lips with her fingers, but as J.W. moved to kiss her, she pulled back. "It's getting late, J.W."

"Yeah. Look, you need some sleep. Let me call Brandi. She'll let you stay there."

J.W. introduced Sharra as Dr. Aysa Nur, but Sharra shook her head. That's all over with. I've taken my maiden name, Thabit. I am Sharra Thabit."

Brandi insisted Sharra sleep in her bed. Though Sharra protested, she was so exhausted, she allowed Brandi to walk her into the bedroom. Brandi emerged a moment later, closed the door gently, and said sadly, "She's already asleep. God, she's beautiful. I've never seen eyes like that before. She's so gentle."

"Don't tell me that. Tell me she's a dog, will you please?" J.W. laughed. "Tell me it's just a phase. Brandi, I'm scared."

Brandi handed J.W. a mug of coffee, and as he watched her female hands, he thought of Sharra's, and how close he had come to touching her body, and how impossible that was. His eyes glanced at Brandi's watch—it was nearly midnight. J.W. ignored that, sure it was many hours earlier, but the clock on the wall bode the same ill news, and he jumped up to call Krista, to make up another lie, to apologize for being late, to dig the pit even deeper.

"You sure you want to call?" Brandi asked. "I mean, feeling like you do and all?"

He hugged her and drove the thirty miles to Cedar Springs in a haze of fatigue, fear, and confusion. The only certainty was that his life with Krista had changed forever.

CHAPTER FORTY-TWO

Along the highway, before Black Granite and through Black Granite, J.W. thought only of Sharra, though as he passed the war memorial, there came the daily reflection about Viet Nam, about Lieutenant White, and about his promise. While a year-and-a-half in the shadow of his friend's grave had passed, J.W. still hadn't called the lieutenant's parents. How easy it would have been to brighten the lives of an old man and an old woman, but J.W. had thought only of himself, awash in the melancholy of his odyssey and the storm whose energy deepened every day.

At the clinic, Sharra's chair still sat by his desk, as if she had really been there, as if it had been more than just a hallucination; the patient charts, all forty of them, also sat there, as blank as the moment Sharra had reappeared in his life. J.W. trembled, realizing he would see Sharra that day, in ten minutes or an hour. Would she call first or come by and surprise him? Would J.W. cancel his patients and sneak off with her? Would he hold her hand, kiss her fingers? Would she whisper, "I love you"?

At 8 A.M., the staff began to trickle in, and his fantasy faded with each ring of the phone, with each slam of the front door as patients entered seeking his healing magic. His co-workers took their ordinary places in the grand scheme of clinical medicine, scheduling x-rays, lab tests, and CAT scans. J.W. wrote the usual prescriptions for antibiotics and anti-inflammatories, and did acupuncture on patients with back pain and headaches, and on one frantic man with the relentless, maddening, itching cancer that was consuming him. Every few minutes, J.W. excused himself and checked with the A.M. receptionist. "Any calls, any messages?"

J.W. sutured the daily parade of chainsaw-lacerated loggers, rehydrated an infant languishing with chronic diarrhea, and sat for half-an-hour with a three-hundred pound, weathered, long haul trucker who bawled uncontrollably that his wife of fifteen years had just told him she had found another man. J.W. talked and talked, and the driver cried and cried.

"Look man," J.W. preached, "you're gonna be okay Look at you. You're a good-looking, muscular guy. You make a great living. Where's she gonna find a man like you? You got the world by the balls, my friend."

He stared at J.W. inquisitively. "You really think so, Doc?"

"For sure!"

"Yeah? Yeah!" He bellowed as he marched out of the exam room and hooted, "No woman's worth it!"

The waiting room regulars looked down embarrassedly as he pranced past the part-time receptionist, though their attention was soon drawn to the pair of European sports cars that rolled up to the front door.

Kara's BMW was an older model; her mother's, though, was the sports coupe, a pale, reddish brown that complemented her coifed, auburn hair. She was statuesque, disarming, even cute from a distance when she scrunched up her nose as J.W.'s trucker brushed past, grunting, "He's right. She ain't gonna find no one like me."

Kara was seventeen. Her mother, on closer inspection, was a great deal older, sporting badly pockmarked skin and a drooping lip on the left, compliments of a facelift gone awry. She did all the talking. Kara was an aspiring model but was gaining weight. She had been to half-a-dozen doctors for pills, but had been turned down pointblank at every turn. Then mom heard about acupuncture. It was touted to be effective for weight loss, but she dismissed it when she learned the practitioners were almost exclusively Chinese. When a neighbor told her about Dr. Weathersby—the only Caucasian medical doctor in the county licensed to use the needles—she called the clinic, demanded an immediate appointment, and had Brandi call her insurance company to confirm the treatment would be covered.

Kara's mother was a businesswoman, owner of a posh commuter air service. Her eyes darted along the quaint walls of the country clinic, her distrust building until she growled, "What assurances can you give that your treatment is going to work?"

"Assurances, ma'am?"

"Yes. Are you going to stand behind your product?"

"Ma'am, this isn't a fast-food shop. A doctor can't guarantee a cure."

"Look, this is a big deal. I want twenty pounds off her in four weeks so she gets a job that's going to pay for college. If you can't produce, say so. I'll fly her somewhere to someone who can."

"Ma'am, I'll do my best, that's all I can do, but no guarantees. If that's not satisfactory, you need to get her to the Mayo Clinic or Harvard." J.W. barely heard himself, his thoughts were so scattered. He cursed under his breath at the stupid woman and stalked out of the exam room.

With still no word from Sharra, J.W. started to dial Brandi's number, but Kara's mother appeared at his desk and stood over him, waiting until he dropped the receiver. "Go ahead and do whatever it is you do. This is for her career."

Kara took her treatment well. Actually, she said nothing. Her eyes were elsewhere, as if drugged. While J.W. was trying to concentrate on placing the hair-thin needles, her mother stood above them, negotiating price and a weekly slot for Kara. J.W. conceded and offered to come early on Monday mornings so Kara wouldn't miss school. But he had just broken a cardinal rule of clinical medicine. Once a rift had been opened between patient and doctor, no manner of compromise would rescue the relationship. It was an invariable maxim.

J.W. left the room during Kara's therapy, to let the needles work for twenty minutes. He asked if there had been any calls. While he was gone, Kara's knee began to ache at the site of the most important point for weight loss. She flexed and extended it until the fine metal of the acupuncture needle fatigued. A one-inch section of needle broke off in the girl's leg. Her mother shrieked as the delicate needle handle plinked on the floor. J.W. ran back to the room.

"Where's the rest of the needle?" she demanded.

"Well, ma'am, looks like it's embedded under her skin, doesn't it? That's good news, actually. That happens to be one of the latest techniques from China."

"China?"

"Yes, ma'am. Leave the needle at the painful spot. It's not going anywhere. It can't. Good joss, that."

"Good joss? What the hell are you talking about, you quack?" She dragged Kara, limping, from the clinic howling, "You will hear directly from my attorneys, and in short order!"

There was still no word from Sharra, and his mind blanked, not comprehending he was about to break another cardinal rule of emergency medicine, the second that day—never leave the clinic unattended, even for the twinkling of an eye. The instant the doctor walked away, that ER transformed into a grand magnet, cosmically attracting every medical shipwreck in the valley.

He left through the rear door with not a word to the staff. As he backed the Buick out of the driveway, he spotted the nurse, receptionist, and lab tech lined up at the window, staring sadly, silently. The image clutched his chest, and the Buick hesitated. A moment later it crawled back into its parking spot. J.W. tried the phone again. No answer.

Brandi arrived for the afternoon shift, tired, unsmiling, wearing only a daub of patchy makeup. She marched directly to J.W.'s desk, took him by the arm, led him outside to her car, sighed exhaustedly, and began. "This is crazy. She got up in the middle of the night and made a phone call. She was talking in some kinda language, so I don't know what she said. Then she started to cry, like she was screaming. I saw her taking pills. Then she took a shower and left the house. She called me a little while ago and said she was sorry for bothering me, that she had made a long-distance call and was going to pay me back."

"Did she mention me? Leave me a message?"

"Yeah. She told me to tell you she was going to Canada to look for a job. That she was going to be with a friend."

CHAPTER FORTY-THREE

Walking through the door at home that night, J.W.'s heart leapt into his mouth as he focused on the note on the living room floor, a secret note from Sharra, J.W. prayed and feared. His hand uncovered the terse message slowly. "Call Dust Man."

Bernie's voice was tired, scratchy, morose, yet driven, carried by a pressure of speech J.W. had not heard since the psychiatry rotation at St. Augie's. J.W. asked if he was high, but Bernie swore he hadn't fallen off the wagon. "How's Bobbie Jo?" J.W. inquired stiffly, formally, against his better judgment. There was a long silence.

"She's not home. Out working, I think. Got a bit of trouble with the ICC over the hospital beds. Some little old lady in Cape Coral, Florida, got squashed by the product. One of the worm gear drive units shorted out. Cranked for hours, maybe days, 'til they found her."

"That's not your problem, is it? It's a corporate matter."

"That's the problem. See, the headquarters division was just a postbox."

"So?"

"It was registered to one Ishmael Sogup."

"Ah, for God's sakes, Bernie, you used my fraternity alias. You were the founding father of the corporation, weren't you?"

"I didn't think you'd mind if I borrowed a name. Hey, think about it. You borrowed it yourself. So, meanwhile, I moved into this smaller house, my cousin's place on Staten Island. Hell of a lot less crime here. Mostly cemeteries. I told you about Cousin Leon, didn't I? Yeah, I'm sure I did. He's the undertaker. You remember. Hey, he lets me help him with the embalming. Lotta dead bodies waiting around. I saw this one suicide. Shotgun. Closed coffin, if you know what I mean. I mean, what does it take to pull the trigger with a 12-gauge sitting in your mouth? Think about it. Those last microseconds, man. It's too bizarre. Leon let me do a lot of work on the guy; put him in a suit, nice shoes, felt hat. That was his idea, the hat. I thought it was pretty funny. Hey, the guy didn't know, did he? You're a doctor. Think he was feeling any pain? No, he wasn't real anymore, was he? Guy was dead…"

J.W. interrupted brusquely, "Sounds like great fun, Bernie. Wish I could've been there. Hey, I better let you go. Everybody's asleep. I'll give you a call during the week, okay? Say hello."

The first fifteen minutes of the late news were over, the usual potpourri of drug arrests, arson, and the latest on the wonton killing of goats down in Woodside. J.W. popped beer number three during the commercial, and it, too, was gone by the time the network flashed pictures of cachectic, fly-encrusted children dying of thirst in an African famine. As J.W. settled back to suck down a fourth beer, his eyes nearly closed. He did not want to fall asleep on the couch again and wake stiff and tired at dawn, but he could draw neither the strength nor motivation to move. He resolved to gather the concentration to lift himself in three minutes, at the next commercial, and go upstairs to bed, but his eyes closed, and he drifted away. Every few minutes he regained semi-consciousness, Sharra always his first vision, but the alcohol did its job, and he lapsed back into a troubled sleep.

In a dream, he heard a familiar voice but could not place it. For an instant, he was back in Hong Kong, in the apartment, or perhaps it was the hospital, and he was doing surgery, but maybe it was medical school. J.W. sensed a warmth he had not felt in a very long time as the familiar voice became more distinct and soon filled the room—it was coming from the TV. A network reporter was interviewing a thin, gray-haired, old man. The face was foreign, and J.W. was sure he had never seen him, but the drawl and the toughness that it echoed culled a sense of sadness and longing all at once. He listened harder.

Dr. Harlan Flowers stood in the Sahel of East Africa, an emissary of the Mission Church sent to reckon the needs of the wretched. In his alcoholic haze, J.W. must have called out to him, for Krista ran from the bedroom just as Dr. Flowers faded from the screen.

She counted the empties, silently but precisely, and asked, "You crying because of the alcohol, or is there something else?"

J.W. tried to tell her what Dr. Flowers had said, how he looked, how he had aged, but it came out flat, so he stopped.

Another night of tossing and wondering drained him, hours that passed slowly, painfully. He thought how much easier life was for starving refugees, the focus of their existence the pursuit of the next hour's food, a sip of muddy water, a stick of firewood. They worried not about malpractice suits or would-be lovers from far corners of their continent. They were in the fight together, J.W. imagined, those ancient people, with a tribal spirit, a psychic talisman that had allowed them to cope for the millennia. J.W. wore no such armor.

At dawn, he stole down to his little office and called the network. The first receptionist listened impatiently, as did her supervisor. Her boss, however, granted J.W. thirty seconds with the correspondent who had interviewed Dr. Flowers. At the end of that half-an-hour conversation, she invited J.W. to be at Kennedy Airport to welcome him back from Africa.

J.W. said, "No," afraid to let Dr. Flowers see what had become of his dreams and the years of effort. An hour later, however, the network called back and offered to pay for his trip to New York. It also paid for the dinner in Dr. Flowers' honor at the Water Club on the East River, and for the crystal martinis that J.W. guzzled during the evening's conversation. Dr. Flowers and J.W. talked until nearly dawn. J.W. told him about Sharra.

"Do what you think is right, J.W. Do you want me to remind you there's snares along the path?" He shook his head sadly "They're also opportunities. Sometimes they look the same, 'cause a body sees what he wants to see. But just like the rest of us, you can't know 'till it's said and done."

CHAPTER FORTY-FOUR

J.W. found a cryptic note in his pigeonhole at the clinic on his first shift back from New York. He called the number in Stanton. Sharra hesitated but finally asked if there was any chance the clinic would hire her part time. He had not seen her since the night, weeks before, that she'd waited in the rain. He asked her to come to the clinic to talk, but she cried that she couldn't see him, that she had an intense fear of destroying his life.

"How could you hurt anyone?" J.W. asked, "You are a beautiful child. You've never harmed any creature, just yourself."

"I've done it a hundred times," she wept. "I should go back to Iran and let them stone me to death. At least I would die knowing I was being punished for my sins."

"Stop that. I will call the Medical Director and get you an interview. There's reciprocity with California, so that isn't a problem. Everything's gonna be okay. I promise."

She came to the clinic that night. J.W. took her by the hand, leaned forward, brushed her lips with his fingers, and kissed her as tenderly as he had ever caressed a woman. They breathed each other's scent and let their faces touch until J.W. started to cry. "Please Sharra, I want to be with you. Just once. Please, could we?"

"I'd like that. I'll call you tomorrow." She touched his lips and ran from the clinic.

⭤ ⭤

When Brandi walked in to start her afternoon, she stopped short at the backdoor. J.W. looked up to see her draw in the perfumed air and quickly look away.

Sharra did not call that day, or the next. J.W. was afraid she wouldn't come to her interview with Braunwald, but she drove up in a rented car on Thursday; and as they walked to the office, she slipped J.W. a piece of smudged, creamy stationery on which was scribbled a date a week later, his day off. "I don't know if I can wait that long," he whispered.

Sharra and Braunwald spoke for only minutes before he offered her a position. She accepted immediately, though announced to Braunwald that she had a special engagement in a week in Stanton, and would begin after that.

The days that followed held the deepest, blackest anxiety, and the most profound excitement, J.W. had ever felt. Nothing had ever so gripped his consciousness and his dreams. He kept telling himself it was a victimless crime, but his fear peaked each time he started to dial Sharra's number, and he dropped the phone into its cradle.

A nurse from his internship owned a summer home along the Salmon, not far from Mr. Shelton's trailer. Obsequiously, J.W. explained why he was asking to use her cabin, and she agreed on the condition he promise to think about meeting her up there sometime. J.W. was surprised how easy it was to agree, and mean it. Just another in his string of victimless crimes, he laughed sadly to himself.

The sexual gnawing in his gut ground constantly that week. He ran his four miles every night but found himself stopping and walking, touching himself, thinking about Sharra. By the night before their meeting, J.W. was so crazed with desire, he sensed no guilt—he sensed nothing but the dream of the moment he'd love her. They were to meet at 1 P.M., a few blocks from the clinic, behind the tavern. Sharra would follow him along the Salmon to the cabin. As an alibi, J.W. stopped at the clinic and sat at his desk, returning messages, answering questions, and chatting calmly with the on-call doctor.

The top note on his desk was from Herbee Rizzo, director of the Black Granite Medical Center, who had asked for a call-back at J.W.'s convenience. That usually meant one of the clinic's patients, on whom they had missed an important, and usually bizarre diagnosis, was gravely ill, and had come under the aegis of the Black Granite Medical Center. The patient was probably screaming malpractice, and Rizzo just wanted to let them know, as a courtesy, though the conversations with him always seemed to end with a gloating snicker.

"You've done a good job up there, Dr. Weathersby. Some of our physicians are impressed. Ever thought of leaving the clinic and joining our side? Lot more professional. Good back up. There's the haves and the have nots coming in medicine. I think you know which category the Black Granite Medical Center sits in."

The wall clock, that had moved with such lethargy for a week, now read nearly one. "Can I get back to you in a couple of days?" J.W. mumbled nervously.

"Let me ask you a question here. Just take a minute. I know you're busy. Look, tell me about your residency. Over in Cedar Springs, wasn't it? How'd that go? Any problems?"

"Got an emergency patient to see. Let me call you back."

"This afternoon, if you can."

J.W. tore out of the clinic. The x-ray tech commented under her breath, "Where's the fire?" Brandi said nothing, but J.W. saw her standing by the window as gravel flew from the Buick's tires. He sped to the rendezvous in the alley, skidding up to the corner. Sharra was not there. Perhaps she had come and gone; maybe she was just late, like J.W. But as the minutes ticked away, he accepted that he was, once again, the fool.

J.W. waited for half-an-hour before driving toward Brandi's house. He passed Sharra and turned around to follow her. When she finally saw him in her mirror and pulled over, she flushed, apologizing for being so late. "I'll follow you," she offered, but lagged so far behind she became lost, and J.W. had to turn and search for her half-a-mile back up the road.

At the cabin, Sharra emerged from her car with a bouquet of spring blossoms, waving them happily, freely. She took J.W.'s hand and pulled him inside the cabin. Her reed-thin body moved without disturbing the sheer fabric of her silk dress. She touched his face and offered the flowers. Her skin was pure, perfect

"Do you really want to do this?" J.W. asked tremulously. "I mean, what's going to happen if we like it, and I can't stop wanting you? What then?"

"We'll deal with it. All I know is that I need you more than any man I've ever wanted."

She did not vacillate as she let her dress slip from her shoulders. She was wearing thin, black panties and a black lace bra. J.W. was breathing so hard, he was afraid he'd scare her. "Are you sure?" J.W. demanded. "I don't want to hurt you. I love you."

"Don't talk. I just want you in me."

J.W. fumbled through the clip on her bra and beheld the breasts he had dreamed of for years. He drew her nipples into his mouth, delicately brownish pink and already hard. He touched her so gently she shivered, until J.W. kissed her there. She moaned for a few moments then pulled him onto her. After the first instant of being in her, everything faded; the burdens, the decades of desolation, the dread of the next failure, all of it gone; maybe it was for hours or just minutes, but all time was lost in a blur. He was weightless for the first time in his life, aware of nothing but their motion.

Sharra came to a breathless end, over and over, trembling the last time, breaking into sobbing tears. J.W. wrapped himself around her and they slept. He awoke overwhelmed by her aura, her scent, her power. He murmured, "I will never let anyone harm you."

She nuzzled him and whispered, "Now, I know why it's called making love." She was silent for a moment, though soon vowed through tears, "I swear I will love you for eternity," And that afternoon, J.W. believed her.

CHAPTER FORTY-FIVE

"Where have you been?" Krista asked when J.W. called home. "Everyone's looking for you!"

"I told you. I was having my yearly physical. The goddamn Buick broke down. Boy, do I have news for you. What a crazy day. Did I ever tell you about the Black Granite Center?"

"Yes, you did, and they're the ones who called," she interrupted.

"Who, Rizzo? Is he nuts?" J.W. interrupted. "I was just there! I just talked to him. Let me give 'em a call and find out what the hell's going on. I'll be home in an hour."

J.W. hung up before he plunged deeper into the mire. He smeared engine grease on his skin and on his clothes, to obscure Sharra's scent, and sped back to Cedar Springs. He ran into the house with his filthy hands in the air, as if surrendering. "Don't touch me. I'm dirty, and I stink."

"Don't worry," Krista assured.

That night a magnum of Mums champagne vaporized in an hour. J.W. crawled to the bedroom, falling asleep in his clothes. At dawn, Krista did not move. She was curled in a tight ball facing away from him. He woke to a sense of rustling outside the house and wove toward the front door, trying not to jar his head, appeasing the headache that tore at his scalp. The neighborhood was silent and empty. J.W. crawled back to bed.

When he went to his car to leave for work, though, he found a note pushed through the crack he'd left in his side window. The writing was tiny, down sloping. "*Sobh bekheir esh ghe man.* Good morning my love."

⇥ ⇤

"She knocked on my door at 3 A.M. She looked awful," Brandi shook her head, "as if she hadn't been to bed. She was wearing the most beautiful dress I've ever seen. Oh, and that guy, Rizzo, from the Black Granite Medical Center. He called again. So did that jerk, Braunwald."

"You mean the owner, Brandi, your employer?"

J.W. called Braunwald first. "We're impressed with your friend. Can't seem to find her number. Why don't you give it to me so I can call her and get over to Cedar Springs to sign a contract. By the way, her application was incomplete. Let's see here. Is she attached, married? Any children?"

"I better ask her if she wants to fill in the blanks. You know how some people are about their privacy these days. Anyway, I'm the local medical director. I'll be glad to give her a call and tell her she's got the job."

"Don't get so defensive. I just want to see if she needs to put her family on the medical plan, okay?"

"I'm not being defensive. By the way, I don't remember you guys offering *me* a plan."

"Different situation. You needed work, remember? Sharra can write her own ticket. Nothing personal. Just business."

"Well, I'll let DOCTOR Thabit know."

"That's what I've heard. You know a lot about her."

At noon, he ran from the clinic. Sharra was asleep at Brandi's. As J.W. touched her face, she woke and drew him toward her, tugged at his belt, wet him with her mouth, and pulled him onto her.

When they were done, she whispered, "Why are you here?"

"They're going to give you the job."

"We'll be closer, *esh ghe man*, my love."

"Sharra, they know all about us. Everyone does. Who did you tell?"

"No one!"

"Who was it, Sharra?"

"Please don't yell at me. I didn't want this to cost you your family. Maybe you shouldn't have come here. Maybe you should go home before it's too late."

"I'm sorry. I'm just scared. I won't lose my family. And I won't lose you. I'll figure it out. I will not lose this time."

"Yes, you will. You know nothing of losing yet, how it gets easier, and harder, each time." She faced away from him, ripped the covers back, and ran to the bathroom. The lock snapped loudly; the shower soon hissed.

Before J.W. left, he put a note on her pillow. "I won't abandon you. Never." But his writing was tiny and sloped downward.

CHAPTER FORTY-SIX

J.W. accepted the offer from the Black Granite Medical Center. The next day, Krista asked to meet him for lunch and see his new office, but J.W. lied that, for the next weeks, he had meetings with the power elite of the Center every noon. It wasn't, however, the Center that consumed the middle of his days. Sharra and J.W. met to talk by the river, to hold hands, and to make promises.

On his third day at the Center, Sharra appeared at his office door after-hours. "I just want to sit and look at you. I won't bother you. Promise." She relaxed quietly in a corner, staring at the memorabilia and degrees from Princeton left behind by the departed senior physician into whose office J.W. had been placed. Dr. Christensen had left the Center for a much better paying job with a pharmaceutical company, or so the scuttlebutt had it. It must have been an exceedingly good offer, for his coffee cup was still sitting on the mahogany desk with a dried puddle of black mud at the bottom. Next to it was his prescription pad. It was as if he was still there—but it was only the shadow he had cast upon the Medical Center that lingered.

Sharra asked what had become of Dr. Christensen, why J.W. had been granted his large, airy office. He told her he had no idea. Rizzo had just grumbled, "Don't worry about it. Move your things in. Consider this your home for the foreseeable future."

J.W. took down the degrees and put up pictures of Viet Nam, Hong Kong, and Khai. On his fourth morning, J.W. left Cedar Springs before dawn, as in the old days, and drove to the cabin on the Salmon. He gently dug up and potted ferns from the forest outside the window of the bedroom in which he had loved Sharra and placed them in an arc on his desk. He was surrounded by lush green, and by the fragmented symbols of his long path to medicine. When everything was in place, J.W. hung the two Purple Hearts above his desk, lest he forget.

━+ +━

Dr. Flatury, a cardiologist in Greenfield, the town next to Black Granite, and chairman of the local medical disciplinary board, had J.W. come by the golf club to welcome him to the county. Over lunch, along with several other of the county's new doctors, J.W. was treated to an inventory of Flatury's unending board, committee, planning, financial, and civic meetings, and the colorful summits with movie stars who had sought him out as a doctor. While only a few years his senior, Flatury's baldness, six-foot-seven frame, and dour bearing made him seem an elder, of another generation, distended with wisdom. J.W. wondered if Flatury had ever slipped from the path as far as had J.W.

As coffee was served, Rizzo appeared with a packet of forms, W-2s, W-4s, life insurance, and, finally, a magazine-like application for privileges at the local hospital. "There's been a little bit of opposition to hiring a doctor who hasn't finished his residency, but I think it'll be okay Just keep your nose clean." He paused.

"You're married, aren't you? Have a family if I remember correctly? You said that, didn't you, when we first talked?"

J.W. was afraid his face had flushed as deeply as the warmth he felt pour over him. "Yes, of course. Why?"

"That must have been your wife here last night. Well, we're glad to have you both. Just keep in mind what I said."

⊨⊨ ⊨⊨

Sharra called that afternoon. J.W. began the conversation. "They think we're married. Can you believe that?"

Sharra replied tersely, "I have to talk to you. Meet me at the alley tonight. No sex. Please. Okay?"

Khai promised she would tell Krista that J.W. had to work late. Sharra was on time. She stared at the street lamp, hardly able to speak. Finally, she choked, "I don't know what to do. Something is so wrong. I can't eat, I can't sleep. I should be so happy. What is wrong? Please help me. I know you can. I don't want to die."

J.W. touched her face gently. "Welcome to the club. You're depressed. You're stressed out, Sharra. Does that shock you? Neither of us rested after pre-med, after getting into medical school, after internship. You're a world away from your people. It's not natural, Sharra, all that shit with J'Aveed. Both of us need to take some time off. Why don't you go home and have a glass of wine? Relax. I'll bring you some medication in the morning. Everything's going to be okay."

"That's the problem; it's what I'm trying to tell you," she cried harder. "I am drinking so much. I am Baha'i; it is forbidden, but I can't stop. It was the only way I could get through the night, and now I can't survive the day without it. Please help me!"

Her face was as soft as the finest silk, but the color was gone. She struggled from the car and stood outside breathing heavily, waiting for J.W. to drive away. He watched her in his rearview mirror, staring at a sliver of the woman who had been so shy, who had hidden so much that first day of medical school. He loved her, he thought, more than life, even if she was just a hallucination, even if he was allowing the mirage to destroy him.

On the way home, J.W. began to shiver as if the temperature had fallen to zero, and the Buick's heater had died yet again. He was lost, trudging another world, oblivious to the present. It was a miracle that he was able to drive the tortuous country highway unscathed. There was no emotion in his mind beside Sharra. He quaked harder and pushed impatiently on the heater buttons, but they were already on full. He opened the window to save himself, gulping fresh air as the sides of the car closed in on him, but his breathing was so fast, his hands began to tingle. He missed the turnoff for home and sailed north on the interstate before regaining a sense of where his journey was to finish.

At the driveway, he was still shaking and soaked with sweat. Krista met him at the door and put him to bed. "Goddamn flu," J.W. cursed. "Maybe I need to take some time to rest."

In the morning, J.W. dressed and told Krista as he was leaving the house that he felt much better. He drove away before dawn, hiding the bottle of antidepressants for Sharra in his lunch bag. But Sharra did not call that day, nor the next, and on the third day, J.W. phoned Brandi, who had taken the week off. She would not answer the phone. He drove to her house. He had to wrest it from her. "Sharra left a couple of days ago. I don't know where she is. I shouldn't be telling you this. She made me promise I wouldn't tell you."

CHAPTER FORTY-SEVEN

J.W. was thankful for Sharra's silence, the cleansing power of time, he assured himself. His new colleagues loaded his schedule with a collection of less than stellar referrals: problem children, chronic back pain, abdominal pain, and headache sufferers, many fending for themselves on the street with no insurance and fewer means. Rather than with resentment, J.W. viewed these people jealously, for their lack of attachment to reality.

Sharra did not call, and she did not call, and Brandi was steadfast in not answering his messages. J.W. passed Rizzo in the hall. "Dr. Weathersby, Jees, you've lost some weight, haven't you? Wish I could. By the way, the staff's pleased. You've got a good attitude. See anyone who wants to be seen, as long as they can crawl or get carried in. I like that."

"I came here to work, not screw around. And anyway, I got a lot of years to live and a lot of bills." J.W. answered with a forced a laugh. "You know Herb, when I think about Viet Nam, this ain't work—it's a game. Just keep 'em coming."

Rizzo slapped J.W. on the back and turned to leave but hesitated and laughed. "Keeping your nose clean?"

⇥ ⇤

When Black Granite's athletic director showed up in J.W.'s office complaining of back pain, J.W. realized he was being evaluated, no longer by the Center, but by the town. The AD asked about J.W.'s time playing football at Sterling College. "It was college football—a business."

"The AD laughed, "Not that much different at high school level anymore." He locked J.W.'s eyes. "But how'd you like to get involved again?"

At first, J.W. thought he was going to ask him to coach the city's high school team, and J.W. felt his face flush with fear, but also excitement. Hesitating for a moment, J.W. admitted, "Jees, Coach, I'm flattered, but I've never coached any sport."

"No, no, not coach. We'd like you to cover the stadium for us—be the team doctor. Could you do that? We can't pay you, but I bet you miss it. Don't you? Gets in your blood."

J.W. thought for a moment before answering. "You know, Coach, football was a lot of hard work, and I wasn't all that hot. Good memories? I don't remember any, to tell you the truth."

He stared at J.W. hard, disappointedly, like a coach, and J.W. interjected, "But that's not your problem. Sure. I'll be glad to cover a few of the games for you"

The AD popped off the exam table, shook J.W.'s hand hard, like a coach, and left the room without having had his back examined.

⇥ ⇤

As J.W.'s practice evolved, Rizzo assigned him a permanent nurse. Monique had been a trusted member of the Center for a dozen years, but she also made J.W.'s solar plexus grip. Her breasts were taut with nipples that spent a good deal of the day poking through the tight nylon of her blouse, surely a factor in her longevity at the Center. With each breath of her perfume, J.W. thought of what he was missing, of how badly he needed to feel Sharra's body again. By week's end, J.W. sat in his office trying not to give in, though as it had so many times over the last month, his hand took the phone and dialed the Clinic. He asked for Dr. Thabit, but Brandi told him, "J.W., I love you like a brother. Sharra came back. Said she was sick, and now she's gone again. Sick at home."

"I need to see her. Brandi, I love you. Please tell me where she is." J.W. begged.

"I can't tell you. She made me promise."

"What's her number, then?"

"I can't tell you that, either. Please don't hate me. She told me I couldn't give it to anyone."

"I'm not anyone. Tell me where she's living, goddamnit!"

"Don't yell at me. I can't," Brandi choked through sobs.

"Well, then fuck you!" he screamed at her and hung up angrily.

J.W. ordered Monique to call the medical licensing bureau and find Dr. Thabit's home number, but the bureau released only the Clinic's address. J.W. called Braunwald fawningly, asking for help finding her, to inform her of an emergency medical situation with one of her patients. He hung up on J.W.

J.W. besieged a police-officer patient to see if he could find her address, but the man laughed, "Hey, Doc, sounds like you're thinking with the wrong head. Doctor needs to keep it in his pants."

J.W. boiled at his desk, licking the wounds. By the end of the morning, Sharra would be aware he was searching for her, and she would call to demand that he stop his stalking; though J.W. believed, perhaps, she wanted him to chase her, to prove that he wouldn't abandon her as had every man in her life. J.W. needed to hear her say, *"Esh ghe man,* my love," one last time.

J.W. managed to keep his hands off the phone for long periods, but each hour became dreadfully more painful, infinitely more difficult than the last. It was after a pitiable patient, a forty-year-old street person who had been bashed by a jailer, that J.W. finally collapsed and touched the "O," declared a medical emergency, and ordered the operator to connect him with Dr. Thabit immediately. The operator hesitated, and J.W. threatened that if she didn't carry out his demand, and his patient died, she would be held to account for the loss.

"Call the Black Granite Medical Center and ask for Dr. Weathersby if you don't believe me," J.W. shouted into the phone; though the next sound was a gruff voice J.W. thought he recognized. "Yeah? And who the hell wants to talk to her?" the voice demanded. J.W. was sure it was Braunwald.

J.W. hung up gently, laughing perversely that he had paid in his heart for the foolish mistake.

Every night for the rest of that week, he lay on the couch, in front of an ignored television, so intoxicated by his thoughts, he often forgot to finish the fourth and fifth beers. Krista had given up pulling him to bed at midnight, and J.W. slept fitfully, his fatigue deepening, until he was sure everyone at the Medical Center knew about the immense chasm in his heart, and the wind that stormed through his soul like a violent hurricane.

J.W. arrived at the Friday night high school football game with Khai holding his hand, a distraction, his last friend. He hoped she would someday remember being so close to him and the gladiators. After the National Anthem, J.W. placed her right hand over her heart for the Pledge of Allegiance, and he watched her, standing so proudly at attention, glaring at the football players who chattered disrespectfully. He wondered if she would commit the same dreadful mistakes he had, or if she would escape the hard road and arrive at her destination with fewer scars.

His beeper sounded seconds after the kickoff. "Thank goodness you got right back to us, Doctor!" the page operator declared nervously. "We received a call from a lady. All I could get from her was that someone was missing. She had an accent. I'm sorry, doctor, I couldn't get her name. Please talk to her. I'm worried about this one."

The operator patched him through to a phone that rang with the sickeningly familiar sound. A woman answered so softly, through such sobs, J.W. could barely make out the accent.

"Sharra?"

"*Doctori,*" and it became even harder to understand her. He became angry at the ignorant foreigner. How long had she lived here and not bothered to learn English? All J.W. discerned through her tears was a plea that J.W. do something.

"Talk sense, woman!" J.W. shouted into the phone, so scared he was trembling. "What are you calling about?"

"Sharra is gone. Everything is stolen from her."

"Ma'am, who are you? How do you know Sharra? Where is she? Tell me where she is, and I'll find her. I'll help her. Where is she?"

"Maybe with her boyfriend. I don't know." She was crying so hard, J.W. dropped the phone back and called Brandi.

"You tell me where she is. I'm scared. You tell me!"

"She's living at Braunwald's summer home on Lake Jaffee."

"Braunwald?"

"Yeah, Mr. Pinkie Ring, your former boss. He's giving her drugs—in trade. Sharra's mother came out from LA to be with her, to get her away from him, to take her home to Iran. She said America was worse than the ayatollahs. She said it would be better to be sentenced to death there than keep dying here little by little. J.W., you need to do something. Sharra can't talk. She can't work. I'm so worried, I can't sleep. And you be careful. Braunwald's crazy. He carries a gun, and he hates you. Please take care."

⊨⊨ ⊨⊨

J.W. drove Khai home and lied to Krista that one of the football players had been hurt. He retraced the fifty miles to Lake Jaffee, aware and dreading that it would all soon be over, that Krista would learn of the blunders, piled one upon the other, each a gray stone in a wall behind which J.W. had now completely enclosed himself.

Sharrazad Thabit's mother answered the knock. She seemed not surprised when J.W. introduced himself, and took his hand as gently as Sharra had the first time they'd touched. Her skin was warm and soft, like a woman's, like Krista's, like Sharra's. He suddenly felt the grand fool, a stupid man who had torn his life asunder for the touch of a woman's hand. But when J.W. looked into Mrs. Thabit's face, he saw the treasure, the same delicate, soothing features that had captured his soul. Even through the sadness that engulfed Mrs. Thabit's eyes, the jewel-like clarity of Sharra's spirit survived. J.W. shook in dread that Sharra would not live long enough to sparkle as beautifully.

Mrs. Thabit sat quietly, aware she was losing what was left of her life. Perhaps she knew what Sharra and J.W. had done, perhaps she believed they were just friends. She did not say. J.W.

wondered if her anger would suddenly erupt, if she would accuse him of having drawn her daughter out of her home, in the Turkish enclave, where, at least, the enemy was recognizable. He kept his heart steeled for the onslaught, probably with a gun or knife, then laughed wryly to himself that he would not fight back if she sought to kill him. Mrs. Thabit walked back into the room armed only with a tray and two cups.

"Sharra says you like tea."

"She's a very special person," J.W. said after an interminable silence. "I just think she needs some help getting J'Aveed back."

Mrs. Thabit did not answer. Finally, she looked up and mumbled, "They will never give her the child."

"Why is that?"

She looked down, sighed deeply, and urged, "You must go home to your wife and your daughter. Sharra is chattel, like me. We are worthless. Hassan's family has money and position in the new government in Persia. I am sorry. I should never have asked you to come. I was just so scared."

J.W. looked again for some trace of anger, but her face was calm. Though she hugged him warmly at the door, J.W. knew she never would again.

At dawn, J.W. snuck down to his office in the basement and called Mrs. Thabit. Sharra had come home in the middle of the night, her clothes torn and dirty. She had wept drunkenly for hours. He asked to speak to her, but Mrs. Thabit wanted to let her sleep.

On Sunday morning, the phone woke them. Krista handed it to J.W. with a groaning, "Patient."

"Dr. Weathersby, could you meet me at the alley? In an hour? Please."

"I'm sorry, I can't prescribe drugs over the phone. You'll have to call the office first thing tomorrow morning," and he hung up before she could respond.

CHAPTER FORTY-SEVEN

The glass after glass of cheap wine J.W. guzzled, unsavored, after Krista went to bed that night, was more an insult the next morning than during the room-swirling, sleepless night. If he could just get to the Medical Center, the force of the workday would mute the fire in his heart. The predictable cast of patients would smooth the torpid waves of confusion and fear driving him. He sought drowning himself in the intensity of his work, hopeful for an hour's reprieve before the fidgeting began again, before the breathless wait for Sharra's call would crush the tranquility of the day's battles. It made him laugh that no one at the Center, in his family, or in his shrinking circle of friends had ever mentioned his secret, the deceitful life he had carved, though they knew, everyone did. Surely, they, too, saw the increasingly gaunt face that stared back in the shaving mirror each hung-over morning.

Driving to the Center, J.W. forgot the curves where the police sat waiting for speeders. His radio was turned up, blaring tortuous hard rock to drown out all that was left of his thoughts, anything to escape the constant grinding in his head, his heart, and his gut. He was too busy wiping away cold tears to worry about cops when the tandem semi ahead skidded to a stop. He looked up at the last minute to see the brake lights of the phalanx of cars to his front. The hood of the Buick glided in slow motion, approaching the truck's tailgate. J.W. saw his own escape, a chance to undo his seat belt before the crash, but the Buick lost traction on a tiny lake of black ice and skidded onto the muddy shoulder, crashing through wispy, winter-dried weeds. It came to rest four feet from a State Police cruiser.

The trooper jumped out of her car, staring at J.W. intently as she approached him, hand on her service revolver. But she suddenly about-faced and ran back to her car to listen to the radio. She picked up the microphone and screeched out of her lair with lights and sirens screaming. Sweat poured from J.W.'s face and a wave of nausea overwhelmed him. Surely, someone recognized the man in a tie and jacket kneeling by the side of road, vomiting in public, but no one stopped.

His plan was to saunter past Monique to the bathroom, wash his face, brush his teeth, and wait for Sharra's call. He would moan to Monique that he had come down with the flu and let his guilt and fear lose itself in the comic drama of his work.

Monique was at her station, pouring over a letter. Without turning toward him, she murmured, "Administration wants to see you right away." She flipped the letter at him, a blistering missive from Mrs. Westwong, the central theme of which concerned her husband, and his inability to make love to her anymore, ever since the motorcycle accident.

J.W. remembered the case. Rolph Westwong rocketed away from his house in a fury over his spouse's carping that he was, once again, drunk. He was found by the police, prostrate and unconscious, on the aspirin aisle of Evan's Drug Emporium, barely a block away from home. His Harley was wedged in the store's front window.

That had been many months before, shortly after J.W. had begun at the Center, and one of the surgeons, Wilbur Saloy, called him in the middle of the night ordering him to the hospital to assist in suturing together what had been gathered of Mr. Westwong.

"Hey, Will, love to, but I don't have hospital privileges yet," J.W. groaned in mock disappointment.

"I'll take care of it with the staff. You've applied. That's good enough."

They drove a metal rod into what was left of Mr. Westwong's shattered femur, removed the Bic pen that had pierced seven inches into his other leg, stopped and watched while the G.I. surgeons laced the tear in his liver, and stood by when the neurosurgeons were summoned to drain blood from his skull. The marathon ended the next afternoon. J.W. and Saloy had not left the room in over twelve hours. J.W. admitted to Will he hadn't felt so tired or so exhilarated since the OR in Hong Kong. Saloy promised more surgery, time away from the grind of the office, and an opportunity to get back into real medicine.

As Will Saloy and J.W. were changing out of scrubs, the surgeon smiled, "J.W., let's have you stop by and write a note on Westwong's chart every three or four days. I'll have the physician assistant do all the post-op care, so all you need to do is say something like, 'Patient progressing well under care of GI and neurosurg. I'll stop by once every couple of weeks and cosign the notes. Nurses see a real doctor involved from ortho, keeps their feathers from flyin' around. Also, frees up a lot of time for me to do surgery—that's where the bucks come from, and that keeps Rizzo off our asses, *and* makes sure you stay employed."

Mr. Westwong's recuperation was not uneventful. Medically, he did fine, as long as his wrists and ankles were restrained, and the nurses kept him lodged in the isolation room, sparing the rest of the dying patients the screaming fights with Mrs. Westwong. The staff christened her "The Angel of Death," for the Tupperware vats of home cooked goulash she carted into the unit Wednesday evenings. The odor sent Mr. Westwong into a reflexive rage, and the other patients into mad groping for emesis basins.

When they finally discharged him, Mr. Westwong could stand for a few seconds but repeatedly toppled to his left. He lay on the floor screaming that God had cheated him, that just once, he wanted to fall to the right.

Mrs. Westwong finally packed him home, leaving the ICU with threatening words, promising legal retaliation for the discharge that was forced upon the family against her judgment. She groused, as her husband was wheeled to the front door of the hospital, that he was too sick to be turned away, and he, himself, warned that he'd be dead in two days from her cooking.

"You haven't heard the last of us," she yelled as she dumped him into the rear seat of their rusting '67 Dodge.

Rolph blathered, "The next time I see you, I'll be dead."

Mrs. Westwong's handwritten, coffee-stained missive insinuated that while her husband had survived, poor medical technique had left him in such a vitiated state, he was unable to function properly. "He can't get it up no more, if you know what I mean," she wrote in very small script. She went on to refuse to pay the twenty-five dollars a month the Medical Center had agreed to accept for the bill which hovered over the two-hundred-thousand mark. Apparently, Mr. Westwong had let his medical insurance lapse right around the time he'd let ethanolism sabotage his career as an airplane mechanic installing avionics in SkyCo's hybrid aircraft.

At the end of the letter, Mrs. Westwong went on to subtly drop the name of the attorney she had retained to look into retribution

for the Center's second-rate care, describing her counselor as, "…
the best malpractice lawyer in the country." This was the part of
the letter that had piqued the interest of the Center's administration, and for which J.W. had been summoned to the penthouse
of the brand new administration wing.

J.W. met with Rizzo and the Chairman of the Board, Dr. Patel.
He was happy for the hour's reprieve before facing patients.

"We'll confer with counsel," Rizzo said with a poker-face, after listening to J.W.'s version of the Westwong saga.

"Are you going to be talking to Saloy?" J.W. asked. "It's his
patient. I was just helping out."

"Saloy says it was your patient. You were supposed to keep an
eye on him, get consults and the like, before he was discharged."

"You mean to see if he could *produce* a discharge."

Rizzo laughed but the smiled passed quickly, and he stared
into J.W.'s eyes. "Just keep your nose clean."

Monique asked if J.W. was ready to see patients. She came closer
for the answer, a few inches from his face, nostrils flared, sam-
pling the air. J.W. sucked a breath in slowly through his teeth.

"Look, Monique, I'm really sick. I feel like hell. Please, don't
get on my case. I need a minute to get warmed up."

Her intense eyes did not leave his face, except for the few
times they darted, almost imperceptibly, to his crotch. When she
looked back into his eyes, it was expectantly, but a wave of nausea
hit him, and J.W. sprinted to the john to wretch out whatever
was left in his raw innards. When he came back to start seeing
patients, she was on the phone, but hung up quickly when he
came around the corner. Rizzo stopped by a couple of times that
morning to chat with Monique, but ducked into the stairwell
when J.W. came out of an exam room.

CHAPTER FORTY-EIGHT

At noon, J.W. left a patient to take a call from a doctor. It was Sharra. Her voice was so weak, J.W. could hardly hear her. He snapped at her to speak louder, "Stop making me crazy," but that just weakened her monotone. The intensity of her despondency, even deeper than Sunday morning, blasted through the phone. There was, however, no longer a desperation for help; just the flat sound of a bitter winter mountain, where all life had been buried in glacial ice.

They met that night by the lake in a darkened corner of the marina parking lot, where they sat silently watching boats bobbing in the uneven, frigid waters. J.W. held off as long as he could, anticipating that first touch of her body, but when he could not stand it any longer, and their fingers met, her skin was cold and waxy. He kissed her, but her lips were no longer soft. He wanted to pull away and see if it was really her, but she groaned, "I need you. Make love to me."

J.W. pulled her sweater up. She had lost so much weight, and her areolae had become so dark, her nipples looked like fingertips compared to the flattened, empty, wrinkled breasts. Stretch marks made him wonder if she had been pregnant since they had made love months before. She wouldn't let him fondle her.

"I want you in me now. Fuck me! And don't talk."

She faked an end with none of the breathless shuddering that had sealed the ecstasy in the cabin on the Salmon. J.W. also pretended.

"Sharra," J.W. asked after they pulled on their things, "did you ever do anything in your life that you really regretted? I mean, if you could take back anything?"

"Are you saying you would take all this back?"

"I would never take it back, but I need to know if you would. I love you. I mean it. But is love supposed to be so painful? I'm going to lose my daughter and my wife soon, even if you and I never see each other, never touch, again. I'm going to be throwing a lot of years away, Krista and me. And what the hell is there to show for it? I certainly don't have you."

"I'm sorry." She paused for a moment, began to cry, then sat bolt upright. "No, I'm not sorry. Maybe I should never have come, but I'm not going to say I'm sorry. That's all I've ever done, apologize. It wasn't me who screwed up everyone's life. They did it to themselves. Not me. Do you hear? Not me!"

She shot from the car and headed toward the dock. J.W. was afraid she would throw herself into the freezing water, but she held onto a pole, composed herself, and waved him away. He left slowly—though this time, he did not look back.

⊨≺+ +≻⊨

"Just take the hit and shut up. Don't dive deeper into the crater, asshole," J.W. screamed aloud in the car the next morning, but as he neared the Center, he became more incensed for the condemning insinuations and the crazy patients. He charged into Rizzo's office. "Where do you get off grilling me about Rolph Westwong's care? You're not a doctor, Herb. Go ask Saloy what went wrong. He's the surgeon. Leave me the hell alone."

"Calm down, Dr. Weathersby. You're a good doctor, but you're not board certified. Remember? You're the one the attorneys are going after. You have a weak defense. That's why they haven't even named Saloy in the suit. You're not trained. Low hanging fruit. It's no contest, a no-brainer."

"Are you saying I'm a liability for the Center?"

"I'm only saying, Doctor, that you're the one named in the suit. I don't write the rules."

J.W. stormed out as violently as he had entered. At the first phone, J.W. called Saloy at the hospital. He was in an operating room. When Saloy returned his call late in the afternoon, he advised, "Look, J.W., you spent a lot more time with him than I did. People don't sue doctors they like. That's a rule. And another thing, just a word of friendly advice old boy. You remain aloof.

"What?"

"Just stay away from the staff. Don't get involved with the girls who work here." When J.W. did not answer, Saloy went on, "Gotta run. Got another case to do."

He hung up before J.W. could ask again what he was suggesting. While Saloy's warning ate at him for an hour, Sharra's despondency resurfaced. He tried to call her, but Mrs. Thabit whispered nervously that Sharra had driven off before noon and had not come back or called. She was worried because Sharra had pressed her new nightgown, folded it perfectly, and placed it at the foot of her bed. She had also washed the sheets, and even the mattress cover, but left the bed unmade. Only her wine glass was gone.

"You know, my Sharra, I don't think she ever wore the nightgown I made for her."

A sense of bottomless dread gripped him, but J.W. reassured Mrs. Thabit that Sharra had a lot on her mind; he lied he had spoken to her a couple of hours before. "She was fine. Not to worry," he added with false bravado, "she knows what she's doing."

He could barely hear her sigh, "Thank you for being Sharra's friend."

＊＊＊

J.W. lay in bed the next night, every second a dagger, aware the time had come to tell Krista, to face his penalty for the transgression he had so easily rationalized for years. The phone rang; Krista got out of bed and went to the bathroom, closing the door forcibly, shaking J.W.'s concentration. "Mrs. Thabit," he whispered, "please don't worry. Sharra's just doing a lot of thinking. I know I'm right. She's okay, I can feel it."

With Krista still in the bathroom, he went to the basement and called Brandi, but she had not heard from Sharra for weeks. Brandi had been fired for refusing the polygraph all of the staff had been ordered to undergo to discover who had been stealing Demerol from the clinic's narcotic drawer. J.W. called Braunwald's home, but there was only an answering machine in his wife's voice. J.W. slammed the phone down and climbed out of the basement to bare his soul, but each time the truth roiled into his mouth, just as he was about to make the final words of his marriage real, a terrible, heavy vise gripped him. He cursed himself as he climbed the stairs. "You don't even have the balls to do that right."

He lay silently, far to his side of the bed, staring at the ceiling. Krista pretended to read *For Whom the Bell Tolls*, and his *Dr. Zhivago* was opened to the middle, but it lay face down on his chest. Neither of them spoke, and she fell asleep first. J.W. turned off the lights and kissed her gently, aware it would be their last.

J.W. stole into Khai's room and kissed her as well, telling her as she slept how sorry he was for hurting her, and asked her to forgive him, hoping someday she would understand, but he knew there would be no way to explain.

CHAPTER FORTY-NINE

Monique was already whispering on the phone when J.W. dragged in. She hung up and stared until J.W. growled, "Yeah, what disasters you got cooking for me now?"

"Rizzo's looking for you. He wants to see you upstairs. Give him a call first. He wants the others there, too."

Though J.W. was convinced, as he trudged to the penthouse, to Rizzo's office, that the administration had finally uncovered his other life. It was Patel who began the session. "Our attorney is concerned that you were at the hospital without privileges when you ran afoul of the Westwongs. Why is that, Dr. Weathersby? You knew you didn't have privileges, you knew the other doctors knew, and you knew a doctor may not practice medicine in any hospital, anywhere in the world, I might add, without privileges. What were you thinking?"

"*You* knew I was there. Mr. Rizzo knew; Saloy knew. The hospital administration knew. I wasn't writing prescriptions or signing orders, just looking in on Westwong. The PA and Saloy were doing *all* the prescribing. So were the G.I. guys and the neurosurgeons. Hey, Dr. Patel, you even saw me at the hospital in the hallway, maybe a dozen times. How many times did you ask me how my 'mad motorcycle man' was doing? You thought it was funny. Remember?"

"I didn't think it was funny at all. But the problem is that your applying for privileges, by itself, was an embarrassment to the Center. We didn't really need to advertise that we had a doctor on our staff who hadn't finished his residency."

Rizzo had been quiet, but when he took a breath to begin, J.W. interrupted. "Maybe I shouldn't have applied, but Herb, you handed me the forms at lunch that day at the golf club. Look, I was just trying to do what you told me to do."

Rizzo's breath deepened, and his lips tightened. "Well, that's water under the bridge. Let's do a little damage control. Did you write on the chart at the hospital?"

"No. Well, yes, but not orders. Saloy had me write notes and not sign them. He came by a couple times, put down the date, and scribbled his name under them. My name is nowhere on the chart, except maybe in the nursing notes, like 'Dr. Weathersby stopped in to see patient.' You're gonna tell me I'm getting sued for stopping in and seeing a patient, a friend I was interested in following?"

Rizzo turned back to his desk and mumbled the usual about conferring with counsel and bringing it up to the Board of Directors. As J.W. walked out, Rizzo added, "Just stay out of the hospital."

J.W. went back to his office and picked up the phone to call Mrs. Westwong, to tell her how sorry he was things had not worked out. But he remembered the proscription against ever delivering a word of atonement to a disgruntled patient. The attorneys at the quarterly meetings had warned repeatedly, "Ladies and gentlemen, an apology is tantamount to admitting culpability. Never bare your soul, and never, ever, ever, utter the words, 'I'm sorry.'"

"The hell with it, anyway," J.W. mumbled to himself, "She was FN, fucken' nuts, to start with; they're all nuts." He had more pressing things on his mind. He asked Monique to call Mrs. Thabit and find out if Sharra had come back, but there was no answer.

"Well, then call again, goddamnit!"

The rest of the staff looked up from their desks, and Saloy came out of his office as far as the doorway. When J.W. glared at him, Saloy disappeared back inside and closed the door gently. J.W. saw the red light over Saloy's private extension light up on the common phone in the hallway, and J.W. went back to his own office and slammed the door.

Mrs. Thabit still didn't answer. He tried to call Monique's extension to find out if they had a patient, but her line was busy.

At noon, J.W. left the Center and drove to Sharra's. The door of the bungalow was open and he walked in, refusing to look at the floor, afraid of what he might find lying there. The TV was blaring, dialogue from one of the soaps booming meaninglessly. The door to Sharra's room was shut. He hesitated before violating the shred of privacy left her, but he was drawn into the room that still held her scent. It was empty, save for the nightgown so perfectly arranged at the foot of the blue, stained mattress. He started to write a note to leave under Sharra's pillow, to let her know he had been there, to punish her for having tortured him, but J.W. knew it would fall on a deaf heart, and he left without touching her possessions.

J.W. had time to drive back before the first patient of the afternoon, but as the Buick neared the Center, the wheel seemed to lock, refusing to turn off into Black Granite. He realized nearly an hour later he had driven all the way to Cedar Springs. J.W. called Krista at the neighbor's and asked her to come home right away, that it was urgent. Then he called the Center and told Monique he was too sick to finish the day. He hung up before she spoke.

J.W. watched as Krista rushed down the street, her face tight with a weight and dread he had only seen in the expression of the parents called back to the hospital to say good-bye to their children for the last time. "Please sit down. I've screwed up, big league. I have no excuse. I'm sorry."

J.W. thought she knew, but she started to cry and demanded, "What the hell is happening? Tell me!"

"Krista, you remember Sharra Bakhtian from medical school? She's missing. I think she's dead."

"And?"

"And I've got to do something. I love you, but I fucked up and fell in love with her, too. I don't know what to do. I can't ask you to help me. I've got no one to ask for help."

"Like I do? How long has this been going on?"

"I screwed up. I'll leave if you want."

"Do whatever you want to. You always have."

Instead, Krista left the house. In a little while, Khai walked home from school. She stared at her father, sunken into the chair from which he had not moved.

"Where's Mom?" she asked in a frightened voice.

J.W. tried to answer, but his weak reply was absorbed by the uncaring floor long before it ever had a chance to hurt his daughter. Khai ran out into the street to look for her mother.

CHAPTER FIFTY

The dinner of soup and sandwiches J.W. had made was sitting on the table when Krista and Khai returned. He waited in the basement office for the footsteps in the kitchen to fade before coming upstairs to do the dishes. The food lay on the table untouched, but the gallon bottle of burgundy from which J.W. had guzzled two nights before was gone. Krista's wine glass was broken, shards lying in the sink. His glass was still on the shelf.

The phone rang. J.W. waited, but Krista did not answer. The foreboding in his heart deepened as he lifted the receiver, but before he spoke, his eyes reddened. He felt a tear trickle onto his cheek.

"Hello, *Doctori*." It was Mrs. Thabit. "I am sorry, sir. The coroner has called. Sharra is gone. They found my child in a motel in Black Granite. They want me to come see her. Maybe you would come with me? I am sorry to bother you, but she said you were her friend. I love her so much."

"Mrs. Thabit! I am so... Please. I want to be with her. Please, listen to me. I will come to help you."

J.W. dropped the phone and began weaving around the room as if he had consumed the last half-gallon of the wine. He ran up the stairs and stood at the bedroom door.

"Sharra's dead. I don't know what to do."

J.W. ran back downstairs. Krista followed. She had carried the bottle of wine, poured a large glass of the burgundy, and shoved it in front of his face.

"Drink this!"

J.W. gulped twelve ounces and gagged at the burning in his throat. She poured a second. Halfway through, J.W. dropped the glass and watched it shatter on the kitchen floor. He started to cry, choking at first, then harder and harder, breaking down in wails as Krista stood in one spot, swaying as if in mourning. J.W. ran through the front door to the neighbor's house, but Loren did not answer, and J.W. smashed the window with his fist, crawled into the living room, and found a bottle of Stolyna Vodka. J.W. swallowed as much as he could before the nausea clamped his gullet shut.

Vodka trickled down his chin onto his arms. The bottle dropped to the floor and smashed, the colorless, pungent poison tracing a river path along the canted floor. He stumbled around searching for a towel, but when he found one, he couldn't remember why. The next memory was of lying in a ditch along a jogging path. An old man walking his dog asked, "You okay?"

"Leave me alone!" The dog growled, and J.W. bellowed, "Shut your goddamn dog up, mister!"

The dog bared his teeth and growled more fiercely as J.W. crawled out of the culvert toward his house. The doors were locked. A police car was across the street at Loren's, its blue and red lights flashing off the windows from which Krista was staring. She unlocked the front door but ran up the stairs without waiting for J.W. to come in.

J.W. loaded the backseat of his car with the pile of clothes Krista had splattered next to the car keys on the living room floor. It did not matter that the cops were right there, watching as J.W. reversed, jerking drunkenly out of the driveway. The Buick stalled. Police lights flashed in the rearview mirror as J.W. weaved out of the driveway to fumble his way toward the on-ramp for the interstate. Though he had made that trip hundreds of times, he became lost and doubled back several times, until he found himself lurching up the highway. The lights of Cedar Springs disappeared behind him into the fog. With the window open to keep him awake, it was harder to hear the sobbing and screams of rage.

Passing through Black Granite, J.W. thought of stopping and visiting Lieutenant White's family, to show them that he, too, had died, and now it was J.W.'s parents' turn to grieve. But he just shouted out the window at them and continued south. At the bungalow, a dim light glowed in the tiny bedroom. Mrs. Thabit sat motionlessly on the end of Sharra's bed, her delicate hand resting on the nightgown.

"They have called again. I must go to see Sharra. They want me to make sure it is her. Please, Doctor, I should not ask, but maybe you would go with me? You were her friend."

As J.W. opened the car door for her, he waited for the enmity to explode, though she uttered nothing as they drove south toward the morgue in Black Granite, and she remained rigidly silent as the coroner peeled the covering from a nude body. There was a small, white sheet wrapped around Sharra's hair, as if she had just come out of the shower, calm, still magnificent, no inkling of the contorted pain J.W. remembered on the corpses in Viet Nam. Sharra looked more like Lily, his medical school cadaver, no soul, only wax.

The coroner pulled J.W. aside and whispered that it had been a drug overdose, a suicide. Sharra had injected Demerol, hundreds and hundreds of milligrams, intravenously. She had faded off to sleep and stopped breathing. He asked if J.W. knew where she got the drugs, but J.W. mumbled he had no idea.

"She had a hell of a lot with her. There were still a few un-opened vials in the motel. Couple bottles of wine, too. Empty. There was a broken wine glass by her bed. Can you believe that? A doctor! I can't figure how she could have loaded the syringe with the Demerol, as shit-faced as she was."

The coroner glanced at the wedding band on J.W.'s hand and asked, "How did you know her?"

J.W. took Mrs. Thabit by the arm and walked her out of the morgue without answering. At the bungalow, she struggled out of the car and closed the door behind her. She still hadn't spoken.

CHAPTER FIFTY-ONE

J.W. drove back to Cedar Springs, parked in the driveway, and slept in the car. Every few minutes he woke, startled out of a fitful sleep by the freezing cold and the same nightmare, over and over: Sharra's face shrouded in white linen. Then an ancient Vietnamese woman appeared, peeled away the cloth, shook it menacingly at him, and screamed in Vietnamese, "You foreign bastard. You ran over my daughter with a truck."

"Don't blame me. I didn't do it. She jumped in front of it by herself," J.W. moaned in his sleep, "I didn't do it!"

Suddenly, his father appeared in the dream and intoned, "You can't watch *Victory at Sea*. You have to go to jail. I told you you'd wind up in prison. I'll always love you, son, but you have a debt to pay now. It's the law; it's always in effect, even when you pretend it isn't."

"No!" J.W. screamed in the car, waking himself, "I told you I didn't do it. She did it. No! I'm not going. I didn't kill any little girl in Viet Nam." He peered through the steamed windows of the car and saw the image of Sharra's face in the shroud. The dream played itself out a hundred times, until J.W. didn't know if he was dreaming it or remembering it.

At first light, J.W. snuck into the basement and washed in the utility sink. He moved the Buick down the street and waited for Khai to walk by on her way to school, but when she appeared, Krista was holding her hand. They passed, solemn-faced strangers.

——◄┼ ┼►——

Saloy had left a note on J.W.'s desk. "Give me a call when you get in." Monique breezed into the office and handed J.W. an envelope marked "Personal and Confidential."

"Please meet with Dr. Saloy and me at 7 A.M. tomorrow at Denny's." It was signed, D.J. Flatury, M.D., Chairman, Medical Disciplinary Board.

J.W. called Flatury's office in Greenfield to ask why he had summoned J.W. to the meeting, but his nurse said, "Doctor wants to discuss a personal matter with you."

J.W. phoned Saloy, who allowed only that there was a problem, and warned again that J.W. was to stay away from the staff. He added, "Patients are off limits, too. I'm sure you must have heard that somewhere. Like in medical school? We'll talk about it tomorrow morning."

Monique called into J.W.'s office to ask if he would be willing to see an add-on patient for back pain, but J.W. retorted that he wasn't seeing anyone extra, ever again. "Don't bother me with that shit," he hollered into hallway.

J.W. tried to call Mrs. Thabit, but there was no answer. Monique called on the phone this time to tell J.W. there was a scheduled patient waiting, but as J.W. was about to leave his chair, the phone rang. It was Sharra's aunt. Everyone was gathering in New York for the funeral, and she asked if J.W. would deliver the eulogy on Saturday. The instant after his agreement, J.W. realized he had forged in stone the demise of his family.

The Medical Center was abuzz with the news that Dr. Weathersby was in hot water with administration. Monique's entire day was consumed with whispered conversations and absences from her desk. Long, thick, maddening stretches of time passed between the ten patients on his schedule. He secluded himself in his darkened office, the door shut firmly, a chair wedged into the handle, locking out the toxins that sought to slither in and watch the slaughter of the cocky doctor, the great football player, the war hero.

Late in the evening, his attention turned to where he might pass the night. He drove the streets of Cedar Springs for hours, but finished in Krista's driveway. A little past 2 A.M., he woke from a new dream. Now, there was only a shrouded body. He peeled off layer after layer of cloth, but with each, the color darkened and the material shredded until it could no longer be unwrapped. He pushed on the body, but there was no mass, only matted, threadbare, soiled cloth. He yelled aloud, "I know you're in there, Sharra. You are in there. I'll find you, goddamnit."

J.W. jumped awake again, realizing it had all been just a dream—Sharra's death, the meeting with Saloy and Flatury. He felt such relief as the warm glow poured over him, he swore he would forget Sharra, never see her again, renew his affection for Krista, and let the past fade. It was a magnificent sensation to recognize the nightmare had just been that, a dream. He had been warned and given a reprieve. The apprehension in his heart and the tautness of his muscles melted away, and for a few seconds, he had his life back.

But an unfamiliar lump under his head caught his attention, the makeshift pillow on the backseat of the car. The windows were fogged, and wispy, fern-shaped ice crystals had formed on the glass. It was so cold, J.W. felt as if he were in hell, or in a re-frigerated body tube in the morgue, next to Sharra.

CHAPTER FIFTY-TWO

Flatury was late for the breakfast meeting. J.W. sat with Saloy silently, staring at the early-morning traffic creeping past, puffs of exhaust drifting in swirls out of the frigid engines. J.W. was cold and stood to get a cup of coffee. Saloy suggested, "Why don't we wait until Flatury comes? I think he's bringing Rizzo. He may want to do this somewhere else."

"Do this?" J.W. snapped. He stood to walk out of the restaurant and leave for the mountains. He'd sit there for a few days, alone, too grieved to eat or build a fire. And if he died in the cold, it would not matter, for he was still on the staff at the Center—his life insurance policy would care for Krista and Khai forever. He was finally free.

As J.W. turned to savor the look on Saloy's face, Flatury and Rizzo rounded the corner for the door. Their expressions were serious; they moved with such determination, J.W. had no choice but to stop and retake his seat.

Flatury began. "There are a couple of things we need to discuss. I know your patient died, but that happens to all of us, sooner or later. It's something you're supposed to learn in residency."

"What do you mean, 'patient?' What is going on here? Cut the shit and tell me what's going on."

"We have information that a patient of yours committed suicide. If that isn't true, let me know right now."

"She wasn't a patient. She was a doctor. I went to medical school with her, and she replaced me out at the clinic when I came here. Who told you this?"

"What we understand is that you were seeing a member, actually two members, of the staff. This patient found out about it and killed her...took her own life."

"That's not true..."

"What's more," he interrupted, "you are being accused of sexual innuendo with the staff. I'm not making it up, J.W., I'm just reporting what I've been told by some...a lot of, reliable sources. Did you ever ask one of the female staff to meet you at her summer cabin? And they said you spent a night at a motel with one of the nurses."

"Who are *they*? I want to know, damnit."

"That's not important. The Board of Directors got a hold of the information, and now they have no choice but to look into it. It's our job. It's not personal. We need you to cooperate so we can get to the truth."

"The truth? What do you want from me? What are you saying? I didn't do a thing. I haven't gone out with anyone from the staff. Who told you this?"

"I told you I can't reveal that information. It was given to us in a confidential agreement, J.W. And it looks like, if you're not going to cooperate, we're not going to get anywhere. We all have patients to see. We'll meet again tomorrow. I'll see what I can do about getting some more information."

"You mean you don't have all the information, and you're doing this to me?"

Not one of the three offered to pay for the coffee. J.W. ended the meeting by jumping to his feet and glaring at them in a fit of righteous indignation. He flipped five dollars on the table, walked across the street to the Center, and ordered Monique to pack her purse.

"Get out of my practice. I'll see you in court."

She spat back, "You'll never make it stick," flipped him off, stared directly at his crotch, dropped her white coat on the floor, keeled around, and strutted off snickering.

J.W. grabbed charts and started seeing patients. In fifteen minutes a new nurse appeared at Monique's desk, a stubby, older creature, her polyester white nursing pants crusted with little nubbins on the inner thighs, where they had rubbed together for years. She tidied the disheveled desk, unearthing a pile of lab results J.W. had been asking about for days. None of his CAT scans had been ordered, none of his referrals made, perhaps a hint why there had been so many angry patients calling and demanding to speak to him, every one of whom Monique had transferred to administration.

Suddenly, his new nurse was calling him five and six times an hour, not ten times over the entire day, the fare for the past weeks. The days progressed so quickly, J.W. forgot for moments at a time about the hurricane. There was work to be done, and J.W. amazed himself at how fast he was recovering. He was reminded that, like all trouble, this, too, would pass.

J.W. was gathering his papers and his thoughts to leave for his night on call at the emergency room, but the phone rang. The Center operator said it was his wife. He was mortified that Khai had been hurt—there was no other reason Krista would call.

"I'm sorry to bother you, but I have some bad news. I just got off the phone with Bobbie Jo." Her voice cracked. "I'm sorry, but Bernie's dead. He committed suicide."

"You're doing this to hurt me. He's not dead. You're lying."

"I'm afraid I'm not. He died with the nineteen-year-old prostitute he'd been *fucking*."

There was a long pause, and J.W. thought she was about to ask him to come home and talk about all that had happened. A bucket of tears poured from him. She heard his sobs but was silent.

"Could you forgive me? Twenty-two years. So much has passed under our bridge. Kris, there isn't an airport in the Northern Hemisphere we haven't held hands and struggled through. Customs, taxi rip-offs to third-rate hotels. What about eighty jets a day scraping the paint off our roof in Hong Kong? How 'bout Mao the Diarrheic Sheep, and toilets that sprayed water at midnight on New Year's Eve? How many years did we fight through the next course, the next Abraham Cohen, and the next Cicely?"

She finally spoke. "We? Bobbie Jo and I also talked about what happened. She thinks it would be better if you moved out completely."

"*She* thinks? Who the hell is she? She really did a great job holding her life together, didn't she? She's the one advising you?" There was again a long period of silence, and J.W. knew Krista well enough to agree, "Okay, if that's the way you want it, there's not a whole lot I can say, is there?"

"Nope."

"I just need to see Khai. I can't live without her."

"We'll make an arrangement." The phone clicked down.

J.W. felt no need to serve his emergency shift that night, no point in staying at the Center. Everything had ended so quickly, over forty years gone in a couple of days. The Vietnamese in his village of My Co were right. He remembered their axiom: The individual man is but dust, blowing on the red-clay roads of the ancient provinces, across the hectares of rice—nothing but dust.

The daze into which J.W. dropped anesthetized his pain; it numbed the life out of him, and he sat frozen, catatonic. The phone rang again. He prayed it was Krista, but Sally, the page operator, announced, "Kara's mother."

"Who the hell is Kara?"

"Dr. Weathersby, she's threatened to sue me if I didn't put her through. And she's going to sue you, too, she said."

"Don't you worry, Sweet Pea. I know who it is now. I apologize. I didn't mean to snap at you. Got a lot on my mind. And no one's going to hurt you. Put the old bag through."

"Dr. Weathersby," a woman's voice commenced before J.W. said hello, "my husband and I would like to settle with you on the matter of our daughter's permanent disfigurement. She would have had a career in modeling if it weren't for the broken acupuncture needle in her knee. Our attorney said if you agree to pay for her college tuition and expenses for four years, or until she graduates, we will drop any further proceedings against you. I think that is rather fair."

"Ma'am, it has been a pleasure not hearing from you for so long. Apparently, though, you're not going to fade away. You see madam, at this point in my life, I have a twenty-four-year-old car, no furniture, not even a pot to piss in. I have nothing, and you'll get nothing. Speak to my attorney. And in the interim, madam, kiss my ass!" He slammed the phone down, happy for the wrath that had arced the tiniest bit of ardor into the life that had drained from him so violently. He leaned back and waited for the next call, for another loss, but a peculiar sensation washed over him.

"Jesus. I could sit here for another twenty years and wait for the next blow. What are they going to take? My job? My family?

My house? I got nothing. So, I got nothing to lose. Nobody can take anything away anymore." There was a perception of freedom he had never before felt. He could do as he pleased, run into a burning building and save six children, or fly at VNE, "velocity never exceed," plus ten knots, just to see what really happened when you passed the limits. He could go back into the Rockies, live in a cabin near Mr. Shelton, and fend for himself, for real this time. It was the first beat of his life in which there was nothing J.W. Weathersby *had* to do because someone else had told him to, and was watching to make sure he did. He sat back in his chair, feet up on the desk, and surveyed what was left of his world. The Purple Hearts were there. They hadn't moved. They made no demands. He was free.

CHAPTER FIFTY-THREE

The phone rang again. Rizzo asked, "You plan to grace the emergency room with your presence tonight? We're countin' on you. We're short a doc."

"Uh huh." It mattered not where J.W. spent the evening hours. The Center was warm and the coffee and toast were free.

He saw the usual coughs and colds that night, but there was one patient who blew in and asked to be seen immediately. She was in a good deal of pain in her groin after a jazzercise session. J.W. nodded in agreement when he was told it was one of the nurses from the Center. She bounced into the exam room and touched J.W.'s shoulder to thank him for seeing her so quickly. She was sweaty, smelled awful, and was wearing the tightest pink leotards he had ever seen or dreamed of. They were riding so high into her crotch, J.W. had to blink to see if she was wearing anything at all.

She hopped up on the table, spread her legs, and pointed to the pulled muscle in her groin. "I'm sorry I'm so wet down there." He wouldn't touch her, suggesting she point a finger, but she grumbled, "You know, I'm not really sure where the problem is."

He prescribed ibuprofen and left the room at a jog.

After clinic, J.W.'s Buick crawled the streets of Black Granite, mesmerized by the sparkle of headlights through the drizzle, passing the same cops, and the same corners, over and over, stalling for hours before heading east to the driveway in Cedar Springs, and the frigid, hard bed of the Buick's back seat.

With an income soon to evaporate, a career ravaged in its nascence, J.W. could see no further than the prospect of a month or a week in a hotel consuming the bulk of his meager savings—even a single night in a rented room was, at that moment, a luxury.

Despite the car heater that whined on full, the cold seeped into his bones so deeply, it was difficult to recognize the chirp of his beeper trying to wake him. The first two roadside pay phones had been smashed, their black receivers dangling from unwoven spiral silver cords. The third booth was soaking wet with rainwater puddling on the shattered glass. The page operator put him through to a detective in Black Granite.

"Lieutenant Hoyt."

"It's Dr. Weathersby, sir."

"I need to meet with you in your office tomorrow morning. Pick a time between ten and eleven."

"Excuse me, who are you?"

"I am Lieutenant Bosco Hoyt, homicide, Black Granite Police, and I need to talk to you about the death of Sharrazad Thabit."

"What about it, and why can't we do it now, over the phone?" J.W. asked through chattering teeth.

"Pick a time, Doctor. Like I said, I'm flexible."

J.W. drove back to the Center and stole into the laundry area. There were no clean scrub suits, but a bin full of dirty ones. He found a large without blood stains, and went to his exam room and onto the Naugahyde table with its crinkled, grease-stained paper from his last patient. The night passed, punctuated by dreams of cops laughing down at him as they dropped him into a cell with a homeless drunk. The nightmares were bookended by restless hours and incessant visions of Sharra in her shroud.

Though they had agreed upon ten-thirty, Detective Hoyt appeared in the waiting room at nine-fifteen. The receptionist found his business card persuasive, especially the HOMICIDE in raised, gilded letters. She showed him into J.W.'s office without controversy, glancing over her shoulder every few steps at the six-foot-six detective in the ten-gallon hat and snakeskin cowboy boots. Halfway down the hall, a stocky, undercover officer in worn jeans caught up with them. He ignored J.W.

The interview with Detective Hoyt began pleasantly.

"Doctor," he drawled, "We can't release the body to the family until we've determined the exact cause of death. There's a lot of unanswered questions 'bout this whole affair."

"Where you from, Detective? You're not a local boy."

"Texas. Let me ask you. Do you know where Miss, ah, Doctor Thabit, got the Demerol that was found in her motel room?"

"Haven't the slightest."

"Well, Doctor, the DEA tracked those vials down for us. They were signed out in your name, every last one of 'em. How do you explain that?"

"Hey, look. I never gave her or anybody else drugs. I've never taken any and don't know anybody who does. I don't believe in that shit. And I signed for all the medicine at the clinic months ago. I was the medical director. It was my job to make sure we had the proper amount of narcotics in the safe for injured patients. If they didn't transfer the record to the new medical director, that's their problem."

Hoyt scrutinized J.W.'s eyes, searching, as if he were reading a crystal ball. "Doctor, we're not accusing you of anything. We just want to get things tidied up before we close the book on this one. It seems Miss Thabit had begun to use cocaine, but where she was getting it is a mystery. Can you help us with that?"

"What are you talking about?"

Hoyt's eyes pried deeper, shooting barbs tormentingly. "I'm not trying to upset you, but you need to help us. She had three bags of that shit sewed into the lining of her purse, just in case. We talked to her latest boyfriend, the one who was living with her when he could get away..." He stopped abruptly.

"Did he have a pinkie ring?"

"I'm not at liberty to discuss that. She made him try the coke, and he did it, just so he wouldn't lose her. We promised we wouldn't arrest him 'cause he only did it once, only for her, and he swore he'd never do it again. Must 'a been some kind 'a woman." Detective Hoyt waited for J.W. to recover then stood and told his partner, "We got enough here to call it a suicide. Let me ask you one more question, Doctor. And you don't have to answer, if you don't want. Were you romantically involved with Miss Thabit?"

Again he waited, but not long enough for J.W. to consider his options. "Well?"

"Yeah. I was nuts about her. I wish I'd died instead of her, or maybe with her. Is that what you wanted to hear? I'm not afraid to say it anymore."

Lieutenant Hoyt stuck out his hand, smiled disinterestedly, grabbed his silent partner by the sleeve, and left.

An hour later, Sharra's uncle called the Center to tell J.W. the funeral would be held that Saturday as planned. The body had just been released.

At the eulogy in New York, it took some time for J.W. to compose himself. As he looked up from the pulpit, finally ready to speak, J.W. saw Marshall Seltzer at the back door, pushing a wheelchair. J.W. focused on the woman with the drab, greying, curly hair sitting in it. Her arms writhed awkwardly as she fought to wave at J.W. They were the only ones to smile when J.W. related the adventure of the also-rans, the fraternity of wild cards accepted from the bottom of the heap, but finished at the top. He spoke of Dr. Ronald MacDonald who had instructed, "Miss Bakhtian's hands are gentle. You need that when you're around kids. She has grace. Watch her. Learn from her."

J.W. went on. "Sharra used to wonder if she'd ever make it, ever become a doctor. She did. Higher than the rest of us."

A few late mourners drifted in, but there was no J'Aveed. He was already back in Tehran. Mrs. Thabit sat quietly, draped in her usual black. While J.W. spoke, he looked at her only once, out of the corner of his eye. Her brothers surrounded her, and even after the ceremony, J.W. could not get close enough to face her.

⊯ ⊱

The night J.W. returned from New York, he found a room in a garage in Braxton Falls, a hundred dollars a month and no heat. The toilet was frozen in the morning, and there was no water for a shower. It was miles from Krista and Khai. The cost for the two electric space heaters going around the clock and the hot plate came to over fifteen dollars a day. That made it cheaper to guzzle wine in bed than keep the garage livable. Each night, the level of Chianti in the tumbler crept a fraction higher, while the time to fall into a coma shortened. At 4 A.M., he dragged himself to the sink and gagged on his toothbrush. It became less challenging simply to chew a glob of toothpaste and use his finger to brush, and soon easier just to forget the whole thing.

Existence at the Center dragged slowly, waiting the endless hours to drive home and fill the first glass with his blood-red salvation. He was visiting the liquor store every other night, usually just to grab a half-gallon of wine, but one night, the store was very warm, and walking the aisles was free. On a poster near the hard liquor section, a magnificent, black-eyed, enigmatic woman with silken, ebony hair sipped an exotic liquor steeped at the other end of the Earth. The crystal goblet that touched her lips had the slightest veneer of ice, while waves of heat from the bleached sand beach upon which she stood shimmered off the glass. Her cheekbones were as majestic as Sharra's, her lips as perfect.

J.W. bought a bottle and hurried along Braxton Falls' manicured roads toward his hovel on the far side of the lake, eyeing the brown paper bag on the passenger seat, wondering if he should open it and get started right then and there. The bottle found its way into his hands and to his lips before the end of the next block. The first few sips burned like hell, though the fire in his throat stopped the shivering. A few more gulps, and there would be no need to spend money to warm the little room, if he got that far. He would be able to slip under the covers, wake at dawn, splash icy water on his face, and drive back to Black Granite.

J.W. lay in bed, sipping from the bottle still keep secret by the paper bag. As his intoxication bloated, he took a full swallow. "Screw 'em, all o' you bastards!" Abruptly, he screeched, "I'm my own man. You have no power over me. Who the hell are you fuckers to treat me like that?"

J.W. called Krista. "Fuck her, too," J.W. shouted, but when she answered, he started to cry, and all he could do was try to hide his desperation. In the haze, he heard her remind, "One reaps what he sows, and buddy boy, you is reaping a big harvest."

At the Center, a letter marked "Personal and Confidential" sat on his desk. It made his chest tighten and his palms sweat. He laughed about the old days, a few months before, when he assumed any letter so marked carried the best of news: admission to medical school, perhaps a match with the best residency program in the nation. Now, all human interaction was doomed to result in another loss. Dread underpinned every encounter. There could be nothing positive in the letter sitting on his desk, only more trouble and deeper pain.

J.W. thought about tossing it away. Why open a new wound? But why not? It couldn't get worse, only funnier. He stared at the address and postmark: Los Angeles. Certainly, it was something to do with Sharra, even more reason to throw it away, and more to open it and keep it forever. On the light blue linen paper was a letterhead of darker blue print: "Ramona Thabit – Attorney at Law"

> Dear Dr. Weathersby,
> "I have taken the liberty of writing to you. I am Sharra's sister. I just want you to know that I do not blame you for what has happened. As I am sure you guessed, Sharra had been cursed from the day she married that monster. There was nothing we could do.
> We were surrounded by such desperation in New York. She was the brighter of us, and prettier. Maybe I was jealous. When she took up with Arthur, I begged her to stop, but she so wanted to be an American. He told her everyone was doing the things my mother and I hated. We did not speak for many years. I knew the demons would catch up with her, but I prayed they wouldn't consume what was left of our family.
> I did not come to the funeral because if I had, the Iranian spies would have kidnapped me, raped me, and, if I lived through it, put me in a wooden box and shipped

me back to Tehran to be tried and stoned to death for not having turned in my sister.

But now I feel so guilty. It was a mistake.

I hope you will understand. My mother says you are a kind man. There may be a day we can meet as friends, but right now, I am having hard enough time forgiving myself.

Sadly,

Ramona

J.W. brought the letter to his face. It was the scent of Ramona Thabit. Though his hands shook, J.W. dialed the number embossed on her stationery. A woman answered the phone. She spoke softly, with a familiar timbre, and a profound sadness that was as recognizable. J.W. was frozen in fear. The voice asked who it was in Farsi then in English. His hand dropped the phone back onto the cradle. He had heard Sharra's voice again. It would have to last forever.

⇥⇤

J.W.'s new nurse knocked at his door, opened it cautiously, and stuck her head in guardedly. She asked if J.W. was ready to start seeing patients but backed out on her tiptoes when she saw him head down, weeping into folded arms at his desk.

"Even in the best of families," she mumbled as she walked away.

By late afternoon, those who passed J.W. averted their eyes. In the stairwell, J.W. heard three young voices giggling from floors below. "I heard he's been dragged before the Board for raping some patient."

"Yeah, and they sent that receptionist from ENT to him at the emergency room. Wanted to see what would happen. I heard he tried to ask her out—go to some motel."

Another laughed, "All those Viet Nam guys are crazy."

J.W. went back to his office and closed the door again. He riveted his mind on the Purple Hearts and asked himself over and over, a hundred times, if he *was* crazy, and if he was, when had it begun? J.W. called Krista and begged for help. Her prescription: "Go fuck yourself."

The phone rang. The new nurse asked if J.W. would accept a call from a Ms. Thabit. His gut ratcheted. "Yes. Put her through."

"Dr. Weathersby, it is Ramona Thabit. I think you know who I am."

"Yes, of course. I just got your letter. I wish I knew what to say."

"I have some bad news."

"Bad news?" J.W. asked passively, yet steeling himself for the next dagger.

"My mother is gone." Her voice cracked, and an unbroken eternity of sobs began.

"What do you mean?" J.W. finally demanded, the receiver resonating with the now-familiar tremor.

"Be calm, damn it," J.W. admonished himself, "You've been here before." He leaned back and waited for the onset of another chapter of the macabre dream from which he was waiting to wake.

The choked crying ebbed, and Ramona began. "My mother is dead. She took her own life this morning. Her doctor gave her medication for depression yesterday. It's my fault. I told her to go. She took all the pills. She's dead. Everyone is dead. What am I going to do? What is to become of me? I am cursed. Tell me what I have done. What have I done?"

The phone dropped, and J.W. listened to the sobs in the background for a moment before he gently replaced the receiver.

CHAPTER FIFTY-FOUR

K rista called that evening. He should have told her what had happened, but it would only have culled another strike of venom, another biblical homily about cause and effect. She started, not in her usual tone of righteous indignation, but with a determination that had, over the many years, always meant, "I will not be dissuaded from my decision."

"J.W., I am taking Khai back to Boston. You cheated on me. That was cruel, and I was not surprised, but now my flesh and blood has to live with the shame of a rapist father. I hope they drag you to prison by your balls, if they can find them."

"Not Khai!" J.W. screamed. "What the hell are you talking about? Tell me."

"Januz called. I know all about the rape. I will not allow Khai to go through this."

"Who the hell is Januz?"

"His daughter is on Khai's soccer team. You don't even know that, do you? He works at County Hospital. He's an accountant or something. He said one of the doctors from Black Granite told a resident at his hospital that a Dr. Weathersby had raped a patient.

"I did no such thing. It's a goddamn lie. You already know the full fucking story. Every word of it. I never raped anybody, and I didn't walk out on you. I'll call this Januz, but don't you dare take my child away."

She hung up while J.W. was still talking.

Januz was just repeating what he had heard, and swore one of the board members from the Black Granite Medical Center had come to Cedar Springs because J.W. had done part of his internship there. "Look pal, I don't know you from a hole in the wall, but I want to know who told you I had raped a patient."

"I can't tell you. I don't remember. I heard it in passing."

"Januz, whoever the hell you are, I don't have a lot of time to go, but I promise you, I'll drag your ass into court, or worse, along with every swingin' dick on your staff, if you don't tell me who it was, and I'll..." but the phone jammed down on the other end.

J.W. called Patel at home. "No one is accusing you of rape. The only question is one of sexual misconduct, and, for lack of a better word, of living an alternative lifestyle. The Board of Directors is meeting at seven. The best I can do is plead your side of the situation. They're pretty concerned, but I'll do what I can to buy a little time."

"Look, I haven't done anything that could be construed as sexual misconduct with a patient or with anyone else. There was another woman, but she was a doctor, and she was never my patient. How many times do I have to tell you that?"

"The feeling is, J.W., where's there's smoke, there's fire. I'm telling you, we're very concerned. I'll call you at eleven and give you the verdict."

J.W. called Rizzo and demanded to be told who had been feeding the Board neatly trimmed bits of data, stories about which J.W. had no knowledge. Rizzo wouldn't talk to him. "We are in the middle of an investigation, Doctor."

By noon the next day, Patel had not called, so J.W. phoned his office. He had been by, dictated a few charts, and left for lunch. He was unavailable that afternoon, busy at the hospital in a deposition for a malpractice suit that had been filed against him for operating on the wrong hand, for the second time in as many months.

Saloy had been invited to the Board meeting that morning, and when he arrived back at the Center to see patients, J.W. greeted him, waiting for a hint about his fate. Saloy ran past J.W., calling over his shoulder, "They are very concerned." He flew into his office, slammed the door, and did not emerge until long after the first patient of the afternoon had arrived. The light on his extension glowed the entire time.

Patel called the next morning. "Sorry I didn't get back to you yesterday. I am very busy with important matters. We will allow you to meet briefly with the board members, one at a time. We do not want a situation in which you say we did not grant you due process. So, you must contact them today. We are meeting again in the morning."

It was not easy to discover the Board's composition. No one seemed to be sure, and the few names J.W. was given turned out to be members who had long since left the ranks. J.W. appealed to Rizzo for some hint about his jury, and while the names were provided, albeit reluctantly, only five of the nine members were willing to meet. They came separately to his office late that day and into the evening. J.W. honed his performance as the audience rotated. He revealed the story of the hole that been blown in his heart, the freezing air that rushed through for everyone to see and feel.

But, in truth, J.W. felt nothing. By the fourth interview, he was past master of the art of the wrenching novella. The dropped jaw and gasp each man heaved when J.W. told him of the call from Sharra's sister earlier that day fueled his routine. J.W. told them that he had lost his family. He told them of Bernie He sensed a wave of pity for the sad creature perched, cold, bare, and alone, in front of them. It was as if they were not that far from the abyss themselves. Each of the board members rose and offered his hand before leaving.

J.W. felt a sense of pride in having hidden from the omnipotent his numbness, the dearth of feelings and caring inside him. He had camouflaged the psychosis, the alcohol, and best of all, the plans that had begun to crystallize for his escape. He took succor and caressed a grotesque warmth in knowing the pain would soon end, that there would only be embarrassment for the Center, no longer for him. J.W. sat in the office until midnight, not moving a single bone, staring at the ferns from the cabin on the Salmon. He wondered if they had been alive when J.W. was a child in the Bronx, when his thoughts were foolish dreams of flying off carriers and dying for his country; perhaps they had only started growing years later when J.W. sat at his father's feet and listened to his stories of the war in the Pacific. Were they growing when J.W. passed the years in Asia?

⊨⊨

J.W. called the Center answering service at 5 A.M. and told them to reschedule his patients, that he was too sick to come in. At dawn, he went to Krista's home, pulled his old flight suit out of the garage, then drove to Black Granite, to the Army Reserve Helicopter Detachment at Royal Field. There was an ease to his gait, a pride he had not remembered, and he asked himself if facing another day was sadder than what was to come in the next two hours.

A row of sixteen, dull olive drab, H-Model HUEYs stood in military precision, STRAC, Standing Ready Around the Clock. The military police guard shack was darkened, though a soldier slid the window aside and saluted "Good morning, Captain. May I help you, sir?"

"Morning, Corporal. I'm riding with the Reserve."

The guard saluted smartly and hit the button that opened the gate to the flight line. J.W. pretended to walk toward preflight, but when he was out of sight of the guard shack, he slithered along the tail booms to the center ship. The doors were unlocked, a helmet propped on the cyclic. There would be no need to wear it, no reason to talk to anyone on his final flight. He laughed at the army for having taught him how to fly, and for having allowed him a so many airborne hours. He could start and fly a HUEY in his sleep.

J.W. slipped into the right seat, gently placing the helmet behind the seat. It would not be hard to find Cedar Springs for a low pass over Krista's house, to say good-bye, and then fly west again, fifty feet off the deck, for a couple of passes over the Center. Next, J.W. would roll out and flee farther south along the interstate to the shabby motel in which Sharra's spirit was entombed. Whether he met her there or not, J.W. planned to climb and fly between the peaks for as long as the fuel lasted. When the twenty-minute fuel warning sounded, he would nurse the helicopter as high as it would go, level off at the five-minute fuel siren, and wait until the fuel was exhausted to enter a dive into the granite. There would be no trace of the aircraft or the madman who had flown it, and no proof his estate was responsible for the disappearance.

J.W. found the master switch where it had been two decades before. It snapped on and activated a whir of gyros, the static hum of avionics J.W. had never seen. The fuel pump ticked, and J.W. smelled kerosene being readied to spray into the cans of the turbine engine. He rolled the throttle to the start detent and cleaned away his condensed breath from inside the freezing canopy. There would be little time to dally once the turbine came hot.

The main rotor began its counter-clockwise creep. The slowly pivoting blades entranced him. He discerned every millimeter of their movement for the first time since he had been in a helicopter cockpit. He was entranced until, with his head raised, he perceived the rose glow of a dawn sky over the Rockies as it reflected off the canopy. Maybe Khai was seeing it as she dressed for school. Maybe his dad had seen the same sun two hours before on his morning, five-mile constitutional, and would think about his missing son on those walks for the rest of his life, if he ever again ventured from the house.

Khai would speak of her missing father when she told a boyfriend about how her dad had disappeared years before. Maybe her world would collapse as had Sharra's, searching for the father who'd abandoned her.

The sun brightened. Mount Brickner glowed splendidly. He was surprised that he was still able to fathom natural beauty, that he had the capacity to welcome a morning, a beginning, to see colors. J.W. rolled the throttle shut and flicked off the master switch. The door on the aging ship creaked open, and J.W. crawled out. He dusted off the helmet on his flight suit before propping it back on the cyclic. He left through the same gate he had entered, passing a laughing gaggle of crew cut officers heading toward their ships. The lieutenants saluted, offering a friendly, "Morning sir," in unison. One turned back with an inquisitive glance, the army having long since changed its flight suits, but the lieutenant shrugged and walked on with his buddies.

J.W. stood in the parking lot for a while, watching them board, and as he drove the Buick off Royal Field, the last ship hover-taxied forward. J.W. called the tower that evening. All the HUEYs had returned safely from their training mission. J.W. dialed his dad. He had had a particularly good walk. "Pop, what were you doing early, early this morning?"

"Probably looking into the sky, thinking about you the way I did when you were in Viet Nam, wishing I could help you, Sonny."

"You did, Pop. I love you."

CHAPTER FIFTY-FIVE

Both Patel and Rizzo stopped by the next morning. They did not come into the office. From the doorway, they told him the Board had extended J.W.'s tenure at the Center for two more weeks, but only so they could have more time to deliberate his fate.

"You mean, I'm not going to be fired?"

"You were never going to be fired; we're just not going to renew your contract. It's not the same thing. You've got to understand the mood of the Board. What with the episode before you came, the head of medicine department and all that, and then that pediatrician. We can't afford another scandal. We're not going to let the Center go down the tubes over moral questions. It's that simple."

"I don't know a thing about those guys, except that you gave me the first one's office. No one's ever told me. All I've heard is whispers. Janitors and nurses gossiping. What the hell did he, they do?"

"We can't discuss that, and it's not important. We can convince the Board to shelve the matter for a while, but there's a lot of rumors to look into. Like I said, 'Keep your nose clean.'"

>><<

J.W. saw Krista that evening when he came to see Khai. "How 'bout we go to dinner and talk things over?" J.W. stammered, his eyes reddening, but all she would discuss was a support check. He asked again. "Please, let's talk."

"Why don't you hold your breath!" she laughed sarcastically.

CHAPTER FIFTY-SIX

J.W. called Harlan Flowers and spilled his guts. The old man was very quiet. "It doesn't matter, J.W. It's what's in your heart. You can be sure, Hoss, that this world is a far better place for the few seconds you've spent here. The older I get, the more I am convinced nothing matters but your heart. You were a hero in a war. It got you into graduate school and medical school. The moral of the story is simple: war and killing is good, it is sacred, and it is rewarded with the greatest gifts in life. But to fall in love is profane, and if you do, you will be punished, everything taken away. That is the logic you face when you stick your head above the crowd. Someone will slash at it. That is why I believe in the Lord, and only the Lord. Nothing else makes sense.

"Now, look, you know I love working overseas, but I've begun to realize, probably too late, that there's plenty to do here at home. Remember the story you told me about your army Ranger buddy, the one from the Indian reservation? He's a congressman now, you said."

"Actually, he's a senator."

"All the better. Give him a call. See if the Department of Indian Affairs has an opening on his reservation."

━━◆ ◆━━

Clumps of scarlet mud clung to his old army boots as he trod the last mile to the DIA clinic on the Rosebud Sioux Reservation in South Dakota. When his party finally came to the little settlement, the guide pointed to a wooden shack and bowed slightly. "Doctor, that is your room. You will like to sleep there. It has running water and electricity.

The man walked J.W. to the door, unlocked it, shook J.W.'s hand, and strode away. There was a small room with a wooden bed and a single battered pot sitting on a kerosene stove. A few cans of beans and mackerel in tomato sauce were left in the one open cabinet.

J.W. passed the endless hours waiting for morning, mostly unable to sleep, visions of Krista and Sharra mixing together until he could not tell one from the other. At dawn, a child appeared at his door and presented J.W. with four warm tortillas then ran off as if he had seen a monster.

At dusk, after seeing a hundred supplicants, an orange sun shone through the western haze. It struck J.W. that the same sun had lit his father's life, and would soon shine on Khai. The ladies sat around fires and perked coffee as thick as paint. They shoveled in tablespoons of raw sugar. An old lady brought J.W. a cup, her toothless smile as pure as the air.

J.W. thought back to medical school and the grand matriarch, Mrs. Mahdi, and how a cup of piquant coffee, not terribly different from the one in front of him, had been her last worldly experience.

Late the next evening, tin pots simmered over sparkling open fires as the men drifted back from the fields. The prairie sky spewed flashes of exotic constellations from horizon to horizon. He thought about walking off by himself and shouting at the stars, begging them to tell him what to do to resurrect his life.

━┼ ┼━

For nine months, J.W. sat at a wooden table in his clinic, placing teaspoons of antibiotics into the mouths of the sick children, whiling the hours away, conversing with his patients. He related the story of his sadness, but his new friends wanted to talk about the strong colt that had been born *that* morning, not yesterday's sorrows.

A few letters came over the months, from Khai mostly, and a few from his parents. Krista forwarded one from the Center. It said that upon further investigation, the rumors that had circulated so freely were really the same story told over and over, embellished with each narration. They could find no firm proof that J.W. had done anything worthy of dismissal. They closed by offering J.W. a position when he returned from his sabbatical. It was signed by Rizzo and Patel. They reminded that no actual punitive action had been taken against J.W., and, thus, there was no culpability on the part of the Center for what had transpired. Moreover, there was no need for hard feelings and unseemly, messy retribution. "Let's just get together and talk. I look forward to it."

He received a separate note from Flatury at the Medical Disciplinary Board. It denied liability for the simple misunderstanding.

CHAPTER FIFTY-SEVEN

The Buick rolled quietly along the miles of snow-lined Route 22 until the turn off for the cabin in which he had loved Sharra. The entire area was white, save for the center of the river, which had not yet frozen. It flowed with its usual determination, rapids forever rumbling over black boulders just below.

J.W. took the key from its hole in the tree trunk and went directly to the couch on which he had first touched Sharra. He stared at the walls that had witnessed the surreal afternoon, and he was sure he perceived Sharra's scent lingering in the room. He built a fire. The primordial smoke that curled out of the warped metal door puffed toward the logged ceiling, carrying away with it her last vestiges. Would that he had known when he had held Sharra, so long before, what he knew now. But J.W. allowed himself the crumb of truth—nothing would have changed.

After the fire burned down and the cold began to seep through the cracks of the door, J.W. left for the trailer up the road. The old man was at the window, watching the smoke from the rusted chimney pipe being carried off by the winds of the

Salmon. Now, J.W. understood him. He popped into the trailer and left a twenty on the table. Mr. Shelton looked up then back out the soot-smeared window. Not a word passed between them.

As J.W. drove by a small airport on the way back to Cedar Springs, he noted the sign offering helicopter rides and instruction, though he accepted, as he had over the past twenty years, the impossibility of ever flying again. He laughed and laughed at himself, at the craziness of dreaming he would ever soar above the morass. He was still laughing when he wrote a check for his first lesson that weekend.

CHAPTER FIFTY-EIGHT

The Black Granite Medical Center, now state-of-the-art in technical terms, was also in the midst of an uneasy cultural expansion when J.W. returned from South Dakota. Doctors were being added at a furious pace. With turtlenecks, beards, and long hair, the new generation of healers challenged the logging town's conservative sensibilities.

"It doesn't matter." Rizzo laughed behind his hand. "This is becoming one hell of a yuppie enclave. And they've all got good insurance. We've even added a few lady doctors as an experiment."

J.W. was welcomed back to the Center at a catered luncheon of smoked turkey and sprouts on whole wheat. Herbee Rizzo smiled unctuously as he presented his "package" for J.W.'s scrutiny. "We're offering a generous salary and benefits, like medical, dental, disability, and life insurance. You get a twenty-four-hour answering service, paid vacations, and a pocket dictating machine so that you'll never have to handwrite a patient note again." Rizzo grabbed one of several dozen sparkling waters from the center of the table then stuffed two frilly, truffled pastries past his lips. "We still provide clean white coats, a new one every day if that makes you happy."

With so many new doctors and staff, and so many new buildings, J.W. recognized his history would be lost in the wave of growth. He smiled at Rizzo. "That's very generous of you, Herb. Let's talk here in a minute, see if we can hammer out a plan. But first, I need to visit the john. Be right back."

J.W. stood and walked toward the men's room, greeting old colleagues around the table. He smiled as he passed the bathroom door, and more broadly when walked out of the Center's main doors into the parking lot. As hard as he tried not to, his middle finger rose and wagged as he drove past the main building. He did not try to wipe away the grin.

The next day, J.W. took Khai to a country inn on the Salmon. They talked and laughed about Mao the Cat, and she admitted she had never forgiven herself for letting him escape. J.W. cried. She held him very hard.

J.W. found a cabin on the Salmon. He lived there year-round and worked in Braxton Falls a couple of days a week in an emergency room. It was enough. He bought a used computer and soon found himself spending most of his time away from the emergency room writing. On Wednesday afternoons, after school, he and Khai shared a cockpit in a little Cessna. All she talked about was learning to fly HUEYs.

She also loved the spawn in autumn, but especially the salmon hatch in spring. She told J.W. she believed there was little difference between the lives of the people she knew and the lives of the fish who struggled upriver by the thousands each year just to die.

OTHER TITLES BY
WILLIAM S. GOULD, MD

AT YONAH MOUNTAIN

Brand new Second Lieutenant J.W. Weathersby is on orders to depart for a combat tour in Viet Nam. At a West Point wedding, though, he commits a very public faux pas and is thrust as punishment into a class of 160 select young officers who sweat and freeze through months of brutal training at the United States Army Ranger School. J.W. joins an African American PhD candidate and a Rose Bud Sioux Harvard graduate, the three pushed together to trudge the mountains, forests, and deserts as Ranger buddies. As half the class is weeded out, they share their disparate lives and dreams. J.W. struggles to be cut from the program, and at the same time fights desperately to remain. At Yonah Mountain is a coming of age adventure, an examination of race relations in the military, and an authentic tale of Army Ranger training.

CAPTAIN IRON MUSTACHE

Captain Iron Mustache takes place in 1968 and 1969. United States Army lieutenant, J.W. Weathersby, just out of Ranger School, volunteers for duty in Viet Nam. It is not long before he changes from naïve youngster to hardened soldier. Something about rural Viet Nam, though, captivates him, and he convinces his commanding officer to allow him to live as the sole American in a remote rice-farming hamlet. His mission is to win the hearts and the minds of the peasants. J.W. forms a deep friendship with the village chief, and falls in love with the schoolteacher, Miss Lin. During a mid-night battle, Miss Lin is arrested and tortured as a communist agent. At the same time, the chief is critically wounded, and disappears after being flown out of the village by an American medevac helicopter. J.W. and the chief's wife spend the last month of his tour driving the deadly roads of Viet Nam searching hospital after hospital for the man. Nearly half a century later, J.W. and his wife return to Viet Nam in a surreal effort to find the chief. He also wants to see Miss Lin, but the Vietnamese government is suspicious of his motives, and the days of his sojourn are fraught with struggle and frustration until a simple act of kindness changes his life.

C.O.L.A.

The day his father died, Dr. Solomon Forte promised his mother he would honor the man's memory by dedicating his years as a doctor to the treatment of injured workers. It seemed so clear a decision—his patients would be like his dad, stoic, honest, working class stiffs who sought nothing more from a doctor than an arm around the shoulder, a word of reassurance, and an ally in dealing with the state industrial insurance system. His life at the Whitaker Hospital and Medical Center is, though, the antithesis of his dream. He can't tell which of the roadblocks is most daunting: that posed by his medical colleagues, the threats of S.M.A.C., the State Medical Abuse Commission, the bureaucracy at C.O.L.A., the state's Commission on Labor Affairs, or the duplicitous patients, some of whom spend every waking moment trying to dupe him out of drugs and government benefits. Occasionally, a case is obvious–the worker really was devastated by an industrial accident. It seems to Sol, though, that those are the very patients C.O.L.A. torments. On the other hand, claimants skilled at ripping off the Commission run free for decades. C.O.L.A. also examines the specter of serious medical errors, and how they are so much easier to make on patients whose care is mired in the aggravation of government-sponsored insurance plans. Questions are also raised about the state-appointed morality commissions that determine which doctors relinquish their licenses for treating pain. Finally, it is a disturbing look behind the scenes of a modern, multi-specialty medical clinic.

A HEART WIND FROM THE DESERT

D r. Solomon Forte has lost everything. There is little left but to offer himself to the wretched in war-torn Sudan. Arriving in the desert, heart brimming with hope, it does not take long to recognize that the social and political beliefs that have spawned the war and famine are the very forces that prevent him from carrying out his dream of caring for the dispossessed. At first, despite the warnings of the tiny European medical team left at the refugee camp in Darfur Province, he fights back with typical, strident, American resolve to save the entire population of refugees. The obstacles of central African life, however, soon draw the spirit from him, and he turns his efforts to preserving the lives of his Western companions. He falls deeply for a gorgeous, but outwardly hardened, British nurse. When she disappears from camp, he spends what strength is left searching for her. A Heart Wind from the Desert examines the need in all of us to accomplish something meaningful in the tiny fragment of time we are allotted, and the impossible hurdles faced when trying to change the way people have thought and behaved for the millennia. It is a tale of beautiful, warm children, but also of the stark life in the sub-Saharan Sahel.

RAPHAEL'S BLANKET

Raphael Blumenkopf is born clandestinely at the Bergen Belsen Nazi death camp on the 14th of April, 1945. His birth is an unprecedented miracle, as is the liberation of the camp by British forces that very afternoon. He has only his mother and a few surviving villagers from their home in Checzonovska, Poland. While the majority of the refugees leave Central Europe for Israel and the West, his band travels across Russia to China. A relative has promised jobs in Shang Hai's old Jewish settlement. The journey is fraught with threats from starving Russians, barbaric border guards, and destitute Chinese peasants. Just as the lives of the immigrants begin to normalize in China, the victory of Mao Zedung's communist army forces them to flee, this time to Hanoi. Five years later, the communist movement in North Viet Nam topples the French government, and the Jews run again. They settle in Saigon until the unrest there compels them to emigrate to America. Raphael's years in the U.S. are colored indelibly by the poison that follows him from the Holocaust, and he formulates a plan to extract revenge from a Federal judge with ties to the Nazis. Who could have envisaged the price he'd pay?

LINCOLN FRIDAY

Lincoln Friday is born into nothing, an obscure, dirt farmer's son, destined to live dominated by the jagged edges of two wars. His early years are an endless series of losses, yet he struggles back after each blow, and slowly, a strongbox of dreams emerges from the fog of his hopelessness.

The harshest test of Lincoln's life, though, comes when the effects of his exposure to Agent Orange devastate both his and his daughter's lives. While the Fridays fight back passionately, the courts, Congress, and the VA turn their backs on them.

In the end, his deeds were neither profound nor dazzling, but he left his mark on disparate people in disparate lands. The world he touched chafed less for his quiet dignity.